Nuclear imaging in clinical cardiology

DEVELOPMENTS IN CARDIOVASCULAR MEDICINE

Other volumes in this series:

Nuclear imaging in clinical cardiology

edited by

M.L. SIMOONS, MD
J.H.C. REIBER, PhD
Thoraxcenter
Academic Hospital Dijkzigt
Erasmus University, Rotterdam
The Netherlands

1984 **MARTINUS NIJHOFF PUBLISHERS**
a member of the KLUWER ACADEMIC PUBLISHERS GROUP
BOSTON / THE HAGUE / DORDRECHT / LANCASTER

Distributors

for the United States and Canada: Kluwer Boston, Inc., 190 Old Derby Street, Hingham, MA 02043, USA
for all other countries: Kluwer Academic Publishers Group, Distribution Center, P.O.Box 322, 3300 AH Dordrecht, The Netherlands

Library of Congress Cataloging in Publication Data

Library of Congress Cataloging in Publication Data
Main entry under title:

Nuclear imaging in clinical cardiology.

  (Developments in cardiovascular medicine ;
  Includes index.
  1. Radioisotope scanning--Addresses, essays, lec-
tures. 2. Heart--Diseases--Diagnosis--Addresses,
essays, lectures. I. Simoons, M. L. II. Reiber,
J. H. C. III. Series.
RC683.5.R33N85 1983   616.1'207575   83-13451
ISBN-13: 978-94-009-6746-5   e-ISBN-13: 978-94-009-6744-1
DOI: 10.1007/ 978-94-009-6744-1

ISBN-13: 978-94-009-6746-5

Copyright

Contents

Introduction

In recent years methods have been developed to study cardiac function, myocardial blood flow and myocardial metabolism with radionuclides. These developments have been facilitated through the introduction of new radiopharmaceuticals, the design of special gamma cameras and dedicated computer systems. However, part of the information provided by nuclear cardiology can also be obtained through other investigations such as echocardiography, exercise electrocardiography and cardiac catheterisation with ventriculography and coronary arteriography. Thus the practising physician must select the most appropriate method(s) of investigation for each patient. Such choices should be based on proper understanding of both the value and the restrictions of each method.

In this book the state-of-the-art in nuclear cardiology is reviewed, including *radionuclide angiography* for analysis of left and right ventricular function and for measurement of shunts and regurgitation volumes, *perfusion scintigraphy* and other methods for measurement of myocardial bloodflow and metabolism and *computer processing* of radionuclide images.

Each chapter has been written by an expert from either Europe or the USA, who has contributed to the developments in his particular field. The principles of each method of investigation are described, as well as the precautions that should be taken in order to obtain high quality data. Guidelines are provided for the interpretation of the data based on studies in various centers where the methods were developed and tested.

We hope that this book will help the clinical cardiologist or internist to understand the value and the limitations of nuclear cardiology for diagnosis and functional evaluation of patients with heart disease.

M.L. Simoons
J.H.C. Reiber

List of contributors

Berger, H.J., MD, Yale University School of Medicine, Section of Nuclear Medicine, 87 LMP, 333 Cedar Street, New Haven, CT 06510, USA.

Berman, D.S., MD, Departments of Medicine and Radiology, UCLA School of Medicine, Los Angeles, CA 90048, USA.

Deanfield, J., MD, ChB, MRCP, MRC Cyclotron Unit and Cardiovascular Unit, Hammersmith Hospital, Royal Postgraduate Medical School, Ducane Road, London W12 0HS, UK.

Detry, J.M., MD, Cliniques Universitaires St. Luc, 10 Avenue Hippocrate, B-1200 Brussels, BELGIUM.

Dymond, D.S., MD, Cardiac Department, St. Bartholomew's Hospital, London, EC1A 7BE, UK.

Garcia, E.V., PhD, Department of Nuclear Medicine, Cedars-Sinai Medical Center, P.O. Box 48750, Los Angeles, CA 90048, USA.

Lammetsma, A., PhD, MRC Cyclotron Unit and Cardiovascular Unit, Hammersmith Hospital, Royal Postgraduate Medical School, Ducane Road, London W12 0HS, UK.

Landsheere, Chr. de, MD, MRC Cyclotron Unit and Cardiovascular Unit, Hammersmith Hospital, Royal Postgraduate Medical School, Ducane Road, London W12 0HS, UK.

Maddahi, J., MD, Division of Cardiology, Cedars-Sinai Medical Center, P.O. Box 48750, Los Angeles, CA 90048, USA.

Melin, J.A., MD, Cliniques Universitaires St. Luc, 10 Avenue Hippocrate, B-1200 Brussels, BELGIUM.

Okada, R.D., MD, Cardiac Unit, Massachusetts General Hospital, Boston, MA 02114, USA.

Reiber, J.H.C., PhD, Thoraxcenter, Erasmus University, Dr. Molewaterplein 40, 3015 GD Rotterdam, THE NETHERLANDS.

Rigo, P., MD, Department of Nuclear Medicine & Cardiology, University of Liège, Hôpital de Bavière, 66 Boulevard de la Constitution, B-4020 Liège, BELGIUM.

Selwyn, A., MD, MRC Cyclotron Unit and Cardiovascular Unit, Hammersmith Hospital, Royal Postgraduate Medical School, Ducane Road, London W12 0HS, UK.

Simoons, M.L., MD, Thoraxcenter, Erasmus University, Dr. Molewaterplein 40, 3015 GD Rotterdam, THE NETHERLANDS.

Shea, M., MD, MRC Cyclotron Unit and Cardiovascular Unit, Hammersmith Hospital, Royal Postgraduate Medical School, Ducane Road, London W12 0HS, UK.

Terton, D., BSc, MRC Cyclotron Unit and Cardiovascular Unit, Hammersmith Hospital, Royal Postgraduate Medical School, Ducane Road, London W12 0HS, UK.

Wackers, F.J.Th., MD, University of Vermont, College of Medicine, Section of Cardiology, Burlington, VT 05401, USA.

Wall, E.E. van der, MD, Interuniversity Cardiology Institute and Cardiology Department, Free University Hospital, De Boelelaan 1117, 1007 MB Amsterdam, THE NETHERLANDS.

Wilson, R., MD, MRC Cyclotron Unit and Cardiovascular Unit, Hammersmith Hospital, Royal Postgraduate Medical School, Ducane Road, London W12 0HS, UK.

Wijns, W., MD, Cliniques Universitaires St. Luc, 10 Avenue Hippocrate, B-1200 Brussels, BELGIUM.

Zaret, B.L., MD, Yale University School of Medicine, Section of Cardiology, 87 LMP, 333 Cedar Street, New Haven, CT 06510, USA.

1. Introduction to imaging of the heart:
Contrast angiography, digital angiography, nuclear imaging, echocardiography

Maarten L. Simoons

Introduction

Recent developments in cardiovascular imaging and signal analysis offer the physician a wide range of methods to evaluate the anatomy and function of the cardiovascular system. These include contrast angiography, echocardiography, nuclear imaging, digital subtraction angiography, and in the near future nuclear magnetic resonance. The cardiologist, internist or radiologist must then choose the technique(s) which provide the most useful diagnostic information in a given patient. Such decisions should be based on precise understanding of the strength and limitations of each method. Excellent reviews and books are available which describe the various imaging techniques. However, these focus mostly on the value of one particular technique and to a lesser extent on the questions which should be resolved in clinical practice. In this chapter the value of the various methods to provide clinically useful information on the anatomy and function of the heart, such as cardiac output, ventricular function, ventricular and atrial dimensions, intra-cardiac shunts, coronary anatomy and myocardial metabolism will be analyzed.

It should be realized that in addition to the general aspects as discussed below, the choice of a given investigation will depend also on the availability and costs of various methods and certainly on local expertise.

Cardiac output

Cardiac output, the product of heartrate and stroke volume, is a measure of performance of the circulation as a whole. A wide range of regulatory systems can change cardiac output and, equally important, the distribution of regional bloodflow. Accordingly, determination of cardiac output provides little insight in cardiac performance in a given patient. Actually, cardiac output can be maintained at normal or near normal levels in the presence of even severe heart disease. Nevertheless, measurement of forward cardiac output in conjunction with other data such as blood pressure, ejection fraction and total stroke volume can provide vital information on systemic and pulmonary vascular resistance, left and right ventricular volumes and the presence and degree of valvular regurgitation. Furthermore, repeated determination of cardiac output aids the analysis of the cardiovascular response to stress and other interventions as well as evaluation of the action of drugs in a given patient.

Most methods for determination of cardiac output are based on the indicator-dilution principle. The indicator can be administered continuously or as a bolus. The most widely used invasive method is *thermodilution* with a Swan-Ganz catheter in the pulmonary artery. This method is particularly useful during cardiac catheterization procedures and in the intensive care unit [1, 2]. *Dye dilution* is an older method which is still used for calibration of other techiques. This method requires a central venous or preferably pulmonary artery catheter as well as arterial determination of dye concentration [3]. The *Fick method* is an indicator dilution technique using oxygen as an indicator which is continuously administered to the circulation in the lungs. Here measurement of O_2 uptake is required as well as determination of the oxygen content of mixed venous and arterial blood. This method is most useful if O_2 uptake is also needed for other purposes such as in exercise physiology [4]. *Radioisotopes* can be used as indicator and detected with a gamma camera or nuclear probe. A "first pass technique" can be used which requires a bolus injection in a large central vein or a continuous infusion of a short living isotope such as Kr-81m can be used. [5, 6]. Furthermore, this method can be adapted in the nuclear cardiology laboratory in connection with measurement of ejection fraction to check the determination of ventricular volume. Changes of cardiac output, for example during a stress test, can be determined from "stroke counts" in gated bloodpool studies.

Truly noninvasive methods for determination of cardiac output are the CO_2 *rebreathing method* [7], which is again used in exercise physiology, and *impedance plethysmography*. The latter method has not been accepted widely, probably since its reliability in patients with heart failure or during stress has not been established.

Finally, cardiac output can be derived if *stroke volume* is measured by echocardiography, contrast angiography or radionuclide angiography as discussed below.

Detection of intracardiac shunts

The presence of intracardiac shunts, including open ductus arteriosus is usually suspected on the basis of physical findings. *Contrast echocardiography* can be used to document these shunts. Small left to right shunts can be detected by echocardiography if a glucose 5% solution is injected in wedge position in the pulmonary artery [8, 9]. Quantitative information on shunt flow can be obtained by analysis of O_2 *content* in the blood during cardiac catheterization or by *first pass* radionuclide angiography as discussed in Chapter 8. The advantage of cardiac catheterization is that other data such as pressure measurements can be obtained simultaneously. Angiography as well as contrast echocardiography permits the precise location of single or multiple shunts in patients with ventricular septum defect [9, 10] (Table 1). Both the nuclear procedure and echocardiography can be repeated easily and can thus be used to study the augmentation or reduction of shunt size and to study the presence of a shunt and its size post surgery. Certain precautions should be taken to provide accurate shunt measurements which are described in Chapter 8.

Table 1. Schematic comparison of the value of various methods for evaluation of intracardiac shunts

Detection of (intracardiac) shunts

	Location	Quantitation
O_2 content	+	+++
Contrast echocardiography	++	−
Radionuclide angiography	+	+++
Contrast angiography	++	+

Ventricular volume and stroke volume

Ventricular volume is enlarged in patients with chronic severe valvular incompetence and in dilated cardiomyopathy, due to both coronary heart disease and other causes. There are indications that the size of the left ventricle per se is a determinant of prognosis in patients with aortic incompetence. Accordingly, several authors claim that surgery is indicated in asymptomatic patients with aortic incompetence when significant left ventricular enlargement occurs [11]. However, recent studies from our unit do not support such claims [12].

In the absence of regurgitation, the end diastolic volume and end systolic volume can be calculated from cardiac output and left ventricular or right ventricular ejection fraction. Direct determination of ventricular volumes is possible by contrast angiography, echocardiography and scintigraphy. In principle, ventricular volume is derived from a shadow projection by contrast angiography wherein information on depth is not present. Echocardiography provides a tomographic plane without information on possible incoordinate wall motion outside that particular plane. Both *contrast angiography* and *echocardiography* require a high quality image in which the contour of the ventricle can be traced. Ventricular volume is then obtained from the contour(s) in one or two planes by the area-length method. Errors can be made by such computations if the contours are not properly determined and, more important, if the shape of the ventricle is irregular. Finally these methods do not correct for the volume of the papillary muscles in the ventricle. The use of these methods has been facilitated by the development of computer systems which perform all necessary measurements and calculations, once the contours have been indicated. More recently fully automated systems for analysis of contrast angiograms have been developed such as the Contouromat [13]. The use of *2D echocardiography* for this purpose is limited, since adequate images can be obtained in part of the patients only. In our laboratory echo-volume determinations could be made in 23 out of 29 consecutive patients using Simpsons rule in multiple views and in 34 out of 39 patients with an ellipsoid model in a single plane [14].

Digital angiography does not provide new information in this regard. However, by subtraction methods adequate quality angiograms can be obtained from intravenous injection of contrast, or from injection of small contrast volumes in the left ventricle [15].

The area-length method has also been used in *radionuclide angiography*. However, the determination of the left ventricular contour by this method is not accurate due to the poor spatial resolution of the gamma camera (± 1 cm). Since the radiation is linearly related to the volumes in the heart chambers, the total counts within the left ventricular contour can be used to calculate its volume. This approach does not require any geometrical model, however, corrections should be made for attenuation of radiation in the blood volume and the surrounding tissues. Such correction can be made after measurement of the distance between the center of the left ventricle and the camera and determination of the counts from a blood sample [16–18]. More recently it has been proposed to determine tissue attenuation through measurement of transmission of radiation from the esophagus [19].

Tomography might become the method of choice for determination of ventricular volumes, provided that images can be obtained at such speed that the method becomes insensitive to heart motion. At present such systems are not yet generally available. It is as yet uncertain which tomographic method will yield optimal results at reasonable costs: computed X-ray tomography, nuclear magnetic resonance [20, 21], echocardiography [22], positron tomography or tomography with a rotating gammacamera.

The shape of the left and right ventricle

Details on the shape of the ventricles can readily be observed by all three imaging methods: contrast angiography, blood pool scintigraphy and echocardiography. In addition the latter method usually provides information on the precise thickness of the wall of the left ventricle. Furthermore, *echocardiography* is the method of choice for detection of intracavitary masses such as vegetations, thrombus or intracardiac tumors [23]. In comparison with the other two, blood pool scintigraphy has the lowest resolution, while interpretation of the images is often hampered by overprojection of various parts of the left ventricle or of both ventricles.

Ejection fraction

The ejection fraction is a measure of the pump function of the left or right ventricle. The multitude of papers on ejection fractions at rest and during stress in recent years is largely due to the ease of its determination from blood pool scintigraphy. It should be remembered that ejection fraction is but an indicator of global ventricular function. A normal ejection fraction does not preclude abnormal function of one or more regions of the ventricles. It is dependent on other hemodynamic factors such as heart-rate, ventricular filling pressure or end diastolic volume (preload) and the outflow resistance of the ventricles (afterload). Nevertheless, a wide range of studies have demonstrated that prognosis as well as surgical risk in patients with coronary heart disease are related to left ventricular ejection fraction. Similarly the response of ejection fraction to stress has been proposed as an indicator of timing of surgery in patients with aortic incompetence [24]. Finally a normal response of ejection fraction during stress indicates the absence of severe coronary disease in patients with chest pain [25].

Left ventricular ejection fraction can be computed from end systolic and end diastolic volumes from *contrast angiography*. This method is regarded as the gold standard for other methods. However, it remains dependent on observer variability in the drawing of the contours and it is limited by the model used for volume calculations based on area-length measurements or Simpsons rule. *Radionuclide angiography* offers a direct measurement of both left and right ventricular ejection fraction even without measurement of ventricular volumes. This method is limited by the need to correct for background radiation. Similar to contrast angiography, ventricular contours should be determined. This can be done manually, but recently computer programs have been developed for semi- or fully automated detection of these contours independent of the human observer [26]. The principles of such computer programs are described in Chapter 9.

The *nuclear stethoscope* can provide beat to beat changes in ventricular volume and left ventricular ejection fraction. This method is particularly useful for evaluation of drug responses [27, 28] (See Chapter 7). From a conventional *M mode echocardiogram* ejection fraction can be determined, but often not in a reliable manner since too many assumptions on the shape of the ventricles have to be made. Better results can be obtained by *2D or cross-sectional echocardiography*. However, it is often difficult to define accurately the endocardium in the echocardiogram, while good quality images cannot be obtained in 20–50% of patients, dependent on the subset of patients studied. Those who are familiar with the images can often provide an accurate description of ventricular wall motion from a 2D echocardiogram, although it remains difficult to condensate this description in a single number such as the ejection fraction [29, 30].

In clinical practice, left ventricular ejection fraction can be measured by contrast angiography in the catheterization laboratory or by scintigraphic

Table 2. Comparison of the relative value of three methods for determination of left ventricular ejection fraction

Measurement of left ventricular ejection fraction

	Contrast	Echo	Nuclear
Precise	+++	++	+++
Success rate	90%	50%	95%
Observer variability	++	+	Automated
During stress	+	–	+++
Main problem	Invasive	Low success	Background

methods (Table 2). The advantages of radionuclide angiography for determination of ejection fraction are the success rate, which is close to 100% in all conditions; the ease of application of these methods in sick patients in an intensive care unit and during interventions such as stress testing and the now fully automated measurement of ejection fraction. The methods of first pass and gated radionuclide angiography are described in detail in Chapters 7, 9 and 11.

Ventricular function

The term "ventricular function" is used for a wide range of measurements which reflect either global pump function (stroke volume, stroke work, ejection fraction), regional wall motion or pressure derived indices which supposedly reflect muscle contractility (dP/dt/P, Vmax, mean circumferential fiber shortening) [31]. In some studies more distant indicators of ventricular function are used such as *systolic time intervals* or the *rise of systolic pressure* during exercise. One should remember that such measurements all describe different aspects of the function of the left ventricle. A proper description of ventricular function in a given patient, or changes in ventricular function during an intervention should include multiple measurements, preferably a combination of volume measurements, regional wall motion and pressure derived indices. In addition, changes in heartrate, left ventricular diastolic volume (preload) and afterload should be specified.

Regional wall motion

A *qualitative description* of regional wall motion can again be obtained by contrast angiography, 2D echocardiography and radionuclide angiography. Interpretation of scintigrams can be facilitated by the use of functional images such as Fourier amplitude and phase images [32, 33]. A *quantitative description* of regional wall motion can be obtained from both contrast angiography and scintigraphy. For the former various models have been proposed including shortening of hemiaxes, radial shortening, shortening of the contour [34, 35], analysis of the "true" motion pattern [36], and the regional contribution to ejection fraction [37]. Similar methods have been applied to blood pool scintigraphy. Of these, computation of segmental ejection fraction seems most promising, since it is little

Table 3. Comparison of the features which can be studied by three methods for ventriculography, analysis of the coronary arteries and coronary perfusion

Technical aspects	Contrast	Echo	Nuclear
Resolution	1 mm	1 mm	1 cm
Quantitation	+++	+	+++
Success rate	Invasive	50-90%	95%
Serial studies	−	+++	++
Response to stress	++	+	+++
Costs	+++	+	++

Features to be studied	Contrast	Echo	Nuclear
Wall thickness	+	+++	−
Wall motion	+++	++	+++
Valve structure and motion	+	+++	−
Tumors, vegetations	+	+++	+
Coronary anatomy	+++	+	−
Coronary bloodflow	+	−	+++

influenced by definition of the contours and reflects the principle of radionuclide angiography where counts are related to intraventricular volume and its changes (see Chapter 9).

Coronary anatomy

The anatomy of the coronary arteries can at present be studied only by *selective contrast angiography.* Thus this investigation remains mandatory and is there to stay in patients who are candidates for coronary bypass surgery or percutaneous transluminal coronary angioplasty.

Echocardiography has been used for visualization of the left main coronary artery, however, this has a low success rate and little if any practical application [38]. Attempts to visualize coronary anatomy by *digital subtraction* after intravenous administration of contrast yielded little success so far.

A considerable number of studies have addressed the prediction of coronary anatomy from thallium scintigraphy [39, 40, 41].

Although a reasonable correlation between these methods and the angiogram has been reported, such predictions are not accurate enough to replace the angiogram in symptomatic patients [42]. On the other hand, the value of noninvasive tests for prediction of recurrent infarction or death may be equal to angiography, as will be discussed below.

Coronary blood flow and its distribution

Coronary blood flow can be measured in man by *thermodilution* with a special catheter in the coronary sinus. Similarly flow in the great cardiac vein, draining the anterior part of the left ventricle, can be measured. Regional blood flow in the anterior wall can be measured by the *Xenon washout* method which requires intracoronary administration of Xe and a gamma camera [43]. Both methods can be used to study the effect of interventions or drug administration in a given patient. Fast changes in the distribution of blood flow can be visualized with *short living isotopes* such as ^{91}Kr which are continuously infused either in the coronary artery, or in the aortic root with a special catheter. Further information on measurement of coronary blood flow is presented in Chapter 3.

Thallium scintigraphy has gained the widest application for analysis of distribution of myocardial blood flow, and has surpassed other isotopes with similar biological properties such as ^{43}K. The distribution of ^{201}Tl uptake does indeed correlate closely with the distribution of blood flow [44–46]. However, absolute measurements of total or regional blood flow cannot be obtained with this method. The main indications for thallium scintigraphy are detection of coronary artery disease in patients where stress electrocardiography provide insufficient information, and the detection of exercise-induced ischemia in patients with known coronary disease and atypical symptoms, e.g. after bypass surgery or after myocardial infarction. Finally thallium scintigraphy has been applied with success to illustrate the efficacy of interventions such as percutaneous transluminal coronary angioplasty [47] and to study the value of intracoronary thrombolysis in acute myocardial infarction [48]. In Chapters 4 and 6 in this book the value and limitations of thallium scintigraphy in clinical practice are addressed in detail.

A new approach to visualization of myocardial blood flow distribution is the application of digital angiography. With the aid of such computer systems, the appearance time of dye in the myocardium during coronary arteriography can be analyzed in large number of small areas of the heart. Color displays of the time to peak concentration of contrast have been used to demonstrate changes in coronary blood flow after administration of nitrates or calcium antagonists.

Application of radionuclide imaging, echocardiography and contrast angiography in clinical practice

As will be evident from the previous discussion, many clinical problems can be addressed by all three methods for imaging of the heart. However, the type of information and its quality differ. Accordingly, the physician should specify which information is needed in a given patient and for which purpose. Different investigations may be used in the same patient in order to obtain a diagnosis, to decide whether surgery should be performed, to provide prognostic information or to follow the development of disease. This is illustrated in the following paragraphs on detection of myocardial infarction, quantitation of infarct size and prediction of prognosis in patients with coronary heart disease.

Detection of myocardial infarction and quantitation of infarct size

Myocardial infarction is characterized by loss of blood flow and permanent loss of normal metabolism in the affected myocardium. Thus all methods discussed in the previous paragraph will show abnormalities in patients with acute myocardial infarction. It has been demonstrated that *Tc pyrophosphate* and similar agents, accumulate in a myocardial infarction [49, 50]. However, this infarct avid scintigraphy has only limited clinical value, since the diagnosis can usually be made earlier and in a less expensive manner by other methods. *Thallium scintigraphy* has been studied in large series of patients with suspected acute myocardial infarction [51, 52]. An abnormal Tl scintigram was found in all patients studied within 8 hours after the onset of myocardial infarction, while false negatives were observed in part of the patients with a small infarction admitted after a longer delay (Table 4). However, with this method no difference can be made between areas of old or recent myocardial infarction. Furthermore such investigation is too expensive in comparison with serial ECG analysis and determination of serum enzymes such as CK-MB. On the other hand, thallium scintigraphy can be used to estimate infarct size, and to study the effect of interventions which aim at reduction of infarct size [48, 53]. Possibly more refined analysis of infarct size will be possible through positron emission tomography in centers where such systems are available.

Echocardiography can be used to visualize areas with abnormal wall motion. In a recent series adequate echocardiograms were obtained in 65

Table 4. Time course of the sensitivity of various methods for diagnosis of myocardial infarction. On top time is presented as hours after the onset of symptoms. An elevated CK-MB level is considered to be the "gold standard" and thus reaches a sensitivity of 100%. In some patients no significant ECG changes are observed, for example in very small infarcts or in patients with conduction defects. Serial ECG analysis is superior to a single tracing for detection of myocardial infarction. Thallium scintigraphy has a sensitivity close to 100% within the first hours after myocardial infarction. However, it cannot distinguish old from new infarcts, while we have observed no abnormalities in some patients with very small infarcts.

Time (hours)	0-4	5-8	9-16	17-32	33-64
ECG	+++	95%	+++	++	++
CK (MB)	+	100%	100%	++	+
Thallium	95%	95%	90%	++	++
Tc Pyp	–	–	+	+	80%
Echo	75%	++	++	++	+

out of 80 patients (81%). Abnormal wall motion was present in 31 out of 33 patients with myocardial infarction (94%). Thus the method is successful in approximately $81 \times 94 = 75\%$ of patients with myocardial infarction [54].

Prediction of prognosis in patients with coronary heart disease

The aim of treatment of patients with coronary heart disease is first of all alleviation of symptoms by administration of drugs, bypass surgery or percutaneous transluminal coronary angioplasty. The choice of one or a combination of these methods will depend on the symptoms and other noninvasive or invasive findings in a given patient. In addition therapeutic interventions have been proposed to increase life expectancy in asymptomatic patients with coronary heart disease, for example after myocardial infarction. These include treatment with beta blockers [55–57], possibly treatment with other drugs and bypass surgery. The possible benefits of such prophylactic treatment should be weighted carefully against the risk and possible side effects of the proposed medical or surgical intervention. It should be attempted to *select the most appropriate intervention* in each patient, based on careful prediction of the risk of mortality or reinfarction. Factors which have been shown to be of predictive value include age, sex, a history of smoking, previous myocardial infarction, previous angina, or heart failure [58], estimation of infarct size from electrocardiography or enzyme release in patients with a first infarc-

Table 5. Factors related to the prediction of mortality after myocardial infarction

---

Prediction of mortality after myocardial infarction

— General risk indicators
    age
    risk factors (smoking, hypertension)

— Extent of myocardial damage
    history of previous infarction
    infarct size (ECG, enzymes)
    pump failure (CCU, reconvalescence)
    ejection fraction (contrast, radionuclide angiography)
    exercise tolerance (workload, blood pressure)

— Extent of coronary disease
    coronary angiography (3 vessel disease)
    exercise-induced ischemia (angina, ST, TL-201)

---

tion [59], left ventricular function as determined by radionuclide angiography [60] or contrast angiography [61], extension of the infarct demonstrated by serial 2D echocardiography [62], exercise tolerance during stress tests, changes in heartrate or systolic pressure during exercise [60], exercise-induced myocardial ischemia detected from history, by electrocardiography [63–65], or thallium scintigraphy [66] and the presence of runs of ventricular tachycardia during ambulatory monitoring, exercise testing or after electrical stimulation of the heart [67].

Unfortunately, few studies have compared the relative value of the above mentioned investigations. The few comparisons which have been made indicate that the predictive value of *coronary angiography* and *stress testing* are similar [68] as well as the predictive value of stress testing and measurement of *left ventricular ejection fraction* by blood pool scintigraphy [60]. Further large scale studies are mandatory to further illucidate this problem including the cost benefit ratio of different strategies [69, 70]. At present the procedure shown in Figure 1 might be proposed, using the strength of exercise testing, angiography and blood pool scintigraphy, respectively.

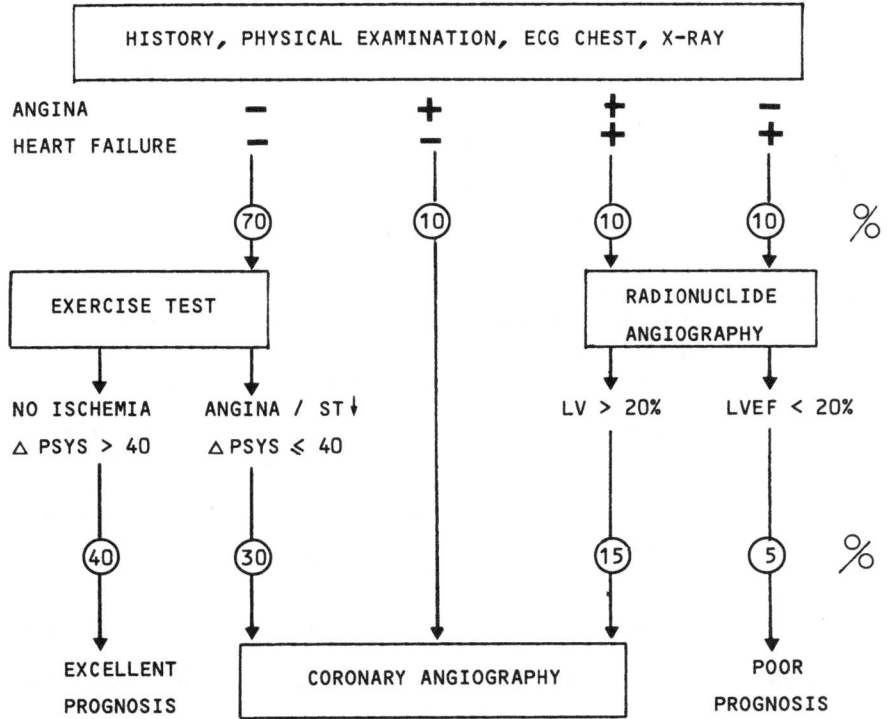

Figure 1. Strategy for evaluation of patients after myocardial infarction based on the follow up experience at the Thoraxcenter [60]. The numbers within the circles indicate the approximate percentage of patients in each category. A symptom limited stress test is performed in all patients except those with angina, heart failure or other limiting factors. Those who show no ischemia and an adequate bloodpressure response (increase systolic pressure greater than 40 mmHg) have an excellent prognosis and need no further investigations. Patients with heartfailure and a low ejection fraction have a poor prognosis, which can most likely not be influenced by surgery and thus do not need angiography. Coronary arteriography is indicated in those with abnormal stress test results or angina, provided that left ventricular function has not been compromised too much.

Conclusion

The clinician has presently several methods at his disposal to study the anatomy and function of the heart and the coronary arteries. For each clinical problem the most appropriate methods of investigation should be selected. Such selection should be based on proper understanding of the data which can be obtained by the various studies. This review of the strength and limitations of various methods might be used as guideline. However, in additon to this general discussion, the ultimate choice will be influenced by cost, locally available equipment and local expertise.

References

1. Branthwaite MA, Bradley RD: Measurement of cardiac output by thermodilution in man. J Appl Physiol 24: 434, 1968.
2. Ganz W, Donoso R, Marcus HS, Forrester JS, Swan HJC: A new technique for measurement of cardiac output by thermodilution in man. Am J Cardiol 27: 392, 1971.
3. Shepherd RL, Higgs LM, Glancy DL: Comparison of left ventricular and pulmonary arterial injection sites in determination of cardiac output by the indicator dilution technique. Chest 62: 175, 1972.
4. Selzer A, Sudrann RB: Reliability of the determination of cardiac output in man by means of the Fick principle. Circ Res 6: 485, 1958.
5. MacIntyre WJ, Storaasli JP, Krieger H et al.: [131] I-labeled serum albumin: Its use in the study of cardiac output and peripheral vascular flow. Radiology 59: 849, 1952.
6. Budinger TF: Physiology and physics of nuclear cardiology. In: Nuclear Cardiology. James T. Willerson (ed). F.A. Davis Company, Philadelphia, 1979, pp. 9–78.
7. Franciosa JA, Ragan DO, Rubenstone SJ: Validation of the CO_2 rebreathing method for measuring cardiac output in patients with hypertension or heart failure. J Lab Clin Ned 88: 872–682, 1976.
8. Roelandt J, Meltzer RS, Serruys PW: Contrast echocardiography. In: Echocardiology, H. Rijsterborgh (ed). Martinus Nijhoff, The Hague, 1981, p. 219.
9. Roelandt J: Contrast echocardiography. Ultrasound in Med & Biol 5: 471–492, 1982.
10. Hagler DJ, Tajik AJ, Seward JB, Mair DD, Ritter DG, Ritman EL: Videodensitometric quantitation of left-to-right shunts with contrast sector echocardiography. Circulation 58 (suppl II): 70, 1978.
11. Henry WL, Bonow RO, Rosing DR, Epstein SE: Observations on the optimal timing for operative intervention for aortic regurgitation. II. Serial echocardiographic evaluation of asymptomatic patients. Circulation 61: 484, 1980.
12. Fioretti P, Roelandt J, Bos RJ, Meltzer RS, Van Hoogenhuijze D, Serruys PW, Nauta J, Hugenholtz PG: Echocardiography in chronic aortic insufficiency: Is valve replacement too late when left ventricular end-systolic dimension reaches 55 mm? Circulation 67: 216–221, 1983.
13. Reiber JHC, Slager CJ, Schuurbiers JCH, Meester GT: Contouromat – A hardwired left ventricular angio-processing system. II. Performance evaluation. Comput. Biomed. Res. 11: 503–523, 1978.
14. Das S, Domenicucci S, Roelandt J, Wijns W, Vletter W, Lubsen J, Simoons M, Reiber, JHC: Comparison of LV volumes and ejection fraction determined by 2-dimensional echocardiography with new 3.5 MHz transducer and radionuclide ventriculography. In: Abstractbook European Society of Cardiology, Working Group on Use of Isotopes in Cardiology, April 14–16, 1983, 5 (abstract).
15. Kronenberg MW, Price RR, Smith CW, Robertson JM, Perry JM, Pickens DR, Domanski MJ, Partain L, Friesinger GC: Evaluation of left ventricular performance using digital subtraction angiography. Am J Cardiol 51: 837–842, 1983.
16. Links J, Becker LL, Shindledecker JL, et al.: Measurement of absolute left ventricular volume from gated blood pool studies. Circulation 65: 82–90, 1982.
17. Wijns W, Reiber JHC, Lie SP, Van Duyvendijk K, Simoons ML: Reliability of radionuclide absolute left ventricular volume measurements. J Nucl Med 5: D 27, 1983 (abstract).
18. Parrish MD, Graham TP, Born ML, Jones JP, Boucek RJ, Partain CL: Radionuclide ventriculography for assessment of absolute right and left ventricular volumes in children. Circulation 66: 811–819, 1982.
19. Maurer AH: Siegel JA, Denenberg BS, Carabello BA, Gash AK, Spann JF, Malmud LS: Absolute left ventricular volume from gated bloodpool imaging with use of esophageal transmission measurement. Am J Cardiol 51: 853–858, 1983.

20. Kaufman L, Crooks L, Sheldon P, Hricak H, Herfkens R, Bank W: The potential impact of nuclear magnetic resonance imaging on cardiovascular diagnosis. Circulation 67: 251–257, 1983.

21. Afidi RJ, Haaga JR, El Yousef SJ, et al.: Preliminary experimental results in humans and animals with a superconducting, whole-body, nuclear magnetic resonance scanner. Radiology 143: 175–181, 1982.

22. Moritz, WE, McCabe DH, Pearlman AS, Medema DK: Computer generated three dimensional ventricular imaging from a series of two-dimensional ultrasonic scans. Comp in Cardiol: 19–24, 1982.

23. Asinger RW, Mikell FL, Sharma B, Hodges M: Observations on detecting left ventricular thrombus with two-dimensional echocardiography: emphasis avoidance of false positive diagnosis. Am J Cardiol 47: 45, 1981.

24. Borer JS, Bacharach SL, Green MV, et al.: Exercise-induced left ventricular dysfunction in symptomatic and asymptomatic patients with aortic regurgitation: Assessment with radionuclide cineangiography. Am J Cardiol, 42: 351–357, 1978.

25. Borer JD, Bacharach SL, Green MV, et al.: Real-time radionuclide cineangiography in the noninvasive evaluation of global and regional left ventricular function at rest and during exercise in patients with coronary artery disease. N Engl J Med, 296: 839, 1977.

26. Reiber JHC, Lie SP, Simoons ML, Hoek C, Gerbrands JJ, Wijns W, Bakker WH, Kooij PPM: Clinical validation of fully automated computation of ejection fraction from gated equilibrium blood pool scintigrams. J Nucl Med 24: 1983 (in press).

27. Berger HJ, Davies RA, Batsford WP, Hoffer PB, Gottschalk A, Zaret BL: Beat-to-beat left ventricular performance assessed from the equilibrium cardiac bloodpool using a computerized nuclear probe. Circulation 66: 811–819, 1982.

28. Strashun A, Horowitz S, Goldsmith S, et al.: Noninvasive detection of left ventricular dysfunction with scintillation portable ECG-gated probe detector. Am J Cardiol 47: 610–611, 1981.

29. Schiller NB, Ports TA, Silverman NH: Quantitative analysis of the adult left heart by echocardiography. In: Echocardiology, Rijsterborgh H. (ed). Martinus Nijhoff, The Hague, 1981, pp. 145–161.

30. Quinones MA, Waggoner AD, Reduto LA, Nelson JG, Young JB, Winters WL, Ribeiro LG, Miller RR: A new, simplified and accurate method for determining ejection fraction with two-dimensional echocardiography. Circulation 64: 744–753, 1981.

31. Kreulen TH, Bove AA, McDonough MT, Sands MJ, Spann JF: The evaluation of left ventricular function in man: A comparison of methods. Circulation 51: 677–688, 1975.

32. Adam WE, Tarkowska A, Bitter F, Stauch M, Geffers H: Equilibrium gated radionuclide ventriculography. Cardiovasc Radiol 2: 161, 1979.

33. Botvinick E, Dunn R, Frais M, O'Connell W, Shosa D, Herfkens R, Scheinman M: The phase image; its relationship to patterns of contraction and conduction. Circulation 65: 551–560, 1982.

34. Brower RW, Meester GT: Computer-based methods for quantifying regional left ventricular wall motion from cine ventriculograms. Comp. in Cardiol: 55–62, 1976.

35. Gelberg HJ, Brundage BH, Glantz S, Parmley WW: Quantitative left ventricular wall motion analysis: A comparison of area, chord and radial methods. Circulation 59: 991–1000, 1979.

36. Slager CJ, Hooghoudt TEH, Reiber JHC, Schuurbiers JCH, Booman F, Meester GT: Left ventricular contour segmentation from anatomical landmark trajectories and its application to wall motion analysis. In: Computer analysis of left ventricular cineangiograms. TEH Hooghoudt, Thesis, 1982.

37. Hooghoudt TEH, Slager CJ, Reiber JHC, Serruys PW, Schuurbiers JCH, Meester GT: "Regional contribution to global ejection fraction" used to assess the applicability of a new wall motion model to the detection of regional wall motion in patients with asynergy. In: Computer analysis of left ventricular cineangiograms. TEH Hooghoudt, Thesis, 1982.

38. Feigenbaum H: Visualization of the coronary arteries by two-dimensional echocardiography. In: Echocardiology, Rijsterborgh H (ed). Martinus Nijhoff, The Hague, 1981, pp. 61–72.

39. Lenaers A, Block P, van Thiel E. Lebedelle M, Becquevort P, Erbsmann R, Ermans AM: Segmental analysis of Tl-201 stress myocardial scintigraphy. J Nucl Med 18: 509, 1977.
40. Rigo PR, Bailey IK, Griffith LSC, Pitt B, Burow RD, Wagner HN, Becker LC: Value and limitations of segmental analysis of stress thallium myocardial imaging for localization of coronary artery disease. Circulation 60: 973, 1980.
41. Massie BM, Botvinick EH, Brundage BH: Correlation of Tl-201 scintigrams with coronary anatomy: Factors affecting region by region sensitivity. Am J Cardiol 44: 616, 1979.
42. Atwood JE, Jensen D, Froelicher V, Witztum K, Gerber K, Gilpin E, Ashburn W: Agreement in human interpretation of analog thallium myocardial perfusion images. Circulation 64: 601–609, 1981.
43. Lichtlen PR, Engel H-J: Assessment of regional myocardial blood flow using the inert gas washout technique. Cardiovasc Radiol 2: 203, 1979.
44. Strauss HW, Harrison K, Langun JK, Lebowitz E, Pitt B: Tl-201 for myocardial imaging: Relation of Tl-201 to regional myocardial perfusion. Circulation 51: 641, 1975.
45. Weich HF, Strauss HW, Pitt B: The extraction of Tl-201 by the myocardium. Circulation 56: 188, 1977.
46. Okada RD, Jacogs ML, Daggett WM, Leppo J, Strauss W, Newell JB, Moore B, Boucher CA, O'Keefe D, Pohost GM: Tl-201 kinetics in non-ischemic canine myocardium. Circulation 65: 70–77, 1982.
47. Wijns W, Serruys PW, Reiber JHC, Brand M vd, Simoons ML, Balakumaran K, Hugenholtz PG: Quantitative coronary angiography in single left anterior descending disease: Correlation with pressure gradient and exercise thallium scintigraphy. Circulation, in press.
48. Simoons ML, Wijns W, Balakumaran K, Serruys PW, Brand M vd, Fioretti P, Reiber JHC, Lie P, Hugenholtz PG: The effect of intracoronary thrombolysis with streptokinase on myocardial thallium distribution and left ventricular function assessed by blood pool scintigraphy. Eur Heart J 33: 433–440, 1982.
49. Stokely EM, Buja LM, Lewis SE, et al.: Measurements of acute myocardial infarcts in dogs with 99mTc stannous pyrophosphate scintigrams. J Nucl Med 17: 1, 1976b.
50. Olson HG, Lyons KP, Aronow WS, Kuperus J, Orlando J, Hughes D: Prognostic value of a persistently positive technetium-99m myocardial scintigram after myocardial infarction. Am J Cardiol 43: 889, 1979.
51. Wackers FJ, Sokole EB, Samson G, et al.: Value and limitations of Tl-201 scintigraphy in the acute phase of myocardial infarction. N Engl J Med 295: 1, 1976.
52. Pond M, Rehn T, Burow R, et al.: Early detection of myocardial infarction by serial Tl-201 imaging. Circulation 56: 893, 1977.
53. Kennedy JW, Fritz JK, Ritchie JL: Streptokinase in acute myocardial infarction: Western Washington randomized trial – protocol and progress report. Am Heart J 104: 899–911, 1982.
54. Horowitz RS, Morganroth J, Parrotto C, Chen CC, Soffer J, Pauletto FJ: Immediate diagnosis of acute myocardial infarction by two-dimensional echocardiography: Circulation 65: 323–329, 1982.
55. The Norwegian Multicentre Study Group: Timolol-induced reduction in mortality and reinfarction in patients surviving acute myocardial infarction. New Engl J Med 304: 801–817, 1981.
56. Hjalmarson A, Elmfeldt D, Herlitz J, et al.: Effects on mortality of metropolol in acute myocardial infarction. A double-blind randomized trial. Lancet 12: 823–827, 1981.
57. Hampton JR: The use of beta blockers for the reduction of mortality after myocardial infarction. Eur Heart J 2: 259–268, 1981.
58. Henning R, Wedel H: The long-term prognosis after myocardial infarction: A five-year follow-up study. Eur Heart J 2: 65–74, 1981.
59. Witteveen SAGJ, Hemker HC, Hollaar L, Hermens WTh: Quantitation of infarct size in man by means of plasma enzyme levels. Br Heart J 37: 795, 1975.
60. Fioretti P, Brower RW, Simoons ML, Das SK, Wijns W, Fels PW, Reiber JHC, Lubsen J:

Prediction of mortality after myocardial infarction from gated bloodpool scintigraphy versus stress testing. In: Abstractbook European Society of Cardiology, Working Group on Use of Isotopes in Cardiology, Rotterdam, April 14–16, 1983, 18 (abstract).

61. Paine TD, Dye LE, Roitman DI, Sheffield LT, Rackley C, Russell RO, Rogers W: Relation of graded exercise test findings after myocardial infarction to extent of coronary artery disease and left ventricular dysfunction. Am J Cardiol 42: 716–723, 1978.

62. Hutchins GM, Bulkley BH: Infarct expansion versus extension: Two different complications of acute myocardial infarction. Am J Cardiol 41: 1127–1132, 1978.

63. Theroux P, Waters DD, Halphen C, Debaisieux JC, Mizgala HF: Prognostic value of exercise soon after myocardial infarction. N Engl J Med 301: 341, 1979.

64. Weld FM, Chu KL, Bigger JT, Rolnitzky LM: Risk stratification with low-level exercise testing 2 weeks after acute myocardial infarction. Circulation 64: 306–314, 1981.

65. Starling MR, Crawford MH, Kennedy GT, O'Rourke RA: Exercise testing early after myocardial infarction: Predictive value for subsequent unstable angina and death. Am J Cardiol 46: 909–914, 1980.

66. Silverman KJ, Becker LC, Bulkley BH, et al.: Value of early Tl-201 scintigraphy for predicting mortality in patients with acute myocardial infarction. Circulation 61: 996–1003, 1980.

67. Moss AJ: Prognostic aspects of ventricular arrhythmias in patients with coronary artery disease. In: Long-term Ambulatory Electrocardiography. Roelandt J and Hugenholtz PG (eds), 1982, p. 155–159.

68. Feyter PJ de, Eenige MJ van, Dighton DH, Visser FC: Prognostic value of exercise testing, coronary angiography and left ventriculography 6–8 weeks after myocardial infarction. Circulation 66: 527–536, 1982.

69. Stason WB, Fineberg HV: Implications of alternative strategies to diagnose coronary artery disease. Circulation 66: 80–86, 1982.

70. Epstein SE, Palmeri ST, Patterson RE: Evaluation of patients after acute myocardial infarction: Indications for cardiac catheterization and surgical intervention. New Engl J Med 307: 1487–1492, 1982.

2. Characteristics of radiopharmaceuticals in nuclear cardiology. Implications for practical cardiac imaging

Frans J.Th. Wackers

Introduction

The recent explosive evolution of the field of nuclear cardiology found its stimulus in technological advancements in three areas. First, the development of mobile gamma cameras made it possible to obtain nuclear studies at the bedside of critically ill patients. Second, the development of dedicated mini-computers and simplified software allowed for reliable and reproducible data processing. Third, most importantly, the development of new radio-pharmaceuticals and new applications of existing radio-pharmaceuticals for cardiac imaging, has contributed to establishing nuclear cardiology procedures firmly in the diagnostic armamentarium of the clinical cardiologist in the 1980s.

In the present review we will discuss the characteristics of the radio-pharmaceuticals employed for cardiac imaging, with an emphasis on implications of their specific physical properties for practical cardiac imaging.

In nuclear cardiology, aspects of cardiac performance are evaluated after i.v. injection of a radiopharmaceutical that emits gamma radiation or photons. These photons are emitted from a large number of source nuclei in all directions. After accumulation of the radiopharmaceutical in the body, some of these photons are absorbed by surrounding tissues by photoelectric interactions, while other photons are deflected from the original course and degraded in energy by the process of compton interaction. Only a relatively small percent of photons will pass through the tissues of the body and reach the scintillation camera with their original release energy.

The gamma camera is designed to detect only the primary (good) photons and to reject the remainder. Furthermore, the camera identifies the origin of those detected primary photons in a two-dimensional space.

The presently used Anger scintillation cameras employ a sodium iodide crystal for photon detection based upon its properties as a scintillator.

Table 1a. Currently used radiopharmaceuticals for cardiac imaging

Imaging purpose	Half-life	Major KeV	Exposure whole body (mrad/mCi)	Total dose (mCi) per study	Administration mode	Comments
Viable myocardium						
201Tl	74 hr	80	10	2	I.V.	Myocardial perfusion. 201Tl washout characteristics differentiate myocardial ischemia from scar and normal tissue.
123I-FFA	13.3 hr	159	30	3	I.V.	Substrate of myocardial metabolism. Disappearance curve differentiates ischemic from normal myocardium.
99mTc-DMPE	6 hr	140	15		I.V.	Myocardial perfusion. Promising in animals. Less favorable results in human subjects.
81mKr	13 sec	190		continuous infusion	Ao	Continuous measurement of dynamic changes in regional myocardial perfusion.
11C-palmitate	20.3 min	511			I.V.	Positron-emission tomography. Evaluation aerobic myocardial metabolism.
13NH$_3$, 13N-aminoacid	9.9 min	511			I.V.	Positron-emission tomography. Evaluation myocardial blood flow.
133Xe	5.3 days	81		5	I.C.	Quantitation myocardial blood flow.
Infarction						
99mTc-Sn-PYP	6 hr	140	13	15	I.V.	Visualization acute myocardial necrosis (24-48 hrs after myocardial infarction)
111In-leukocytes	2.8 days	173;247	1		I.V.	Visualization inflammatory response to acute infarction <24 hrs.
99mTc-antimyosin (Fab)	6 hr	140			I.V.	Highly specific imaging of necrotic myocardium.

Table 10.

	Half-life	Energy (keV)		Dose (mCi)	Route	Comments
Thrombi						
¹¹¹In-platelets	2.8 days	173;247	1	0.05	I.V.	Detection of "active" clot. Highly specific. High radiation dose to spleen (target organ): 12 rad/500 µCi.
¹³¹I-fibrinogen	8.1 days	364	1	0.5	I.V.	Detection of clot.
Cardiac function						
First Pass: ⁹⁹ᵐTcO₄⁻	6 hr	140	13	15	I.V.	Ideal radionuclide for single determination of right and left ventricular function.
⁹⁹ᵐTc-DTPA	6 hr	140	13	15	I.V.	Radiopharmaceutical for repeat first-pass studies. Cleared by kidneys. Maximum: 3 × 10 mCi, separated by 10 minutes.
¹⁹⁵ᵐAu	30.6 sec	262	0.7	20	I.V.	Ideal half-life for first-pass. Limitation breakthrough of ¹⁹⁵ᵐHg (T½ = 41.6 hrs).
¹⁷⁸Ta	9.3 min	60		20	I.V.	Because of low energy photons and high energy background not ideal imaging agent.
¹⁹¹Ir	4.9 sec	129	35	10	I.V.	Ideal for first-pass and shunt studies in pediatric patients. Half-life too short for adults.
Equilibrium: ⁹⁹ᵐTc-RBC	6 hr	140	10	20	I.V.	In vivo and in 'vitro' labeling of red blood cells. Ideal technique for multiple view imaging.
⁹⁹ᵐTc-HSA	6 hr	140	10	20	I.V.	Poor quality studies due to unstable labeling after 35-45 min.
¹⁹⁵ᵐAu	30.5 sec	262		continuous infusion	I.V.	Lesser quality image but reliable assessment of function. Alternating imaging with ²⁰¹Tl is possible.

I.V.	= intravenous;		
Fab	= anticardiac myosin fragment.		
Ao	= aortic root;		
DTPA	= diethylenetriaminepentaacetic acid;		
I.C.	= intracoronary.		

FFA = free fatty acids;
RBC = red blood cells;
DMPE = dimethylphosphinoethane;
HSA = human serum albumin;
PYP = pyrophosphate;

When a photon strikes the sodium iodide crystal and interacts with the crystal lattice, a light impulse is given off proportional to the energy of the photon. The efficiency of the gamma camera is dependent upon this interaction: the higher energy of the photons and, the thicker the crystal, the more efficient radiation will be detected. The present generation of gamma cameras is able to detect photons over a wide range of energy but the ideal range is between 100 and 200 keV. However, lower energy photons, e.g., 80 keV as emitted by thallium-201 (^{201}Tl) or higher energy photons, e.g., 262 keV as emitted by gold-195m (^{195m}Au), can also be imaged satisfactorily. For optimal imaging in these two extreme situations, special collimation and adjusted crystal thickness is required.

From the above, it is evident that the physical characteristics of the radiopharmaceutical employed are of crucial importance for quality of data acquisition. It is fair to say that at the present time no ideal cardiac imaging agent exists. Such an ideal imaging agent should provide information on both myocardial perfusion and ventricular contractility. It should have a convenient half-life so that repeat studies can be performed; it should expose the patient to minimal radiation dose; it should have an emitted energy suitable for imaging with gamma cameras, and its cost should not be inhibitive. Such an imaging agent is presently not available. A great number of radiopharmaceuticals have at one time or another been employed for cardiac imaging (Table 1a and 1b). Presently, the most widely used are ^{201}Tl for myocardial perfusion imaging and technetium-99m (^{99m}Tc) for myocardial infarction imaging and dynamic cardiac studies.

Thallium-201

Currently, ^{201}Tl is the imaging agent of choice for myocardial imaging, in spite of a number of unfavorable physical characteristics of this radiopharmaceutical. Thallium-201 is a potassium analog that, after intravenous injection, distributes over the body as a function of distribution of cardiac output. Consequently, only 4% of the injected dose of ^{201}Tl is accumulated in the myocardium, reflecting regional myocardial blood flow. The myocardial to background (lung) ratio is relatively low and generally will not exceed a value of 2:1. Moreover, in patients with myocardial dysfunction and pulmonary congestion, this ratio may be considerably lower. As far as imaging is concerned, the predominantly emitted photons are of rather low energy (80 keV), therefore, only marginally suited for gamma camera

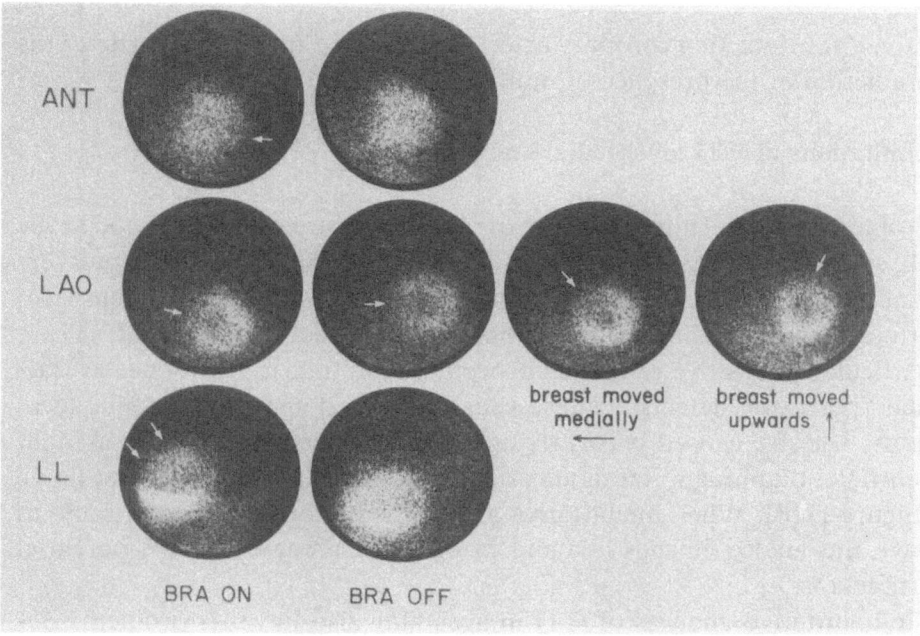

ANT

LAO

breast moved
medially
←

breast moved
upwards ↑

LL

BRA ON   BRA OFF

Figure 1. Thallium-201 imaging in a patient with heavy breasts. The low energy photons of ^{201}Tl are particularly subject to attenuation by overlying tissue which may create artifactual defects. The images on the left are with bra on. Apparent perfusion defects (arrows) are present on all views. With bra off, the defects change in location due to different position of the left breast. On the left-anterior-oblique (LAO) view, defects can be created by moving the breast in different directions. (Reproduced from Ref. 6, with permission).

imaging. A low-energy high-resolution parallel-hole collimator ensures best imaging results.

The worldwide popularity of ^{201}Tl imaging can be explained chiefly because of its convenient half-life of 74 hours which allows for storage on shelf and convenient scheduling of patient studies. In addition, the exercise images usually show better myocardial to background ratio than resting images. A major step forward was made when it was understood that analysis of the myocardial kinetics of ^{201}Tl over time provided insight whether perfusion defects represented transient ischemia or rather scar tissue. Although ^{201}Tl myocardial scintigraphy can be employed to detect and quantitate acute myocardial infarction (which has been shown to provide prognostic information), its major application is in conjunction with (treadmill or bicycle) exercise [1, 2, 3]. Quantitative analysis by circumferential profiles of myocardial activity and the amount of washout of ^{201}Tl from myocardial segments, has considerably improved the sensitivity for detecting coronary artery disease, and in particular allows the prediction of the presence of multi-vessel disease [4, 5].

Limitations of ^{201}Tl myocardial imaging

Problems with the interpretation of ^{201}Tl images are directly related to the physical characteristics of this radiopharmaceutical. The first problem that can be encountered with visual analysis of ^{201}Tl images consist of artefacts due to radiation attenuation. The low energy photons of ^{201}Tl are particularly sensitive to tissue absorption, and thus may produce artifactual "perfusion defects". These usually occur at specific anatomic locations, and are caused by overlying attenuating structures, such as right ventricle, diaphragm, fat tissue and, particularly in women, breast tissue (Figure 1) [6]. When quantitative analysis is performed it is advisable to have the analog images at hand in order to recognize these potential artifacts.

Quantitative analysis of ^{201}Tl images may also have its problem. Because of its relatively long half-life, the maximal dose injected in a patient per study as a rule does not exceed 2 mCi. Only 4% of this injected dose is accumulated in the myocardium. Thallium-201 scintigrams usually are obtained for a total of 350,000 counts in the whole field of view. However, it should be realized that when lung activity is increased, or significant liver or spleen activity is in the field of view, the count rate statistics over the left ventricle may be extremely poor. As a general rule, approximately 50,000 counts should be acquired in the left ventricular region. In order to measure "washout" of ^{201}Tl from segments of the myocardium, the images immediately post-exercise and at delayed imaging (two to three hours later) should be acquired over the exact same time period. Since good count rate statistics in the second set of images are crucial, one has to estimate the time needed for satisfactory count rates in these delayed images. A practical approach we follow in our laboratory is to obtain the first set of images (immediately post-exercise) for eight minutes or 800,000 counts (whichever comes first), and obtain the second set for the same time. Following this protocol, usually satisfactory count rates are obtained. Nevertheless, low count rates can be a problem, in particular, when old myocardial infarction is present in conjunction with exercise-induced, transient ischemia. Small (random) variations of low count rates may change normal washout into abnormal washout. We have established in our laboratory that it is not prudent to evaluate ^{201}Tl washout when mean count rates per segment are below 30 counts.

Although ^{201}Tl, because of its physical characteristics (high attenuation factor and relative poor count rate statistics), theoretically is a poor imaging agent for single photon emission tomography (SPECT), excellent results have recently been obtained using a single rotating detector head and, most importantly, sophisticated computer software [7].

In spite of its limitations, ^{201}Tl has been shown to have distinct practical advantages over other potassium analogs such as: ^{43}K, ^{129}Cs, or radioactive gases as ^{85}Kr and ^{133}Xe, used in the past for imaging of myocardial perfusion. Yet, new radiopharmaceuticals are currently developed for this purpose, as discussed at the end of this chapter.

Technetium-99m

Technetium-99m is the "work horse" of nuclear medicine. Technetium-99m is used as free pertechnetate (^{99m}TcO$_4^-$) or labeled to various biochemical compounds. For cardiac imaging, the following compounds are of importance. Technetium-^{99m}-diethylenetriaminepentaacetic acid (DPTA), ^{99m}Tc-human-serum-albumin, ^{99m}Tc-red-blood-cells, and ^{99m}-Tc-stannous-pyrophosphate. Technetium-99m is an almost ideal radionuclide for imaging with the present generation of gamma cameras. Its energy spectrum is mono-energetic and 140 keV gamma rays are highly abundant (90%), no beta or alpha particles are emitted. The physical half life is a convenient 6 hrs. The radionuclide is easy to produce and readily available in generator form. Importantly, it has the ability to form a complex with many organic or inorganic compounds. Moreover, it is relatively inexpensive. Technetium-99m is the daughter of Molybdenum-99 (^{99}Mo), which has a half-life of 67 hours. Flushing a ^{99}Mo/^{99m}Tc generator with isotonic saline brings ionic pertechnetate (^{99m}TcO$_4^-$) through the column leaving ^{99}Mo behind. The usual dosage for cardiac studies ranges from 10–30 mCi. Dependent on the type of study a general all-purpose or high-sensitivity collimator is used.

Technetium-99m-Sn-pyrophosphate

This technetium-labeled radioactive compound was widely used for bone imaging before it was demonstrated that accumulation in acutely infarcted myocardium of experimental animals occurs. Subsequently, extensive clinical evaluation has confirmed this finding, and the clinical utility of this

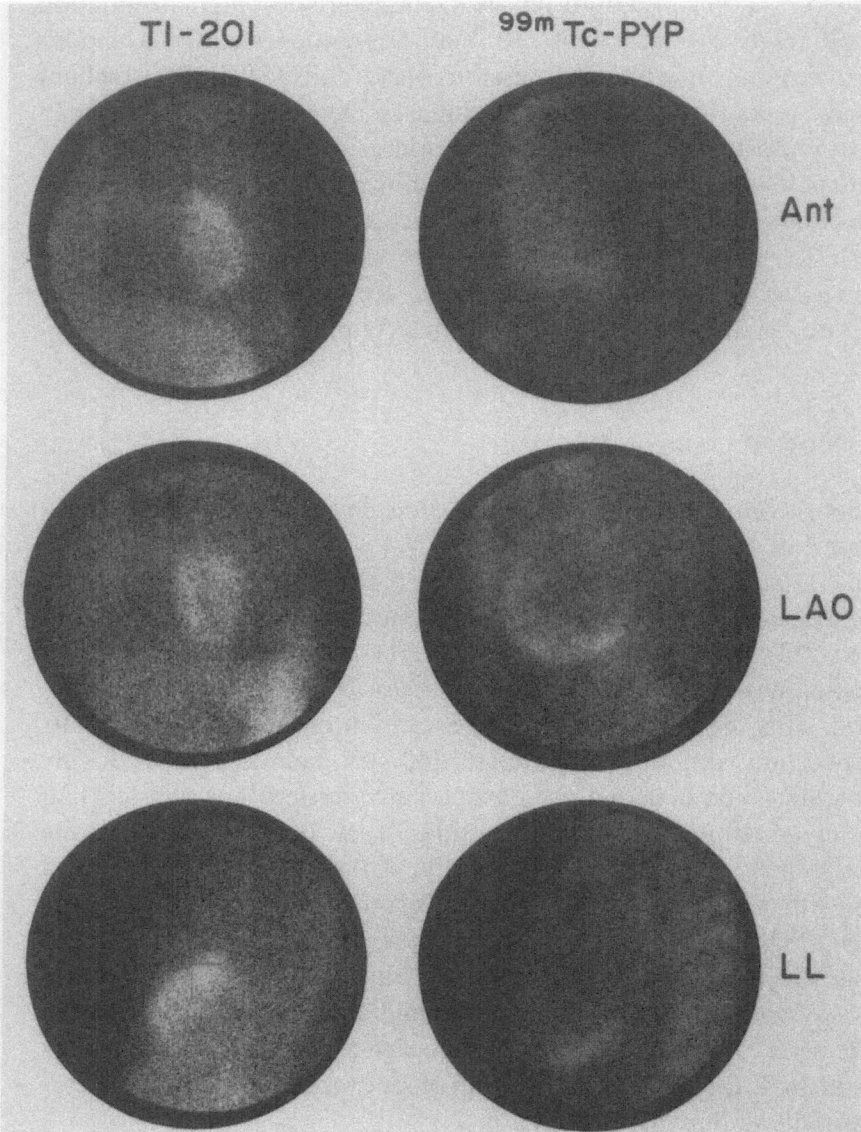

Figure 2. Dual myocardial imaging with ^{201}Tl and ^{99m}Tc-pyrophosphate (PYP). The difference in energy emitted by the two radiopharmaceuticals (and also the difference in dosage) permits sequential imaging. When ^{201}Tl imaging is performed first, imaging with ^{99m}Tc-PYP can be performed without loss of image quality, as shown in this example of a patient with an inferoposterior myocardial infarction and right ventricular involvement. (Reproduced from Ref. 6, with permission).

imaging agent is well defined. In many patients with acute transmural myocardial infarction, intense, discrete accumulation in the infarcted region can be observed (Figure 2). More difficult is the interpretation of less intense uptake which has to be differentiated from residual blood pool activity and diffuse myocardial accumulation. The time of imaging post-injection of the radiopharmaceutical needs to fit into a time window between initial high blood concentration and late marked bone uptake. This usually is between 60 and 90 minutes after injection. Diffuse nondiagnostic activity is the most common problem in analyzing ^{99m}Tc-Sn-pyrophosphate scans. Since inadequate labeling and circulating free ^{99m}Tc-pertechnetate may be the cause, quality control of labeling efficiency is necessary. Delayed clearance of minimal amounts of free ^{99m}Tc may occur as a consequence of severe renal insufficiency, badly deranged left ventricular function or poor metabolic turnover rate of the bone. In these circumstances, it is best to obtain relatively late delayed images, i.e., two to three hours after injection. A second cause of persistent blood pool activity is labeling of the patient's red blood cells with free ^{99m}Tc-per-technetate. This occurs with high concentrations of tin (Sn) and excess free ^{99m}Tc-pertechnetate in injected phosphate compounds. If it does occur, the examination needs to be repeated the following day with delayed imaging two to three hours after injection of ^{99m}Tc-Sn-pyro-phosphate.

Another problem may be posed by abnormal uptake *not* located in the myocardium. In particular, in older patients, abnormal accumulation may be noted in the calcified costal cartilages. This may overlay the cardiac region and lead to misinterpretation. Usually, the activity is then present as bilateral linear structures, converging to the tip of the sternum. Another common source of error (and confusion) may be accumulation of ^{99m}Tc-Sn-pyrophosphate in breast tissue of (older) women.

Occasionally, dual imaging with ^{201}Tl and ^{99m}Tc-Sn-pyrophosphate may be clinically indicated (Figure 2) [8]. In spite of the longer half-life of ^{201}Tl, imaging with this radioisotope should be performed first, to be followed by imaging with ^{99m}Tc-Sn-pyrophosphate. The rationale for this sequence is the low dose and low energy photons of ^{201}Tl, compared to that of ^{99m}Tc.

Infarct sizing employing a computerized reconstruction technique of ^{99m}Tc-Sn-pyrophosphate accumulation from two dimensional images has been reported [9]. This technique, however, is greatly hampered by poor edge definition, and the presence of activity in bony structures. Encouraging results recently have been reported employing single emission photon tomography (SPECT) [10].

Evaluation of cardiac function

Technetium-99m presently is the imaging agent of choice for dynamic cardiac imaging. Cardiac function can be evaluated by two methods: (1) first-pass radionuclide angiocardiography (list-mode or ECG-gated) and, (2) multigated equilibrium cardiac blood pool imaging. The physical characteristics of the radiopharmaceutical employed are of relevance for the reliability of the acquired data.

First-pass technique

For this method the radiopharmaceutical, usually 15 to 20 mCi of ^{99m}Tc-pertechnetate or ^{99m}Tc-DTPA is injected rapidly as a compact bolus into an antecubital vein. Quantitative analysis of the transit of this bolus through the central circulation is based upon the principles of indicator dilution theory. The efficacy and reliability of the first-pass method depends upon obtaining sufficiently high count rates to assure statistical reliability. The sensitivity of photons is determined by the interaction of the radiopharmaceutical employed and the gamma camera (collimation, crystal thickness and gamma-camera electronics). Conventional single crystal scintillation cameras are limited in terms of maximal count rate efficiency. Since the count rate response is linear only up to 50–60,000 cps, further increase of the injected dose will not resolve this problem satisfactorily. Presently, the only gamma-camera systems capable of acquiring sufficiently high count rates are the multicrystal gamma camera and the recently developed digital single crystal camera. These systems are linear up to a count rate of 450,000 and 200,000 cps, respectively.

In addition to the limitation posed by the gamma camera, tissue attenuation plays also a role. Using a conventional single crystal gamma camera reasonably high count rates can be obtained during the passage of the bolus through the right ventricle. However, during the levo phase, because of dilution of the bolus and tissue attenuation, count rates generally are low and inadequate. In order to compensate for the statistical uncertainty of low count rate data, several mathematical manipulations have been proposed for determining left ventricular ejection fraction by first pass technique using a conventional crystal camera [11]. Recently, a combination of first pass technique with electrocardiographic gating has been proposed as a means of determining reliable right ventricular ejection fraction by using a single crystal camera [12]. By this technique, end-diastole and end-systole are not chosen by subjective analysis of a time-activity curve, but by utilizing the physiologic ECG signal as a synchronizing marker, allowing accurate summation of scintillation data.

Multi-gated equilibrium cardiac blood pool imaging

Labeling of the cardiac blood pool can be achieved by two methods: (a) the use of ^{99m}Tc labeled human serum albumin, or (b) *in-vivo* labeling of the patient's red blood cells with ^{99m}Tc-pertechnetate. For the last method, the patient's red blood cells are premedicated with microgram amounts of stannous ion (Sn^{++}). This facilitates intracellular reduction of pertechnetate and achieves approximately 90% labeling efficiency of the patient's red blood cells. Efficient blood pool labeling is extremely important under conditions where degradation of image quality can be expected, such as in obese patients, very small children, or during exercise tests. The labeling efficiency can be improved by *in vitro* labeling or by a recently described variation: *"in vivtro"* labeling. For the latter method, 15 minutes after administration of stannous pyrophosphate, blood is withdrawn and incubated for 10 minutes in a heparinized syringe containing ^{99m}Tc. In this way, high labeling efficiency is achieved already in the syringe. The remaining free pertechnetate together with the labeled red blood cells is subsequently injected into the circulation, where it will bind in turn to other red blood cells.

Counting statistics and calculation of ejection fraction

The clinically most useful parameter of cardiac performance is ejection fraction of right or left ventricle. Ejection fraction is calculated from background corrected counts in end-diastole minus background corrected counts in end-systole, divided by background corrected counts in end-diastole. It is assumed, although probably not entirely correct, that background activity does not change during the cardiac cycle. An incorrectly chosen background may have significant impact on the value of calculated ejection fraction. The effect of error in background on ejection fraction is considerably greater in patients with a normal ventricular performance than in patients with abnormal left ventricular ejection fraction. Therefore, it is important that the method of background determination is well standardized. The background activity usually is significantly higher in

Table 2. Percent statistical error in ejection fraction for different ejection fractions and end-diastolic counts

End-diastolic-counts	Ejection fraction						
	.2	.3	.4	.5	.6	.7	.8
100	88	54	38	28	22	18	15
200	62	38	27	20	16	12	10
500	39	24	17	13	10	8	6.5
800	31	19	13	10	8	6	5
1,000	28	17	12	9	7	5.5	4.5
2,000	20	12	9	6	5	4	3
5,000	12	8	6	4	3	2.5	2
8,000	10	6	5	3.5	2.5	2	1.6
10,000	9	5	4	3	2	1.5	1.5
20,000	6	4	3	2	1.5	1	1
30,000	5	3	2	1.5	1	1	0.8

multigated equilibrium studies than in first-pass studies. We usually employ a crescent shaped area posterolateral to the left ventricle.

In addition, the calculation of left ventricular ejection fraction is affected by counting statistics, i.e., absolute counts obtained in end-diastole and end-systole. Again, the statistical error is related to the baseline value of ejection fraction. The lower the counts and the lower left ventricular ejection fraction, the greater the potential statistical error. A tabulation of the percent error in ejection fraction is given in Table 2. If the statistical error is to be kept within 3% in a patient with 80% ejection fraction, at least 2,000 background corrected counts should be present in end-diastole. For the same statistical reliability in a patient with a 30% ejection fraction, 30,000 counts are required in the end-diastolic region of interest. Fortunately, most patients with low ejection fractions have large ventricles and, therefore, satisfactory counting statistics are relatively easily obtained. As outlined above, the count rates which can be obtained are determined by the technique employed, i.e., first-pass or equilibrium blood pool studies.

Geometric considerations

Radionuclide derived left ventricular ejection fraction has been claimed to be independent of geometric considerations. This is only partly correct. The relative contribution of left ventricular blood pool activity to the total of counts registered by the gamma camera is not uniform, but inversely related to the distance from the detector surface. This is mainly the result of scattering and attenuation of photons within the body. When the contraction of the ventricle is symmetrical and normal, this differential sensitivity for photons from deeper portions of the ventricle will not affect the validity of ejection fraction significantly. However, when significant regional wall motion abnormalities are present, this may have considerable impact on the calculated value for ejection fraction (Figure 3). For example, in the case of an anterior wall aneurysm, the relative contribution of radioactivity from the poorly contracting anterior one third of the left ventricle is far more important than that of the normally contracting remainder of the left ventricle. As a consequence, left ventricular ejection fraction tends to be underestimated in patients with large anterior wall regional wall motion abnormalities. The reverse is true for patients who have significantly posterobasal wall motion abnormalities. The change in count rates observed reflects to a greater extent volume changes in the anterior portion closer to the detector head. Therefore, left ventricular ejection fraction in these patients tends to be overestimated.

In a similar way, the radioactive blood pool of the atria in equilibrium cardiac blood pool imaging affects the calculation of ejection fraction. Whereas, the effect of the left atrial activity on the calculation of left ventricular ejection fraction is minimal because of the greater distance from the detector head, the effect of right atrial activity (which is closer to the detector) on right ventricular ejection fraction is significant and in some patients may lead to gross underestimation of right ventricular ejection fraction.

New radiopharmaceuticals and future developments

Although the currently available radiopharmaceuticals provide valuable clinical information, they are, from a technical point of view, far from optimal. Therefore, investigators have been exploring new radioisotopes with more favorable physical characteristics.

Technetium-99m-labeled myocardial perfusion imaging agents

Since ^{99m}Tc is the radionuclide of choice for diagnostic nuclear imaging, in the last couple of years investigators have explored the possibility of

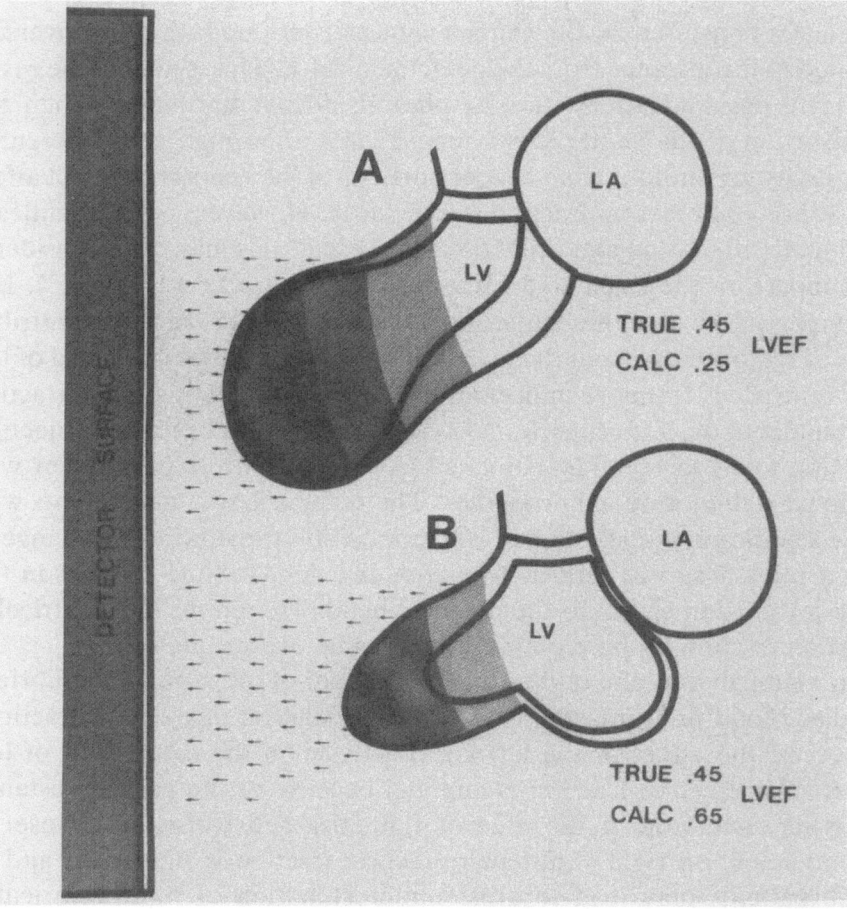

Figure 3. Schematic representation of the effect of location of regional wall motion abnormalities on calculated (CALC) value of left ventricular ejection fraction (LVEF), as compared to true value of LVEF. The detector head of the gamma camera is shown at the left.

A. Large anteroapical area of akinesis. Although the radioactivity is in equilibrium in the cardiac blood pool, the gamma camera will receive a relatively larger contribution from areas closer to the detector surface than from more distal portions. The relative contribution is schematically represented by different shades of gray; the darker the shade the greater the relative contribution to the detected counts. In this example, calculation of LVEF on the basis of changes in count rates (predominantly originating from the anterior portion of the left ventricle) will result in considerable underestimation, compared to the true value of global LVEF.

B. Large posterobasal aneurysm. The well-preserved contraction of the anterior wall will significantly effect the changes in count rates detected by the gamma camera. Since the relative contribution of the abnormal posterobasal segment to detected countrate changes is less, considerable overestimation of calculated LVEF compared to true LVEF will occur.

The differential contribution of photons from the radiopharmaceutical at varying distance from the detector surface is determined by the physics involved in radiation detection, but also by scatter and attenuation of photons within the body.

developing a ^{99m}Tc-labeled radiopharmaceutical that would accumulate in normal heart tissue in a similar way as ^{201}Tl. It is known that radionuclides of the group 1 cations (K^{43}, Rb^{81} and Cs^{129}) accumulate in normal heart tissue. These cations accumulate through involvement of the Na-K-ATP ase system; that is, they function as potassium analogs. Thallium-201 is another such a potassium analog. The concept behind the development of other myocardial agents is that + 1-charged complexes of ^{99m}Tc might mimic the *in vivo* behavior of ^{201}Tl and be taken up by normal heart tissue. Recently, Deutsch and his associates have been successful in preparing a cationic ^{99m}Tc complex with dimethylphosphinoethane (DMPE) which in animal studies showed great similarity to images obtained with ^{201}Tl [13]. The clinical advantage of this new radioactive compound would be three-fold. First, the energy emitted at 140 keV is better suited for gamma-camera imaging and will result in better image quality. Second, because of the shorter half-life of ^{99m}Tc, it will be possible to administer a larger dose to a patient, resulting in better count rates and better image quality. Third, the radiation dose to the patient would be significantly less compared to 2 mCi of ^{201}Tl; 15 mCi of ^{99m}Tc-DMPE would expose the whole body to two times less and the kidney to three times less radiation.

Unfortunately, initial clinical trials have made clear that the favorable results in animals are not reproduced in humans. In particular, the uptake in the liver and also in skeleton is far greater in human subjects than in animals, resulting in rather poor image quality, compared to conventional ^{201}Tl images. Nevertheless, investigators are confident that, along the same track, a technetium-labeled myocardial perfusion imaging agent will be developed in the near future.

Myocardial imaging with free fatty acids

Free fatty acids are substrates for normal myocardial metabolism. In myocardial ischemia, there is an inhibition of free fatty acid uptake in the ischemic myocardium, probably as a result of diminished coronary artery blood flow but also because of a shift to carbohydrate metabolism. Free fatty acids have been labeled with various radioisotopes, ^{11}C, ^{123}I, and, more recently, with ^{99m}Tc. Iodine-123 and ^{99m}Tc are, as mentioned above (Table 1), excellent for gamma-camera imaging. Initial results with free fatty acid imaging demonstrated that images are comparable to those obtained with ^{201}Tl. Moreover, it appears that analysis of the disappearance curve allows for differentiating infarction from ischemia [14].

Thus, although the basic cellular mechanisms involved are quite different, similarities exist between imaging with ^{201}Tl and radio-labeled free fatty acids. Further characterization can be expected in the near future.

Assessment of dynamic cardiac function with short-lived radioisotopes

The relative long half-life of ^{99m}Tc and patient's dosimetry considerations limit the total number of studies that can be performed in sequence, as well as the dose per study (3 studies and 10 mCi, respectively). Recently, short-lived radioisotopes have been proposed for first-pass angiocardiography. Tantalum-178 ($T^{1}/_{2} = 9.3$ minutes) has been proposed as a generator-produced short-lived radionuclide. Although promising results have been reported using this short-lived radiotracer, a limitation appears to be the low energy of the major photon emissions (x-rays at 55–65 keV) and a high level of background activity resulting from a 500 keV photon emission [15]. Another ultra short-lived generator-produced radionuclide that has been proposed is iridium-191m [16]. Although this tracer has optimal photon energy (129 keV) for imaging, its 4.9 seconds half-life is too short for first-pass studies in adults but is probably the radiotracer of choice for cardiac studies in children.

We have recently investigated the use of gold-195m ([195m]Au) [17]. The half-life of 30.5 seconds of [195m]Au appears to be ideally suited for application in adults. In normal adult subjects, radioactivity reaches the left heart chamber within approximately 10–15 seconds after a rapid bolus injection into the basilic vein. This interval may be considerably longer in seriously ill cardiac patients, but rarely exceeds 25 seconds. The half-life of the parent [195m]Hg is long enough (41.6 hours) to allow shipment of the generator to relatively remote places. The yield of this generator is approximately 40%, and adequate dosage (15–30 mCi) of [195m]Au can be obtained per elution. The initial results with first-pass studies using [195m]Au in patients have been extremely satisfactory. The quality of images and the count-rate statistics are comparable to an equivalent dose of [99m]Tc. The advantage of the use of [195]Au is: (1) considerably reduced patient radiation dose: per injection 20 times less to the whole body and five times less to the target organ, the kidneys. (2) The short-lived radionuclide allows for a more differentiated analysis of ventricular function in patients with coronary artery disease. Instead of evaluating ejection fraction only at baseline and at peak exercise, [195]Au allows for rapid serial assessments of left ventricular function at the intermediate stages of exercise. The

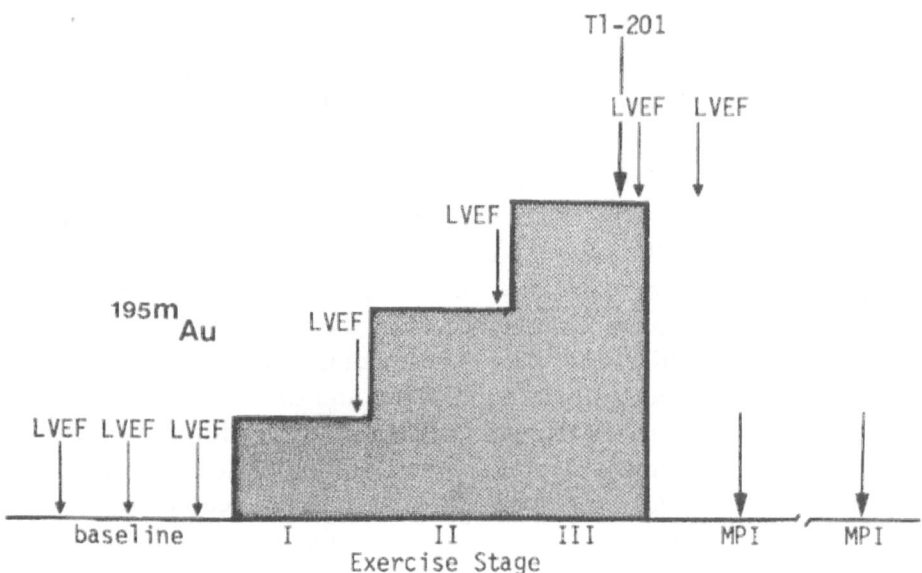

Figure 4. Combined assessment of left ventricular function and myocardial perfusion during one single exercise test is possible using ^{195m}Au and ^{201}Tl. Left ventricular ejection fraction (LVEF) can be assessed at short intervals at rest and during various stages of exercise using short-lived ($t^{1}/_{2}$ = 30.5 sec) ^{195m}Au. At peak exercise, ^{201}Tl is injected. The quality of myocardial perfusion imaging (MPI) immediately post-exercise and 2–3 hours later is unaffected by multiple preceding injections of ^{195m}Au.

pattern of left ventricular dysfunction during exercise may be of relevance for management of these patients. (3) A probably more important practical application is the possibility to combine assessment of cardiac function with evaluation of myocardial perfusion (Figure 4). By obtaining these studies simultaneously, this approach may provide a means of assessing more reliably the functional significance of coronary artery stenosis. This combined technique also has obvious advantages as far as cost effectiveness of patient evaluation is concerned, since only one exercise test is needed to obtain this information. Even with the development of new ^{99m}Tc-labeled myocardial perfusion imaging agents, this combined approach would be feasible because of the difference in primary photopeak of the radionuclides.

For exercise studies, the first-pass technique offers a distinct advantage over multigated cardiac blood pool imaging. Because data are acquired over a short time period, utilizing only three to five cardiac cycles, it is likely that they approximate true left ventricular function during peak exercise more closely than data acquired over several hundred heart beats. In addition, body motion during exercise has a major degrading effect on the quality of equilibrium blood pool studies, which may be reflected in poorer reproducibility of data processing. As discussed above, reliable first-pass studies require instruments with high count rate capability. With the expected further technical development of gamma cameras permitting acquisition of higher count rates, the first-pass technique may well become the method of choice for performing exercise studies. Gold-195m would then become the radionuclide of choice for evaluation of patients with coronary artery disease in conjunction with a myocardial perfusion imaging agent. In this case, consideration will need to be given to medium-energy collimation, detector shielding and adequate crystal thickness to maintain both intrinsic resolution and sensitivity.

In the above, the currently used radiopharmaceuticals for nuclear cardiology studies are reviewed. Understanding of the physical characteristics of the radionuclides employed and the consequences thereof for practical cardiac imaging are important for reliable interpretation of acquired data and images.

References

1. Wackers FJTh, Sokole EB, Samson G, Schoot JB vd, Lie KI, Liem KL, Wellens HJJ: Value and limitations of thallium-201 scintigraphy in the acute phase of myocardial infarction. N Engl J Med 295:1–5, 1976.
2. Silverman KJ, Becker LC, Bulkley BH, Burow RD, Mellits ED, Kallman CH, Weisfeldt ML: Value of early thallium-201 scintigraphy for predicting mortality in patients with acute myocardial infarction. Circulation 61:996–1003, 1980.
3. Ritchie JL, Trobaugh GB, Hamilton GW, Gould KL, Narahara KA, Murray JA, Williams DL: Myocardial imaging with thallium-201 at rest and during exercise: Comparison with coronary angiography and resting and stress electrocardiography. Circulation 56:66–71, 1977.
4. Berger BC, Watson DD, Taylor GJ, Craddock GB, Martin RP, Teates CD, Beller GA: Quantitative thallium-201 exercise scintigraphy for detection of coronary artery disease. J Nucl Med 22:585–593, 1981.
5. Maddahi J, Garcia EV, Berman DS, Waxman A, Swan HJC, Forrester J: Improved noninvasive assessment of coronary artery disease by quantitative analysis of regional stress myocardial distribution and washout of thallium-201. Circulation 64:924–935, 1981.
6. Wackers FJTh, Busemann SE, Schoot JB vd, Samson G, Lewis S, Parkey RW, Willersen JT: Dual imaging in acute infarction. In: Thallium-201 and technetium-99m-pyrophosphate: Myocardial imaging in the coronary care unit. Wackers FJTh (ed). Martinus Nyhoff Publishers, The Hague, Boston, London, 1980, pp. 177–195.
7. Maublant J, Cassagnes J, LeJeune JJ, Mestas D, Veyre A, Jallut H, Meyniel G: A comparison between conventional scintigraphy and emission tomography with thallium-201 in the detection of myocardial infarction: Concise communication. J Nucl Med 23:204–208, 1982.
8. Parkey, RW, Bonte FJ, Meyer SL, Atkins JM, Curry GL, Stokely EM, Willerson JT: A new method for radionuclide imaging of acute myocardial infarction in humans. Circulation 50:540–546, 1974.

9. Lewis MH, Buja LM, Saffer S, Mishelevich D, Stokely E, Lewis S, Parkey R, Bonte F, Willerson JT: Experimental infarct sizing using computer processing and a three-dimensional model. Science 197:167–169, 1977.

10. Holman BL, Goldhaber SZ, Kirsch C-M, Polak JF, Friedman BJ, English RJ, Wynne J: Measurement of infarct size using single photon emission computed tomography and technetium-99m pyrophosphate. A description of the method and comparison with patient prognosis. Amer J Cardiol 50: 503–511, 1982.

11. Berger HJ, Matthay RA, Pytlik LM, Gottschalk A, Zaret BL: First-pass radionuclide assessment of right and left ventricular performance in patients with cardiac and pulmonary disease. Semin Nucl Med 9: 275–295, 1979.

12. Winzelberg GG, Boucher CA, Pohost GM, McKusick KA, Bingham JB, Okada RD, Strauss HW: Right ventricular function in aortic and mitral valve disease: Relation of gated first-pass radionuclide angiography to clinical and hemodynamic findings. Chest 79:520–528, 1981.

13. Deutsch E, Bushong W, Glavan KA, Elder RC, Sodd VJ, Scholz KL, Fortman DL, Lukes SJ: Heart imaging with cationic complexes of technetium. Science 214:85–86, 1981.

14. Wall EE van der, Heidendal GAK, Hollander W den, Westera G, Roos JP: I-123 labeled hexadecenoic acid in comparison with thallium-201 for myocardial imaging in coronary heart disease. Eur J Nucl Med 5:401–405, 1980.

15. Holman B, Neirinckx RD, Treves S, Tow DE: Cardiac imaging with tantalum-178. Radiology 131:525–526, 1979.

16. Treves S, Fyler D, Fjuii A, Kuruc A: Low radiation iridium 191m radionuclide angiography: Detection and quantitation of left-to-right shunts in infants. J Pediatrics 101(2):210–213, 1982.

17. Gold-195m, a new generator-produced short-lived radionuclide for sequential assessment of ventricular performance by first pass radionuclide angiography. Amer J Cardiol 50:89–94, 1982.

3. Myocardial blood flow: clinical application and recent advances

Richard Wilson, Michael Shea, Christian de Landsheere, John Deanfield, Adrian Lammetsma, David Terton and Andrew Selwyn

Introduction

The uptake of oxygen and metabolic substrates by the myocardium is dependent on myocardial blood flow and also on the avidity or extraction of oxygen and substrates by the myocardium. The delivery of oxygen and substrates to the myocardium is therefore an important component in the preservation of normal contractile function. Regional changes in myocardial blood flow frequently occur in patients with coronary artery disease and these are followed by changes in left ventricular function that are transient in angina or permanent in infarction. Because of the morbidity and mortality associated with these changes in ventricular function, accurate measurement of myocardial blood flow is of great clinical importance. Many methods for measuring myocardial blood flow have been described [1]. These can be classified as (1) indicator-dilution techniques using inert gases or thermodilution, and (2) radioisotope techniques using monovalent cations, ammonia, carbon dioxide, water or microspheres. Each of these methods suffers from technical and theoretical limitations of the measurement as well as problems in the clinical applicability. This chapter will review the available methods for the clinical measurement of myocardial blood flow and will discuss their advantages and limitations when applied to clinical problems. Major emphasis will be placed on techniques which are presently in wide use as well as on newer but promising methods.

Methods

Available methods for measuring myocardial blood flow in man (Table 1) vary considerably in their theoretical and technical limitations. In general, however, the majority of these techniques have certain principles and assumptions in common. Many of these techniques are based on the Fick

Table 1. Measurement of myocardial blood flow in man

---

1. Indicator-dilution methods
   a. Inert gases
      i. A-V sampling (N_2O, H_2, He)
      ii. Radioactive counting (Xe-133, Kr-85, Kr-81m, I-131 iodoantipyrine)
   b. Thermodilution
2. Radioisotope flow markers
   a. gamma emitters
      i. monovalent cations (K-43, S-131), (S-129, Tl-201)
      ii. Tc-99m microspheres
   b. Positron emitters
      i. Rb-82
      ii. N-13 ammonia
      iii. Radiolabelled water
      iv. Ga-68 and C-11 microspheres

---

principle. The Fick principle states that blood flow to an organ is equal to the uptake of any substance divided by the A-V concentration difference of that substance. Implicit in this principle are the assumptions that: (1) the system is in steady state during the period of the measurement, (2) the amount of tracer will not affect the transit time, (3) adequate mixing of the tracer with the blood occurs prior to its entry into the system, (4) there is no recirculation of the tracer during the observation period, and (5) flow is unidirectional.

Indicator-dilution techniques

Inert gases

Measurement of myocardial blood flow using inert gases which are not used in the form of radionuclide tracers requires arterial and coronary sinus sampling [2, 3]. The use of radioactive inert gas tracers however may allow noninvasive measurement of blood flow by inhalation of the gas to avoid intra-arterial injection [4]. A-V sampling techniques avoid the administration of radioactivity and minimise the recirculation of the gas since it is removed by the lungs. This technique lends itself to use in the cardiac catheterisation laboratory for studies of global myocardial blood flow only. The venous catheter must be placed well within the coronary sinus (at least 2 cm) to avoid contamination of the sample by right atrial blood [5]. This technique does not adequately sample flow from myocardium which drains directly into the right atrium or other cardiac chambers by the thebesian veins. The period of saturation of the arterial blood by the gas must be long enough to attain the same gas concentrations in normal as well as low flow areas. Similarly the desaturation period must be long enough to adequately sample regions of low flow from which slower efflux of the gas is expected. Unfortunately these gases are highly soluble in fat tissue. The larger the amount of epicardial fat perfused by the coronary arteries, the slower will be the washout of the gas resulting in spuriously low values. This technique has been used with nitrous oxide [2], argon [3], hydrogen [5] and helium [6, 7].

The use of radioactive inert gases to measure myocardial blood flow requires intracoronary infusion of the gas or inhalation of gas with external detection of the emitted radiation during the clearance of dilution of the radioactive gas from the myocardium. This technique lends itself to quantitation of regional rather than global myocardial blood flow. Gases that have been used in this technique are xenon-133 [8], and I-131 iodoantipyrine [10]. Xenon-133 suffers from significant soft tissue attenuation due to its low energy emission (81 KeV). This results in variable count recovery depending on the uneven thickness of the chest wall and breast tissue. In addition, xenon has a high fat: myocardial solubility coefficient so that epicardial fat as well as chest wall fat significantly contaminates the myocardial signal. Since the measurement of myocardial blood flow relies on the monoexponential clearance of the tracer from the myocardium, significant fat deposition of the tracer will effectively slow the apparent myocardial clearance of the gas in an uneven fashion. Intracoronary injection decreases but does not eliminate the problem and may introduce problems related to streaming of the tracer preferentially from the left main stem to one or the other coronary arteries. Although these considerations limit the measurement of absolute regional myocardial blood flow, it does allow serial measurements before, during and after an intervention but only in the cardiac catheterisation laboratory. Use of iodoantipyrine as I-131, I-133 or I-125 has the advantage of lower fat solubility compared to xenon but the I-125 requires an on-site cyclotron for production.

Krypton-81m is a generator-produced short-lived radioactive gas ($t^{1}/_{2}$ = 13 sec) which can be infused in normal saline into the sinus of Valsalva [9]. The high specific activity that can be administered because of the short half-life allows adequate counting statistics during the imaging of the arterial transit of the gas. The very short half-life provides a measure of minute-by-minute changes in regional myocardial perfusion and regions of decreased flow are seen as defects in the perfusion scan. These defects represent a qualitative rather than absolute measure of flow deficit. This technique allows frequent and rapid determination of regional myocardial blood flow especially with disturbed patterns of perfusion seen in patients with coronary artery disease and angina pectoris [11]. Unfortunately the Rb-81 parent in the portable generator has only a 4.6 hour half life.

Thermodilution

This method is based on the changes in temperature of cold normal saline as it passes through the myocardium [12, 13]. The technique is simple, easily used and inexpensive. Its clinical utility is however limited to measurement of global blood flow unless selective catheterisation of the great cardiac vein is performed. Rapid changes in flow can be measured with this technique through repeated infusions assuming that constant infusion rates and adequate time for mixing at high flow rates can be maintained. The measurement favours regions of high flow and cannot resolve regional events in the ventricles with any precision.

Radioisotope flow markers

Gamma emitters

Monovalent cations
A number of gamma emitting monovalent cations have been used to assess regional myocardial blood flow (K-43, Cs-131, Cs-129, Tl-201). Of these the potassium analog currently in widest clinical use is Tl-201. Tl-201 has a high extraction fraction during passage through the coronary circuit. Therefore it is distributed in relation to coronary flow according to the Sapirstein principle [14]. Over a wide range of flows the uptake and the distribution of Tl-201 correlate well with the distribution of myocardial blood flow [15, 16]. However, the uptake of Tl-201 and other monovalent cations is the product of blood flow and the extraction fraction. For Tl-201 the extraction fraction is inversely related to flow [17] when coronary flow is in the normal range. Therefore, at high flows the extraction is much lower and at low flows the extraction is greater. This results in an underestimation of true flow at high flows as well as an overestimation of true flow in low flow states. However, the wall thinning that occurs with ischaemia may improve the detection of a Tl-201 defect. In addition the uptake of Tl-201 may be influenced by cardiac drugs [18] and other

physiologic and metabolic changes [17]. In the case of propranolol, a decreased sensitivity for the detection of coronary artery disease in patients with negative exercise electrocardiograms [19], and with dipyridamole [20] has been observed. This may be due to improvement in regional myocardial ischaemia induced by propranolol with direct or indirect effects on Tl-201 extraction [21]. Exercise-induced Tl-201 defects of the anterior wall are generally better appreciated in the multiple views (anterior, 40°, and 70° left anterior oblique projections) than of the posterior left ventricular wall which may be obscured from view by the left hemidiaphragm [22]. Because of the low energy of the emitted Hg X-rays (80 keV) used in Tl-201 imaging, soft tissue attenuation, such as from the breast, presents a significant limitation. Multiple projections may be helpful in distinguishing an attenuation-induced myocardial "defect" from a true deficit in myocardial Tl-201 uptake. Careful repositioning of the patient for delayed images is necessary to minimise changes in soft tissue attenuation for a given patient.

The clinical utility of Tl-201 imaging is multifaceted. Tl-201 is useful in conjunction with the electrocardiogram during exercise stress testing for the improved diagnosis of coronary artery disease [23, 24, 25], especially in patients with abnormal baseline electrocardiograms and in asymptomatic patients with an ambiguous "ischaemic" ST-segment response on the exercise electrocardiogram [26]. However, the prevalence of the disease in the patient population being studied may alter the predictive accuracy of the test. Tl-201 exercise stress testing may also provide prognostic information in patients with coronary artery disease [27, 28]. Tl-201 imaging may be clinically useful for the determination of the haemodynamic significance of a "50%" diameter coronary artery lesion on arteriography [29]. The use of the redistribution of Tl-201 into a myocardial region may also define the viability of that region [30, 31]. However the extent of redistribution may be decreased if the patient eats a high carbohydrate meal [32] since an intravenous infusion of glucose-insulin-potassium will increase net clearance rates of Tl-201 from transiently ischaemic and normally perfused myocardium [33] and also decreases the extent of Tl-201 redistribution into an area of transient ischaemia [34].

Significant problems exist with the use of Tl-201 as a perfusion marker: (1) the decrease in Tl-201 extraction especially with very high levels of blood flow, (2) the low energy of photons (80 keV) are significantly affected by differences in attenuation especially breast attenuation in women, (3) radiation dosimetry considerations limit the dose of Tl-201 administered and therefore limit count density and image quality. Use of one of the Tc-99m labelled cationic complexes currently under investigation as perfusion agents [35, 36], may improve image quality on the basis of less soft tissue attenuation (140 keV) and higher photon fluxes within current dosimetry restrictions.

Gamma-labelled microspheres

In 1970 the use of I-131 [37] and Tc-99M [38] labelled macroaggregated albumin for measurement of myocardial blood flow in humans was reported. Additional extensive canine studies of the effects of the macroaggregates and human albumin microspheres were also reported [39, 40, 41]. Subsequently over 5000 studies have been performed in humans – confirming the safety of this method [42, 43, 44]. Since the spatial resolution of current gamma cameras including single photon emission tomography does not permit accurate differentiation of endocardial from epicardial myocardium the particle size used is not as important compared to *in vitro* well counting where endocardial and epicardial flows are measured separately [45, 46]. The microspheres require injection into the systemic circulation either in the left atrium via a transeptal catheter or in the apex of the left ventricle to ensure adequate mixing. Currently available planar or single photon emission tomographic imaging systems are not yet able to provide more than a qualitative or at best semi-quantitative measure of flow using microspheres. Absolute quantitation of regional myocardial blood flow using gamma emitting microspheres awaits the development of reliable methods for attentuation correction and corrections for object size (partial volume effect). Because of these as yet unresolved problems, Tl-201 imaging may be preferable by virtue of its noninvasiveness.

Positron-emitters

Rubidium-82

Rubidium-82 (Rb-82) is a short-lived ($T^{1}/_{2} = 78$ sec) positron-emitting monovalent cation which can be used to measure serial changes in myocardial blood flow since Rb-82 uptake is proportional to myocardial blood flow [47]. Rb-82 is eluted from a strontium-82-rubidium-82 generator with minimal breakthrough of St-82 [48, 49]. Due to the relatively long half-life of St-82 ($T^{1}/_{2} = 25d$), the generator can be used for 3–4 months and multiple elutions can be performed for patient studies. The studies are performed with the patient positioned in the positron tomography instrument. A constant intravenous infusion of Rb-82 then provides a steady state arterial concentration during which a 1–2 min scan is performed.

Actual arterial blood samples for Rb-82 activity correlate well with those values obtained from the left ventricular cavity region of interest on the steady state scan. Thus arterial line placement in these patients may be avoided. Following the steady state scan, from which the arterial input is derived, the Rb-82 infusion is stopped. After 30 seconds is allowed for clearance of the Rb-82 from the blood, a "wash-out" scan (120 sec) is performed to measure the myocardial concentration achieved. Appropriate decay corrections are applied to the acquired data. Regional myocardial Rb-82 uptake is then calculated as: regional myocardial Rb-82 activity divided by arterial blood Rb-82 activity times the decay constant for Rb-82 (ml/gm/min extraction). In this manner multiple Rb-82 uptake measurements can be made in a short period of time (4–5 min). Serial images may be obtained in patients undergoing supine bicycle exercise tests as well as other interventions such as hand grip, cold pressor testing, nitrate, dipyridamole or other pharmacologic interventions. Regional changes in Rb-82 uptake in response to these interventions may be appreciated qualitatively as well as quantitatively due to the capabilities of positron tomography. A representative study of a normal patient without significant coronary artery disease is shown in Figure 1. The scans in this figure are the uptake data derived from the arterial input of Rb-82 (steady state scan) and the myocardial scans. A control measurement is performed at rest followed by repeat data acquisition at peak supine bicycle exercise (unless angina or arrhythmias supervene) and during recovery. During and after exercise or other interventions heart rate, blood pressure and electrocardiograms are monitored. The serial uptake scans in this patient show an exercise-induced increase in Rb-82 uptake uniformly in the myocardium which gradually decreases on the recovery scan. Also note the reproducibility of these observations which reflect directionally similar changes in myocardial blood flow with exercise. A representative patient with exercise-induced myocardial ischaemia of the interventricular septum is shown in Figure 2. Gradual resolution of the Rb-82 uptake deficit occurs over the subsequent 45 min, that is, long after the exercise-induced chest pain has disappeared and the electrocardiographic ST-segment depression on exercise has returned to normal. This observation in patients is consistent with the experimental work indicating prolonged recovery of "stunned" myocardium after an ischaemic insult recently summarised by Braunwald [50]. In addition, patients with frequent spontaneous episodes of chest pain and or ECG/ST segment changes can be investigated to determine if these episodes are of cardiac origin and more importantly the response of these episodes to nitrate therapy as well

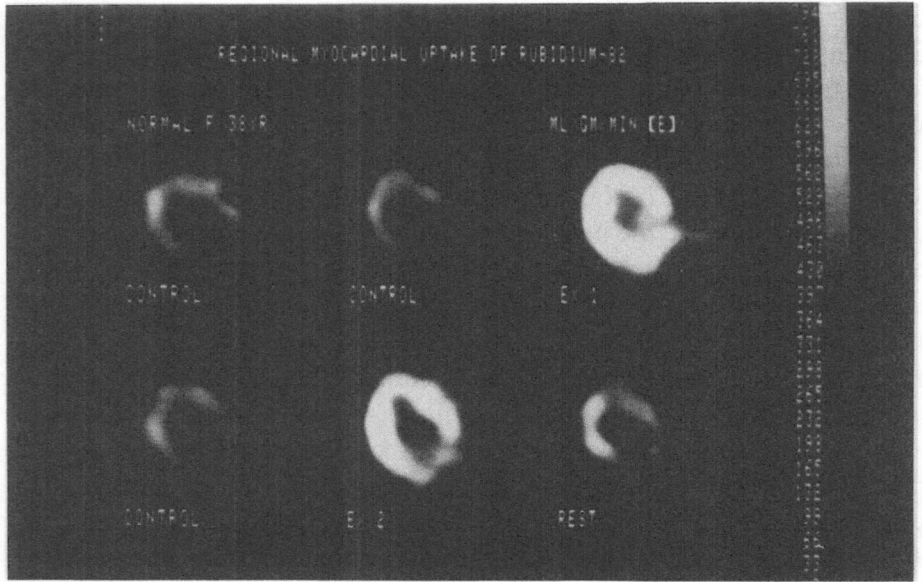

Figure 1. Rest and exercise Rb-82. Myocardial tomogram using Rb-82 in patient without significant coronary artery disease. Rb-82 uptake increases with exercise reflecting exercise-induced increase in myocardial blood flow represented by cation uptake (ml/gm/min × extraction). The tomograms are scaled to the physiological measurements.

as the location and extent of the ischaemia. In Figure 3 a patient with spontaneous episodes of chest pain was initially imaged at rest during one of his episodes of spontaneous ST-segment depression on the electrocardiogram. The evidence of transient ischaemia using Rb-82 lasted much longer than the chest pain or ECG changes. The ECG changes subsequently returned with reappearance of the septal Rb-82 defect. Intravenous administration of isosorbide dinitrate resulted in resolution of the chest pain, ST-segment depression and the Rb-82 septal defect. This sequence of scans illustrates the ability of Rb-82 myocardial imaging to assess the physiologic significance of spontaneous chest pain or asymptomatic ECG changes as well as therapeutic (or provocative) interventions on regional myocardial Rb-82 uptake as a marker of changes in regional myocardial blood flow. Thus Rb-82 is well suited for the extensive investigation into the pathophysiology of coronary artery disease. The major advantages of the Rb-82 generator system are that: (1) it is free of cyclotron scheduling logistics, (2) multiple patients and multiple scans on each patient as his own control can be performed rapidly, (3) high specific activity of the generator allows satisfactory counting statistics and image quality in relatively short imaging times. Although some investiga-

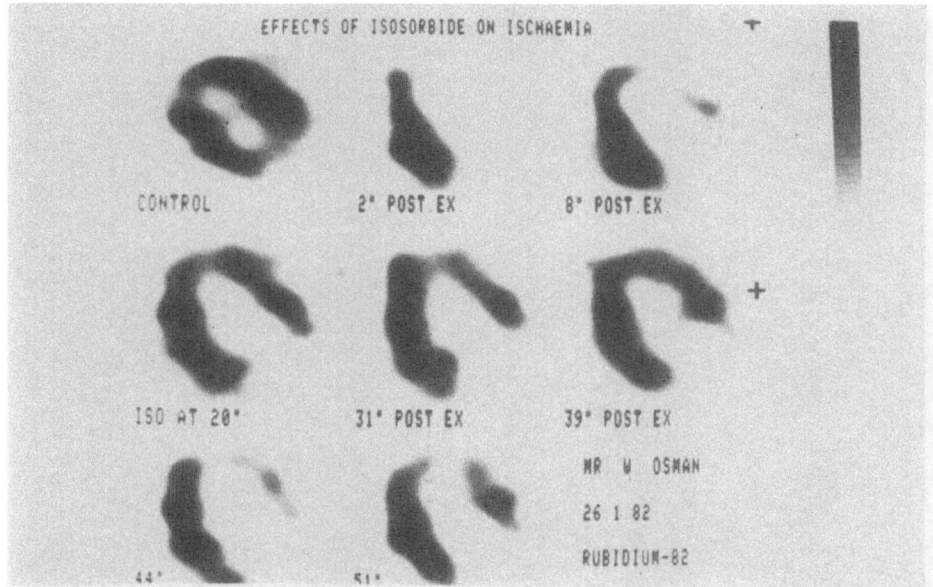

Figure 2. Exercise-induced ischaemia in a patient with significant coronary artery disease involving the left anterior descending coronary flow distribution. Prolonged recovery of the apical septal Rb-82 uptake defect is evident despite more rapid resolution of chest pain symptoms and ischaemic ST-segment depression on the electrocardiogram. The test was repeated to show reproducibility in repeatable measurements.

tors have used Rb-82 with a multicrystal gamma camera [51] for qualitative measurements, at present it requires a positron tomographic instrument. Improved detection of the presence and extent of Rb-82 uptake defects should be enhanced by the developed multi-slice positron tomography units.

N-13 ammonia
N-13 labelled ammonia ($^{13}NH_4^+$) has recently been developed by Schelbert and coworkers [52, 53, 54] as a flow marker which concentrates in the myocardium with an extraction fraction of approximately 70%. Although the directional changes in N-13 ammonia uptake are the same as changes in real myocardial blood flow, these changes are not linear at very high flow rates. Moreover, the uptake of N-13 ammonia by the myocardium is dependent on both blood flow and metabolic trapping catalysed by glutamine synthetase [54, 55].

Radiolabelled H_2O
Recently radiolabelled water can be inhaled as $C^{15}O_2$ [56] or given intra-

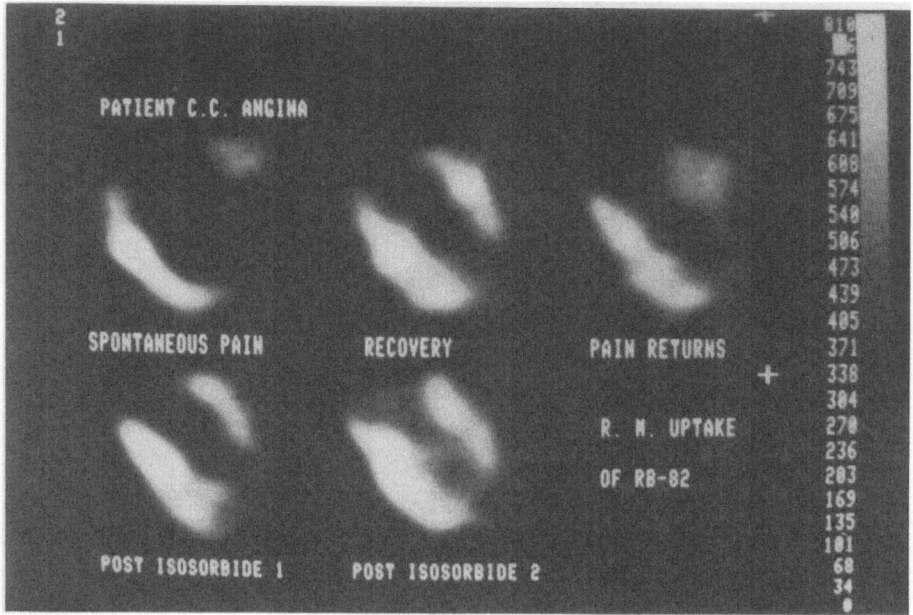

Figure 3. Spontaneous episode of pain in a patient. Diminished Rb-82 uptake in the interventricular septum partially resolves only to return again with renewed chest pain and ST-segment depression which is eventually reversed with intravenous isosorbide dinitrate administration. The clinical state does not show this evidence of ischaemic disturbances.

venous by H$_2$^{15}O [57, 58] and has been used to quantitate myocardial perfusion using positron tomography. Good correlations have been found with regional myocardial blood flow determined by reference gamma-emitting microspheres and *in vitro* well counting. These measurements are subject to a loss of count recovery due to the small object size relative to the resolution of the positron tomography instrument – the partial volume effect. Consequently corrections need to be made for the myocardial wall thickness to measure regional myocardial blood flow in absolute terms. In addition, correction for the significant residual blood pool activity requires an arterial line and is subject to the errors inherent in the blood pool subtraction.

Radiolabelled microspheres
Our laboratory has developed a new labelling process to incorporate C-11 into human albumin biodegradable microspheres [59]. These spheres can be used in a manner similar to the traditional use of reference gamma-

emitting microspheres except that counting for regional myocardial concentration can be done *in vivo* by positron tomography. Four-five million C-11 labelled biodegradeable albumin microspheres may be injected into the apex of the left ventricle at the time of cardiac catheterisation and subsequently positron emission tomographs are obtained. Arterial sampling at the time of the C-11 microsphere injection will provide a reference for calculation of regional myocardial blood flow. Correction for the partial volume effect may be performed by direct measurement of wall thickness (in animal studies), using 2-dimensional echocardiography, or by *in vivo* tomographic determination of myocardial density. To perform the latter correction a transmission scan and a ^{11}CO blood pool scan are obtained. The ^{11}CO blood pool scan is normalised to the arterial blood ^{11}CO arterial activity and then is subtracted from the transmission scan (normalised to peak activity). The resultant image is a measure of the count rate recovery coefficient for a given wall thickness [56]. Therefore, these regional recovery coefficients can be used to correct the C-11 microsphere scan to obtain full count recovery and thus true regional myocardial blood flow. Preliminary work in dogs has shown good correlation between *in vivo* C-11 microsphere determined regional myocardial blood flow and reference *in vitro* gamma microsphere flow determined by well counting ($r = 0.96$). Figure 4 shows a rectilinear scan of a dog after C-11 microsphere injection into the left atrium. The distribution of the cardiac output to the various organs can be appreciated especially in the high flow organs such as the tongue, nose, thyroid, heart and kidneys. Serial C-11 microsphere myocardial images from another dog are shown in Figure 5 to illustrate the stability of the radiolabel by the absence of blood pool activity over time. Blood C-11 activity per gram at 40 minutes was less than 1% of the myocardial C-11 activity per gram and approximately 0.04% of the injected dose was retained in the total intravascular space. Thus no significant loss of the C-11 label from the albumin microsphere occurred over the 40 minute period of observation. This is in distinction to Ga-68 labelled albumin microspheres in which significant losses of the label occur by 20 minutes [60, 61]. The detection of regional myocardial perfusion defects are readily appreciated using C-11 microspheres. Figure 6 shows an apical perfusion defect in a dog in which a transient occlusion of the distal left anterior descending coronary artery supplying the apex had been created. Reference gamma microsphere flow assessed by *in vitro* well counting showed the apical flow to be 35–40% lower than the flow to the left ventricular free wall. Similarly C-11 microsphere flows determined *in vivo* with correction for differences in wall thickness and count rate

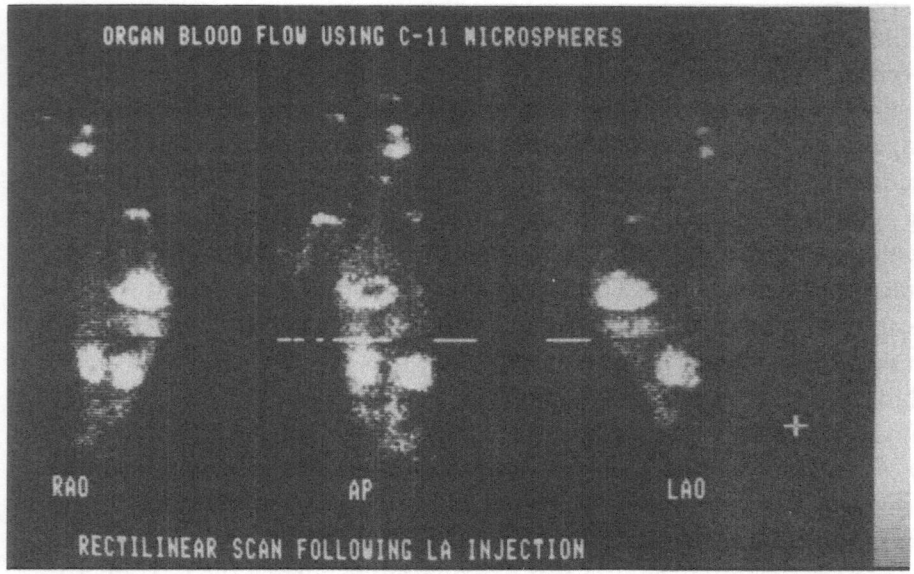

Figure 4. Rectilinear scan of C-11 albumin microsphere distribution in a dog. Organs of high flow include the tongue, nose, thyroid, heart and kidneys. This demonstrates quantitatively the distribution of cardiac output, organ and myocardial blood flow.

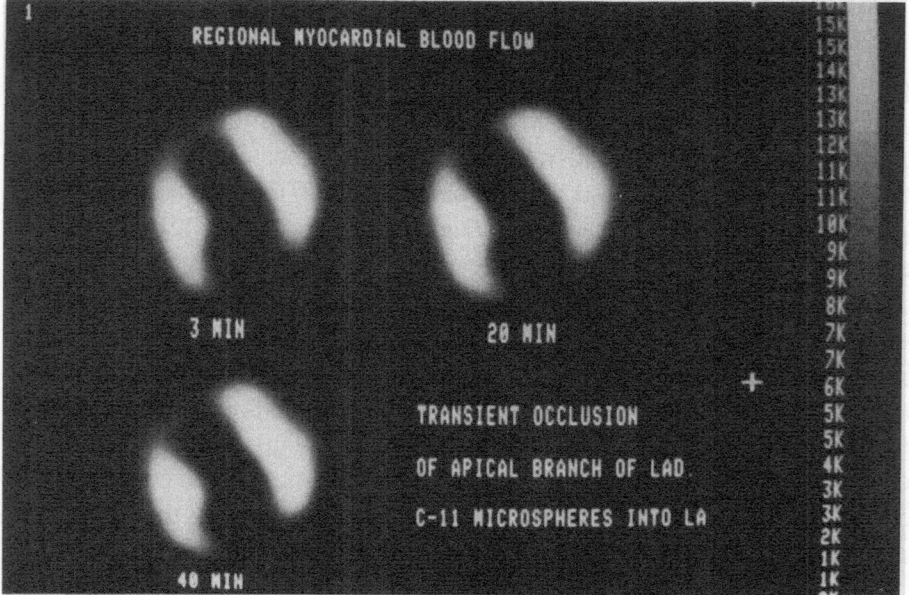

Figure 5. Serial C-11 albumin microsphere images in a dog showing the stability of the radiolabel over 40 mins.

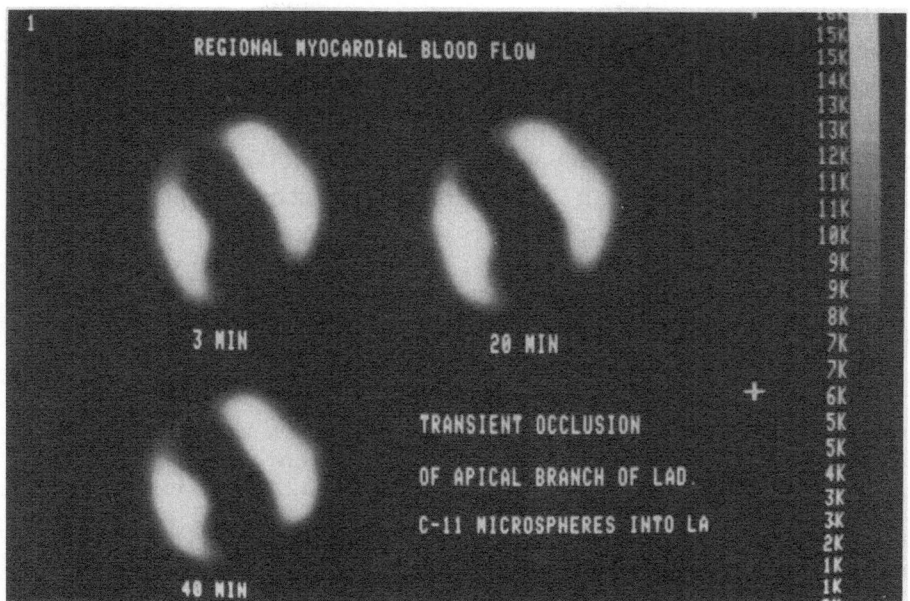

Figure 6. C-11 albumin microsphere detection of an apical perfusion deficit in a dog. *In vitro* gamma microsphere apical myocardial flow and *in vivo* C-11 albumin microsphere apical flow measurements both showed a 35–40% flow deficit compared to the left ventricular free wall.

recovery (the partial volume effect) also showed a 35–40% reduction in flow to the same apical region compared with the left ventricular free wall. Although this technique will be mainly of clinical and experimental research interest and will not easily permit repeated measures of flow, it will allow accurate and rigorous determination of absolute regional myocardial blood flow *in vivo* with few assumptions.

Conclusion

This chapter attempts to briefly review the available techniques for the estimation of coronary blood flow. The clinical scientist must first decide upon the specific questions in clinical and research work with patients. Having chosen a particular approach the limitations of the methodology should be well defined in experimental work.

The qualitative detection of transient ischaemia and single observation of the distribution (not level) of regional myocardial blood flow is most easily performed using Tl-201 and possibly Tc-99m and iodine labelled nuclides in the future. Gamma and positron labelled spheres may well provide the most rigorous and quantitative research tools. Rb-82 offers significant advantages with tomography and provides multiple physiological responses in health and ischaemic heart disease. These methods have documented that ischaemic episodes can occur without clinical symptoms, and that often myocardial ischaemia persists long after symptoms, and ECG changes have disappeared. Such prolonged ischaemia can jeopardize the heart in patients with coronary artery disease.

References

1. Hoffman JIE: Coronary bloodflow. Circulation 62, 1: 187–198, 1980.
2. Kety SS and Schmidt CF: The nitrous oxide method for the quantitative determination of cerebral blood flow in man: theory, procedure and normal values. J Clin Invest 27: 476, 1948.
3. Kochsiek K, Cott LA, Tauchert M, et al.: In: Coronary Heart Disease. Kattenbach M and Lichtlen P (eds). Thieme, Stuttgart, 1970: pp 137–153.
4. Cannon PJ, Weiss MB, Sciacca RR: Myocardial bloodflow in coronary artery disease: Studies at rest and during stress with inert gas washout techniques. Progr Cardiovasc Dis 20: 95–120, 1977.
5. Klocke FJ, Koberstein RC, Pittman DE et al.: Effects of heterogeneous myocardial perfusion on coronary venous H_2 desaturation curves and calculations of coronary flow. J Clin Invest 47: 2711–2724, 1968.
6. Klocke FJ, Wittenberg SM: Heterogeneity of coronary bloodflow in human coronary artery disease and experimental myocardial infarction. Am J Card 24: 782–790, 1969.
7. Klocke FJ, Bunnell IC, Greene DC, et al.: Average coronary bloodflow per unit weight of left ventricle in patients with and without coronary artery disease. Circulation 50: 547–559, 1974.
8. Ross RS, Ueda K, Lichtlen PR, et al.: Measurement of myocardial bloodflow in animals and man by selective injection of radioactive inert gas into the coronary arteries. Circ Res 15: 28–41, 1964.
9. Selwyn AP, Jones T, Turner H, et al.: Continuous assessment of regional myocardial perfusion in dogs using Krypton-81m. Circ Res 42: 771–777, 1978.
10. Krasnow N, Levine HS, Wagman RJ, et al.: Coronary bloodflow measured by I^{131} Iodo-antipyrine. Circ Res 12: 58–62, 1964.
11. Selwyn AP, Forse G, Fox K, et al.: Patterns of disturbed myocardial perfusion in patients with coronary artery disease. Circulation 64, 1: 83–90, 1981.
12. Branthwaite MA, Bradley RD: Measurement of cardiac output by thermal dilution in man. J Appl Physiol 24: 434–438, 1968.
13. Ganz W, Donoso R, Marcus HD, et al.: A new technique for measurement of cardiac output by thermodilution in man. Am J Card: 392–396, 1971.
14. Sapirstein LA: Fractionation of the cardiac output of rats with isotopic potassium. Circ Res 4: 689–692, 1956.
15. Strauss HW, Harrison K, Langan J, et al.: Thallium-201 for myocardial imaging: Relation of Thallium-201 to regional myocardial perfusion. Circulation 50: 641–645, 1975.
16. Chu A, Murdock RW, Cobb FR: Relation between regional distribution of Thallium-201 and myocardial bloodflow in normal, acutely ischemic, and infarcted myocardium. Am J Cardiol 50: 1141–1144, 1982.
17. Weich HF, Strauss HW, Pitt B: The extraction of Thallium-201 by the myocardium. Circulation 56: 188–191, 1977.
18. Hamilton GW, Narahara KA, Yee H, et al.: Myocardial imaging with Thallium-201: Effect of cardiac drugs on myocardial images and absolute tissue distribution. J Nucl Med 19: 10–16, 1978.

19. Pohost GM, Alpert NM, Ingwall, et al.: Thallium redistribution: Mechanisms and clinical utility. Sem Nucl Med 10: 70–93, 1980.

20. Albro PC, Gould KL, Westcott RJ, et al.: Noninvasive assessment of coronary stenoses by myocardial imaging during pharmacologic coronary vasodilation. III. Clinical trial. Am J Cardiol 42: 751–760, 1978.

21. Hockings B, Saltissi S, Croft DN, et al.: Effect of beta adrenergic blockade on Thallium-201 myocardial perfusion imaging. Br Heart J 49: 83–89, 1983.

22. Verani MS, Miller RR, Del Ventura L, et al.: Relation between regional myocardial hypoperfusion, and wall motion abnormalities during rest and exercise in coronary artery disease patients. Circulation 60, II-134, 1979.

23. Bailey I, Burow R, Griffith LSC, et al.: Localizing value of Thallium-201 myocardial perfusion imaging in coronary artery disease. Am J Cardiol 39: 320, 1977.

24. Botvinick EH, Taradash MR, Shamer DM, et al.: Thallium-201 myocardial perfusion scintigraphy for the clinical classification of normal, abnormal and equivocal electrocardiographic stess test. Am J Cardiol 41: 43–51, 1978.

25. Ritchie JL, Zaret BL, Strauss HW, et al.: Myocardial imaging with Thallium-201 at rest and exercise. A multicenter study: Coronary angiographic and electrocardiographic correlations. Am J Cardiol 39: 321, 1977.

26. Caralis DG, Kennedy HL, Bailey IK, et al.: Thallium-201 myocardial perfusion scanning in the evaluation of asymptomatic patients with ischemic ST segment depression. Am J Cardiol 39: 320, 1977.

27. Brown KA, Boucher CA, Okada RD, et al.: Nuclear cardiology: Assessment of severity of myocardial and coronary artery disease. Am J Cardiol 49: 967, 1982.

28. Goldman ME, Horowitz SF, Blake J, et al.: Can a specific pattern of exercise myocardial perfusion imaging predict prognosis? J Am Coll Cardiol 1: 655, 1983.

29. Gould KL: Assessment of coronary stenoses with myocardial perfusion imaging during pharmacologic coronary vasodilatation. Am J Cardiol 42: 761–768, 1978.

30. Maseri A, Parodi O, Severi S, et al.: Transient transmural reduction of myocardial bloodflow, demonstrated by Thallium-201 scintigraphy, as a cause of variant angina. Circulation 54: 280–288, 1976.

31. Pohost GM, Zir LM, Moore RM, et al.: Differentiation of transiently ischemic from infarcted myocardium by serial imaging after a single dose of Thallium-201. Circulation 55: 294–302, 1976.

32. Sullivan PJ, Wilson RA, McKusick KA, et al.: Effects of eating on the differentiation of scar from ischemia on Thallium stress myocardial images. J Nucl Med 23: 19, 1982.

33. Wilson RA, Okada RD, Harris DD, et al.: Influence of eating on serial exercise: Thallium myocardial and lung clearance rates. Circulation 4: 242, 1981.

34. Wilson RA, Okada RD, Brown KA, et al.: The effect of glucose-insulin-potassium of Thallium-201 myocardial redistribution. J Am Coll Cardiol 1: 590, 1983.

35. Sullivan PJ, Werre J, Okada RD, et al.: Comparison of TC-99m DMPE to 201 Thallium biodistribution. Am J Cardiol 49: 980, 1982.

36. Bushong WC, Weintraub WS, Bodenheimer MM, et al.: Assessment of myocardial perfusion using a newly developed technetium complex: Comparison to 201 Thallium and radioactive microspheres. Am J Cardiol 49: 979, 1982.

37. Endo M, Yamazaki T, Konno S, et al.: The direct diagnosis of human myocardial ischemia using [131] I-MAA via the selective coronary catheter: Preliminary report. Am Heart J 80: 498–506, 1970.

38. Ashburn WL, Braunwald E, Simon AL, et al.: Myocardial perfusion imaging in man using [99]m Tc-MAA. J Nucl Med 11: 618–619, 1970.

39. Schelbert HR, Ashburn W, Covell J, et al.: Feasibility and hazards of the intracoronary injection of radioactive serum albumin macroaggregates for external myocardial perfusion imaging. Invest Radiol 6: 379–387, 1979.

40. Poe N: The effects of coronary arterial injection of radio albumin macroaggregates on coronary

hemodynamics and myocardial function. J Nucl Med 12: 724–731, 1971.

41. Weller D, Adolph R, Wellman H, et al.: Myocardial perfusion scintigraphy after intracoronary injection of ^{99m}Tc labeled human albumin microspheres: Toxicity and efficacy for detecting myocardial infarction in dogs; preliminary results in man. Circulation 46: 963–975, 1972.

42. Hamilton GW, Ritchie JL, Allen DR, et al.: Myocardial perfusion imaging with ^{99m}Tc or ^{113m}In macroggregated albumin: Correlation of the perfusion image with clinical, angiographic, surgical, and histologic findings. Am Heart J 89: 708–715, 1975.

43. Jansen C, Judkins MP, Grames GM, et al.: Myocardial perfusion color scintigraphy with MAA. Radiology 109: 369–380, 1973.

44. Ritchie JL, Hamilton GW, Williams DL, et al.: Myocardial imaging with radionuclide-labeled particles. Radiology 121: 131–138, 1976.

45. Buckberg GD, Luck JC, Payne DB, et al.: Some sources of error in measuring regional bloodflow with radioactive microspheres. J Appl Physiology 31: 598–604, 1971.

46. Yipintsoi T, Dobbs WA Jr, Scanlon PD, et al.: Regional distribution of diggusible tracers and carbonized microspheres in the left ventricle of isolated dog hearts. Circ Res 33: 573–587, 1973.

47. Selwyn AP, Allan RM, L'Abbate A, et al.: Relation between regional myocardial uptake of rubidium-82 and perfusion: Absolute reduction of cation uptake in ischemia. Am J Cardiol 50: 112–121, 1982.

48. Yano Y, Budinger T, Chang G, et al.: Evaluation and application of alumina-based Rb-82 generators charged with high levels of Sr-82/85. J Nucl Med 20: 961–966, 1979.

49. Horlock P, Clark J, O'Brien HA, et al.: 1981 J. Radioanal. Chem. 64: 257.

50. Braunwald E, Kloner RA: The stunned myocardium: Prolonged, postis-chemic ventricular dysfunction. Circulation 66: 1146–1149, 1982.

51. Goldsmith SJ, Cochavi S, Strashun A, et al.: Planar imaging of myocardial perfusion with rubidium-82, a positron emitter. Circulation 62: III: 75, 1980.

52. Schelbert HR, Phelps ME, Hoffman EJ, et al.: Regional myocardial perfusion assessed with N-13 labeled ammonia and positron emission computerized tomography. Am J Cardiol 43: 209, 1979.

53. Schelbert HR, Phelps ME, Huang SC, et al.: N-13 Ammonia as an indicator of myocardial bloodflow. Circulation 63, 1: 1259–1272, 1981.

54. Schelbert HR, Henze E, Phelps ME, et al.: Assessment of regional myocardial ischemia by positron-emission computed tomography. Am Heart J 103: 588, 1982.

55. Bergmann S, Hack S, Tewson T, et al.: The dependence of accumulation of $^{13}NH_3$ by myocardium on metabolic factors and its implications for quantitative assessment of perfusion. Circulation 61, 1: 34–43, 1980.

56. Allan RM, Jones T, Rhodes CG, et al.: Quantitation of myocardial perfusion in man using oxygen-15 and positron tomography. Am J Cardiol 47: 481, 1981.

57. Bergmann SR, Fox KAA, Rand AL, et al.: Quantitation of myocardial perfusion with radio-labeled water. J Am Coll Cardiol 1: 577, 1983.

58. Huang SC, Schwaigen M, Carson RE, et al.: Noninvasive quantitation of myocardial bloodflow by 0-15 water and positron emission tomography. J Am Coll Cardiol 1: 578, 1983.

59. Turton D, Brady F, Pike V, et al.: submitted for publication.

60. Wisenberg G, Schelbert HR, Hoffman EJ, et al.: In vivo quantitation of regional myocardial bloodflow by positron-emission computed tomography. Circulation 63: 6: 1248–1258, 1981.

61. Selwyn AP, Allan RM, Brady F: Clin Sci 62: 3, 1982.

4. Value and limitations of myocardial scintigraphy with thallium-201 and long chain fatty acids for the detection of coronary artery disease

Robert D. Okada

Introduction

Exercise electrocardiographic stress testing has long been used as the standard noninvasive test for coronary artery disease. Unfortunately, the sensitivity of the test for coronary artery disease is low [1, 2]. The specificity is reduced in patients with ventricular hypertrophy, intraventricular conduction delay, prior myocardial infarction, hyperventilation, ST-T wave changes at rest, electrolyte imbalances, pre-excitation syndromes, and in those taking various drugs such as digitalis and quinidine. Perfusion imaging with thallium-201 after exercise or dipyridamole has been developed in an effort to improve the diagnostic accuracy for coronary artery disease. Myocardial imaging with positron emitting free fatty acids has been used largely as a research tool due to the limited availability of cyclotrons and positron cameras. However, more recently, fatty acids have been labeled with gamma emitting isotopes suitable for gamma camera imaging. This chapter will discuss myocardial imaging with thallium and gamma emitting long chain fatty acids. The chapter will focus on myocardial imaging in patients with known or suspected coronary artery disease.

Myocardial imaging with thallium

Background

The use of thallium-199 as a myocardial perfusion imaging agent was first proposed by Kawana and associates [3]. In 1976, Ritchie and associates described thallium-201 myocardial imaging with exercise [4]. If the post exercise thallium images were abnormal, the patient returned to the laboratory at least 72 hours later for a study at rest. If the thallium image defect was no longer present, then transient exercise-induced myocardial ischemia was said to be present during the first study. If the thallium image defect was still present on the rest study, then a myocardial scar was said to be present. In 1977, Pohost and associates described a single thallium dose technique for exercise imaging [5]. Thallium imaging was repeated at least two hours after the initial post-exercise thallium images had been collected. If an initial defect were no longer present (transient defect), then transient exercise-induced myocardial ischemia was said to be present during exercise. If an initial defect were still present two hours later (persistent defect), then a myocardial scar was said to be present. This thallium redistribution technique is now universally utilized due to the reduced cost, radiation burden, and patient and laboratory time commitment.

Thallium kinetics

After intravenous thallium administration, blood levels are initially high, but then fall rapidly. Normally perfused myocardial cells initially equilibrate with blood containing the high thallium levels. Peak myocardial activities are attained after 10 to 25 minutes in normal myocardium [6]. The extraction fraction by the myocardium is approximately 85% [7]. The initial distribution after an intravenous injection is related to myocardial blood flow. Thus areas of ischemia as well as scar demonstrate decreased thallium activity initially. The attainment of peak myocardial thallium levels is delayed in ischemic myocardium [8].

After reaching peak activity, myocardial thallium clearance from normally perfused zones is monoexponential and parallels the clearance from the blood [8]. After ischemia myocardial zones attain a delayed peak activity, the subsequent clearance is slowed compared to normal. The thallium clearance from the normally perfused zones at a time when thallium activity is slowly increasing in ischemic zones accounts for the thallium redistribution seen on clinical images.

Exercise thallium imaging

Protocol

Thallium myocardial imaging, after the tracer has been administered during peak exercise, is widely used as a noninvasive test for coronary artery disease. In our laboratory, patients are usually exercised upright on a standard treadmill. Some patients are exercised supine using a specially equipped exercise table to minimize patient movement and a bicycle ergometer. An intravenous line is inserted into a dorsal hand vein and a 12 lead electrocardiogram is obtained. Patients are exercised using a standard graded exercise protocol. Electrocardiographic leads I, II, and III are monitored continuously for arrhythmias and a 12 lead electrocardiogram is obtained every three minutes. Patients are exercised until symptom-limited by either shortness of breath, leg fatigue, or chest pain. At 30 to 60 seconds before the anticipated end of exercise, 1.5 to 2.0 mCi of thallous-201 chloride is injected intravenously into the dorsal hand vein cannula. Imaging begins as soon after the termination of exercise as is possible. A standard gamma camera is used, usually interfaced to a nuclear medicine computer system. We employ a medium sensitivity collimator and a 20–30% energy window around the 68–80 keV X-ray emissions for thallium. Images are collected in the anterior, 50 degree and 70 degree left anterior oblique projections. We recommend image collection for a preset time, usually 6 to 10 minutes for each projection. At least 300,000 counts should be collected in each image. The three projections are collected again three to four hours after the termination of exercise (delayed images).

Various tomographic techniques have been proposed for image collection. Vogel and associates proposed the use of a 7-pinhole collimator and demonstrated an improved sensitivity without loss of specificity for coronary artery disease [9]. Single photon emission tomographic systems have been recently developed; however, the impact of this approach on the diagnostic accuracy of the exercise thallium test remains to be demonstrated.

Image interpretation

Figure 1 schematically demonstrates the three left ventricular projections and the division of each projection into three segments each. After display on a computer screen, the anterior projection is divided into anterolateral, apical, and inferior segments; the 50 degree left anterior oblique projection into septal, apical-inferior, and posterior segments; and the 70 degree left anterior oblique projection into anterior, apical-lateral, and inferior-posterior segments. Each of the nine segments is subjectively scored using a scoring system ranging from zero (absent activity) to +2 (normal activity). The delayed images are then displayed next to the initial images, and then each delayed image segment is scored in a similar manner. A transient defect is defined as an improvement in segmental

58

Fig. 1.

Fig. 2.

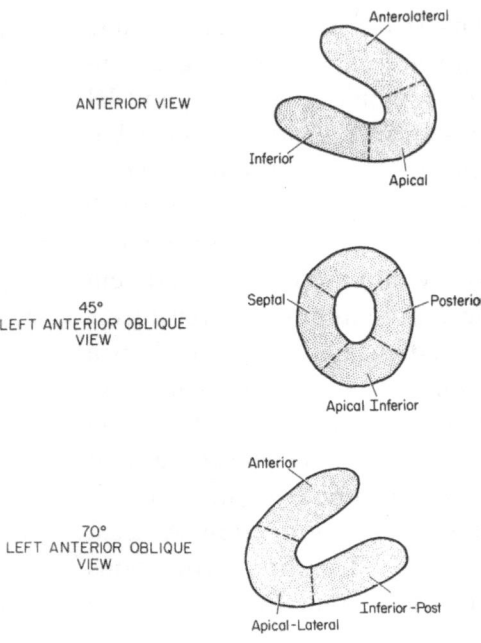

ANTERIOR VIEW

Anterolateral

Inferior

Apical

45°
LEFT ANTERIOR OBLIQUE
VIEW

Septal

Posterior

Apical Inferior

70°
LEFT ANTERIOR OBLIQUE
VIEW

Anterior

Inferior -Post

Apical-Lateral

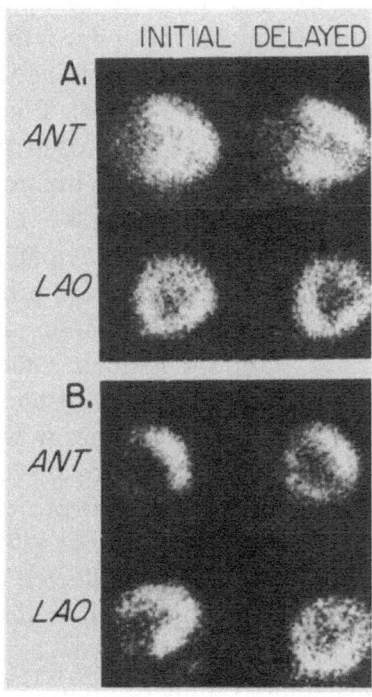

INITIAL DELAYED

A.

ANT

LAO

B.

ANT

LAO

Figure 1. Division of left ventricular myocardium into segments for the qualitative assessment of thallium myocardial images.

Figure 2. A. normal thallium myocardial images immediately after exercise (INITIAL) and 4 hours later (DELAYED). B. abnormal thallium myocardial images. Note the inferior and apical defects in the initial anterior (ANT) view, and septal and apical-inferior defects in the initial left anterior oblique view (LAO). There is complete redistribution into the septal and apical-inferior segments (transient defect), partial redistribution into the inferior segment, and no redistribution into the apical defect (persistent defect). Reprinted from The American Journal of Cardiology 46; 1190, 1980, with permission of the American College of Cardiology.

score of at least one unit on the delayed image. Such a transient defect is thought to represent transient exercise-induced ischemia occurring during the stress test. A persistent defect is defined as an initial and delayed score of 1.0 or less. Such a persistent defect is thought to represent myocardial scar. Figure 2A demonstrates normal thallium images from one patient with normal coronary arteries. Of note is the reduced to absent thallium activity at the base and the normally reduced activity at the apex. Figure 2B demonstrates the thallium images from one patient with coronary artery disease. Both transient and persistent thallium defects are demonstrated.

Thallium lung activity is also qualitatively assessed on the initial ante-

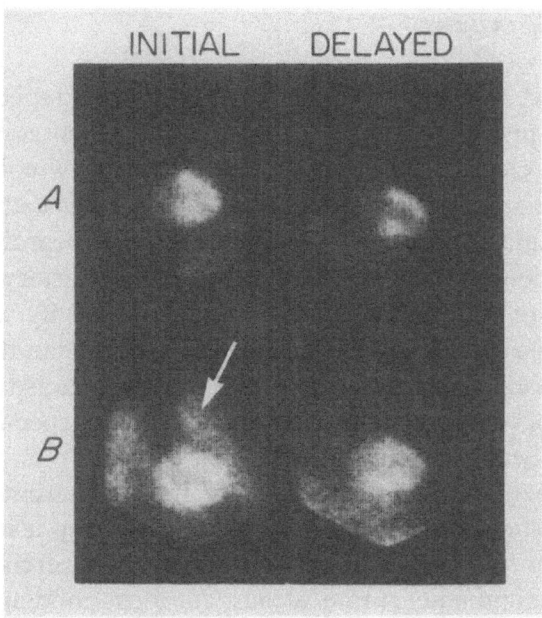

INITIAL   DELAYED

A

B

Figure 3. (A) Thallium images from a patient with normal coronary arteries demonstrating normal lung thallium uptake. (B) Thallium images from another patient with coronary artery disease demonstrating increased lung thallium uptake. Notice that the increased lung thallium activity apparent on the initial images is no longer apparent on the delayed images.

rior projection images. Figure 3 demonstrates thallium images from one patient with normal thallium lung activity (A) and images from another patient with abnormal thallium lung activity (B). Boucher and associates have demonstrated that qualitatively assessed increased lung thallium activity correlates with increases in pulmonary capillary wedge pressure occurring during exercise [10]. It has been postulated that exercise-induced left ventricular ischemia results in increased pulmonary venous pressures and volumes. The resultant increase in pulmonary blood volume may lead to an increase in capillary volume and capillary surface area, thus resulting in a larger net extraction of thallium by the lung. Thallium lung activity has also been quantitated using a light pen and expressed as the lung activity/heart activity in the most normal appearing region. Kushner and associates found that a thallium lung/heart ratio of at least 0.545 predicted 38% of patients with coronary artery disease, whereas no control patient exceeded this ratio [11]. Thus, although the finding of an increased lung thallium ratio is not highly sensitive for disease, such a finding greatly increases one's certainty that coronary artery disease is present.

Sensitivity and specificity

Several studies have examined the relative sensitivity and specificity of the exercise thallium test for coronary artery disease when compared with standard exercise electrocardiography. A recent review collected 1,897 patients from the literature [12]. All patients had cardiac catheterization, exercise thallium imaging, and standard exercise electrocardiography. Of the 1,897 total patients, 1,365 had significant coronary artery disease and 526 did not. The overall exercise thallium test sensitivity was 82% for coronary artery disease. This was significantly higher than the 60% sensitivity for exercise electrocardiography. The overall exercise thallium test specificity was 91% compared with a significantly lower specificity of 81% for exercise electrocardiography.

The large numbers of patients with nondiagnostic exercise electrocardiograms account for much of the improved sensitivity using thallium. Baseline electrocardiographic changes and failure to exercise to at least 85% predicted maximum heart rate account for most nondiagnostic exercise electrocardiograms [13–17]. The presence of conduction defects, ventricular hypertrophy, pre-excitation syndromes, or ST wave changes on the baseline electrocardiogram make the exercise response difficult to interpret. Furthermore, patients taking digitalis or psychotropic drugs and those with electrolyte imbalances are likely to have nondiagnostic exercise electrocardiograms. These factors do not appear to interfere with exercise thallium imaging. Exercise thallium imaging also does not appear to be as dependent on the achievement of maximal predicted heart rate. In a series of 227 patients, Pohost and associates found no difference in the exercise thallium test sensitivity for patients achieving at least 85% maximal predicted heart rate versus those patients who did not [18]. The sensitivity of the exercise thallium test increases as the number of diseased coronary arteries increases, as the severity of the coronary stenosis increases, and in patients with left main coronary artery disease [19–21]. Although the sensitivity of the exercise thallium test is high in patients with left main coronary artery disease, no one image pattern has been shown to differentiate patients with left main disease from those with multivessel disease. The sensitivity of the exercise thallium test decreases as the adequacy of collateral arteries increases and in patients taking propranolol [22].

The improved specificity of the exercise thallium test for coronary artery disease compared with standard exercise electrocardiography is probably due to the many causes for a false positive exercise electrocardiogram discussed above. One special situation in which exercise thallium imaging has been shown to be specific and thus helpful is in asymptomatic patients with false positive screening exercise electrocardiograms [23]. The specificity of the exercise thallium test is reduced in patients with subcritical coronary artery disease (30–45% diameter narrowing). We have found that about 50% of such patients have positive exercise thallium scintigraphy [24]. Although these patients have been thought to have hemodynamically insignificant coronary artery disease, studies using xenon-133 washout techniques have demonstrated perfusion inequalities [25, 26]. Thus the significance of subcritical coronary artery lesions requires further study and patients with such lesions may not actually represent false positive exercise thallium results. Exercise thallium test specificity is also low in females, probably often due to breast attenuation. Positive exercise thallium results have also been described in patients with normal coronary arteries and either aortic stenosis, idiopathic hypertrophic subaortic stenosis, or mitral valve prolapse [27, 28, 29]. Abnormal thallium images have also been described in patients with myocardial bridges and anomalous coronary arteries [30, 31]. These abnormal images may be reflecting a true perfusion inequality in such patients.

Improved diagnostic accuracy of exercise thallium imaging can be accomplished using multiple observers or criteria derived from interobserver analysis of variance. We studied 40 patients with and 10 patients without coronary artery disease [32]. Exercise thallium images were interpreted by four independent observers and each segment scored using the system described above. The interobserver variance was determined for each segment (Figure 4). The variance values were significantly higher for all exercise image segments than for corresponding delayed image segments. Those for the anterolateral and posterior segments in the exercise image were significantly lower than those for the other exercise image segments. The variance for the anterolateral segment in the delayed image was lower and that for the apical segment higher than that for all other delayed image segments. The interobserver variance for the change in score between initial and delayed images was also determined (Figure 5). The variance values for a change in score between exercise and delayed images were lower for the anterolateral and posterior segments than for all other segments, and higher for the apical and apical-inferior segments than for all other segments except the inferior segment. Furthermore, when segmental thallium scores were interpreted by an individual observer using a standard method employing one set of arbitrary criteria, the thallium stress test had a sensitivity of 77% and a specificity of 75% for coronary artery disease. When the scores were interpreted by an individ-

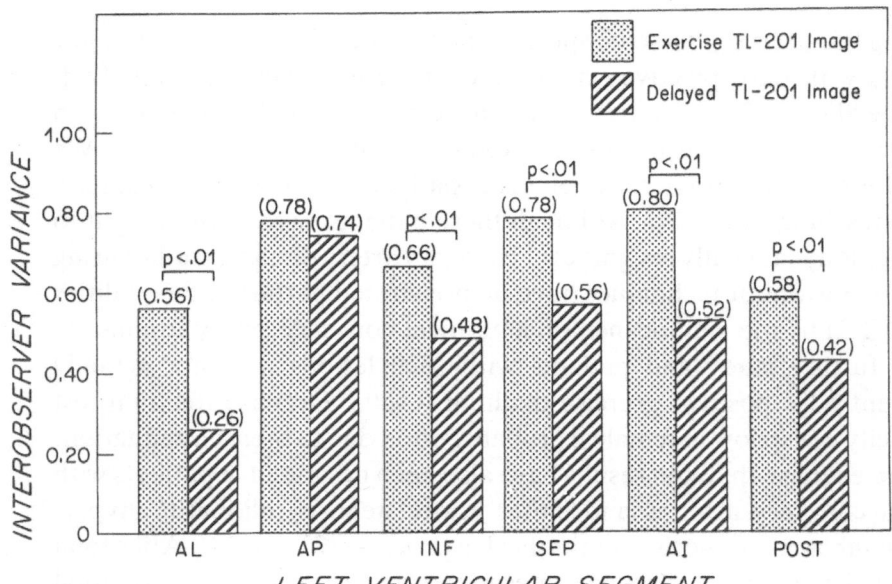

Figure 4. Interobserver variance in the scoring of left ventricular segmental thallium activity for exercise and delayed images, expressed as 2 standard deviations (scoring system from 0 to + 2). Left ventricular segments are anterolateral (AL), apical (AP), inferior (INF), septal (SEP), apical-inferior (AI), and posterior (POST). Reprinted from the American Journal of Cardiology 46; 621, 1980 with permission of the American College of Cardiology.

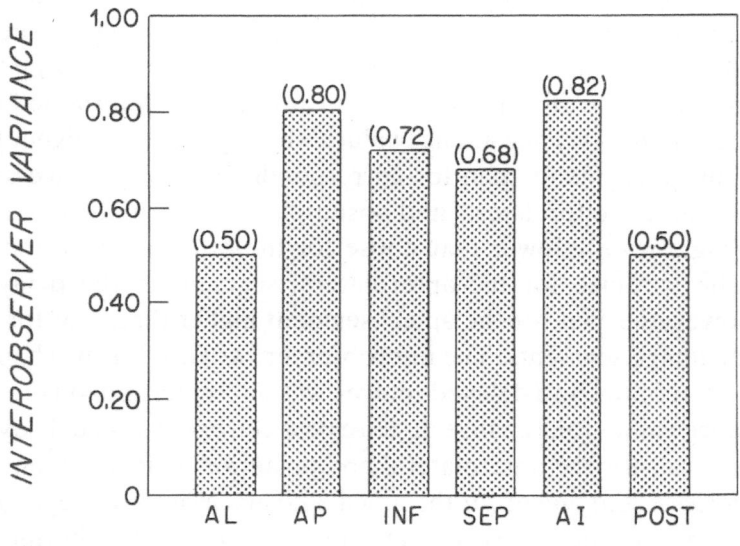

Figure 5. Interobserver variance in the scoring of changes in left ventricular segmental thallium activity in exercise and delayed images, expressed as 2 standard deviations (scoring system from 0 to + 2). Left ventricular segments as in Figure 4 Reprinted from the American Journal of Cardiology 46; 622, 1980 with permission of the American College of Cardiology.

ual observer using criteria derived from interobserver variance analysis, the sensitivity increased to 86% while the specificity (78%) did not significantly change. When multiple observers' scores were averaged and the averaged scores interpreted by a single set of criteria applied to all six ventricular segments, the sensitivity and specificity increased to 90%. Thus, when only one observer is available, diagnostic accuracy is improved by using criteria based on interobserver variance analysis. However, when feasible, thallium stress tests should be interpreted by multiple observers because averaging of the multiple observers' scores maximizes both sensitivity and specificity.

Relationship of left ventricular function to thallium imaging

Thallium redistribution patterns after exercise have been related to rest and exercise left ventricular function [33]. In a series of 61 patients (50 with and 11 without coronary artery disease), left ventricular function was measured by exercise radionuclide ventriculography. In 16 patients with exclusively transient defects, mean left ventricular ejection fraction was 65% at rest and fell significantly to 58% during exercise (Figure 6). In eight patients with exclusively persistent defects, left ventricular ejection fraction did not change during exercise. In patients with normal thallium images, left ventricular ejection fraction increased from 66% at rest to 73% during exercise. Individual wall segments which exhibited transient or persistent defects contracted abnormally, both at rest and during exercise, as compared with segments without defects (Figure 7). Thus, only transient defects, indicative of transient myocardial ischemia, reliably predict worsening left ventricular function during exercise. Furthermore, both transient and persistent defects can be associated with resting dyssynergy.

Right ventricular thallium uptake

In patients with normal coronary arteries, the right ventricle is readily visualized on initial post-exercise images (Figure 8). However, some patients with coronary artery disease may demonstrate defects on initial images. The relationship of right ventricular thallium uptake to coronary anatomy has been examined [34]. Eighty-eight patients underwent exercise thallium testing and coronary angiography. Transient defects of the right ventricle were found in eight patients, all of whom had high grade stenosis of the proximal right coronary artery (Figure 9). Non-visualiza-

64

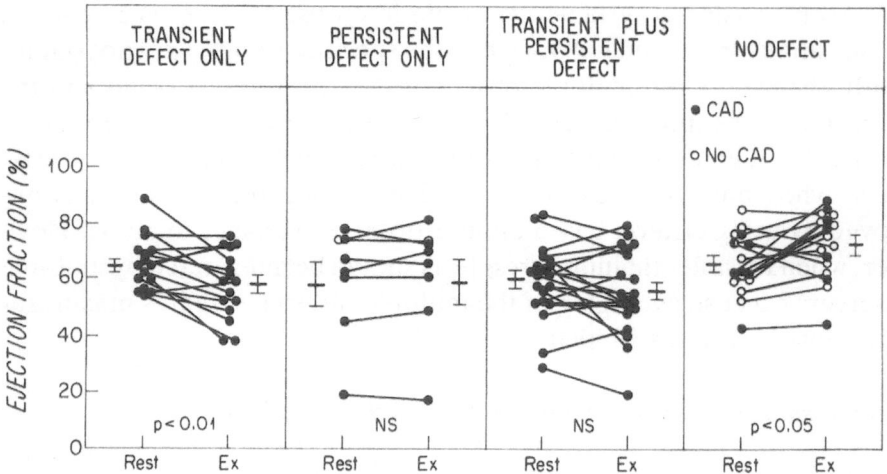

Figure 6. Rest and exercise left ventricular ejection fractions, classified by the results of thallium imaging. Means are listed with bars showing +/− S.E.M. P values represent comparison between rest and exercise means within the same subgroup. Reprinted from the American Heart Journal 101: 734, 1981.

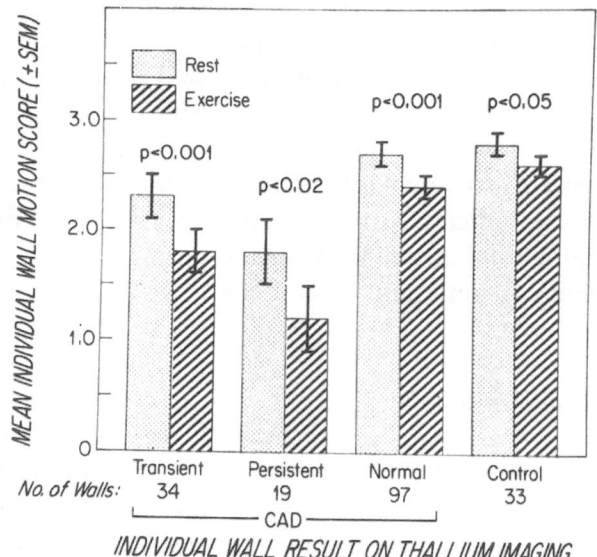

Figure 7. Mean individual wall motion score at rest and with exercise, subdivided by the thallium result for the same wall. P values represent comparison between rest and exercise of the same subgroup. Reprinted from the American Heart Journal 101; 723, 1981.

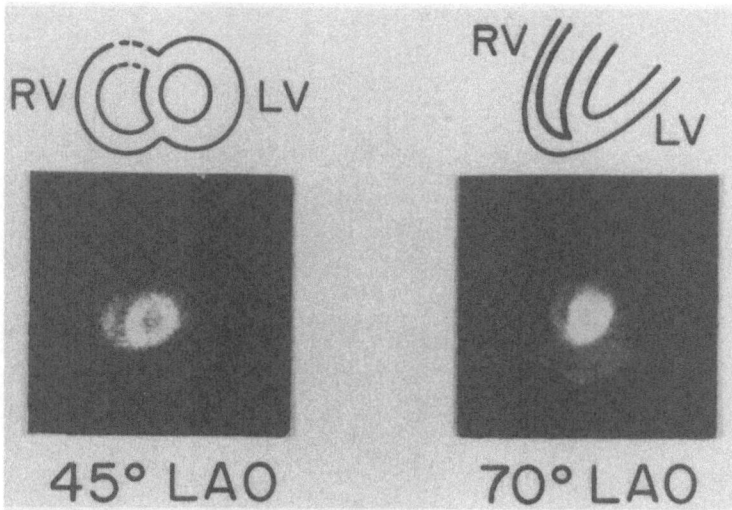

Figure 8. Initial 45 and 70 degree left anterior oblique images in a patient without coronary artery disease, displaying typical right ventricular thallium activity. Above the images is a schematic diagram illustrating the right and left ventricles. Reprinted from the American Journal of Cardiology 50; 1217, 1982 with permission of the American College of Cardiology.

tion of the right ventricle occurred in ten patients, nine of whom had significant disease of the right coronary artery. Thus, either transient or persistent right ventricular thallium defects suggest the presence of right coronary artery disease. Unfortunately, homogeneous right ventricular activity does not rule out right coronary artery disease, since over 40% of patients with this image pattern have right coronary artery disease.

The use of exercise thallium imaging to assess the effect of interventions such as coronary bypass surgery and angioplasty

Exercise thallium imaging has been used to assess the ongoing changes in myocardial perfusion after percutaneous transluminal coronary angioplasty [35]. No distinct defects are recognizable in the region of previously decreased thallium activity after successful angioplasty. Exercise thallium imaging has also been utilized to determine whether coronary artery bypass surgery has improved perfusion, and to follow graft patency after the surgery. Several studies have demonstrated the ability of exercise thallium imaging for detecting graft occlusion [36, 37]. In one controlled prospective study , graft patency was assessed at two weeks and one year after operation. Thallium scintigraphy was 80% sensitive, 88% specific and 86% accurate in detecting graft occlusion at these times. Either

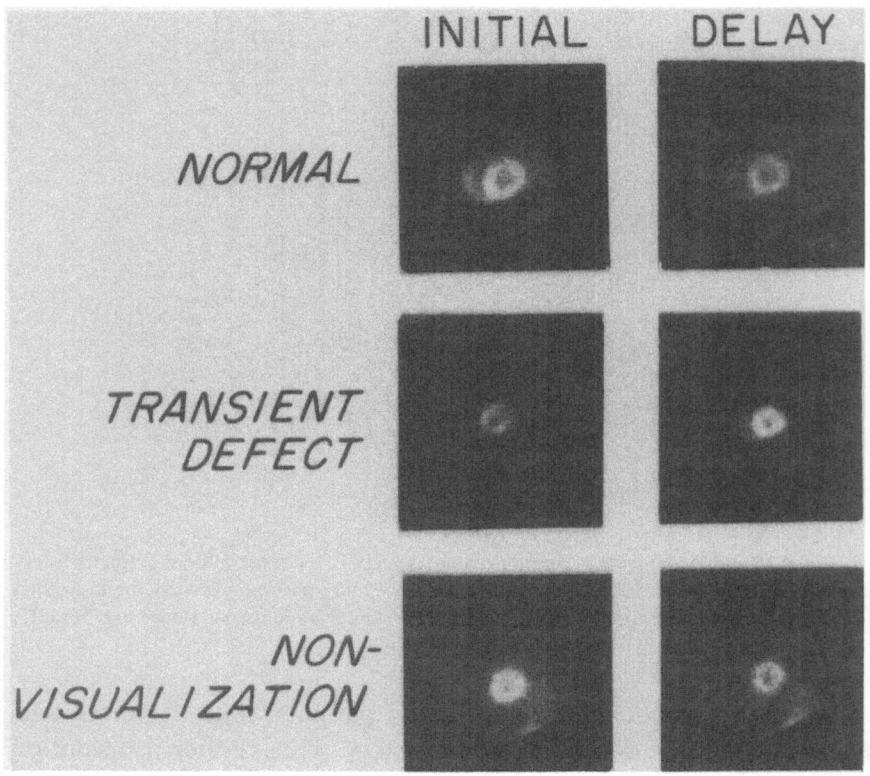

Figure 9. Representative examples of serial 45 degree left anterior oblique thallium images displaying normal activity, transient defect, and persistent defect. Reprinted from the American Journal of Cardiology 50; 1217, 1982 with permission of the American College of Cardiology.

transient thallium defects consistent with ischemia or persistent thallium defects consistent with new scar were predictive of graft occlusion. Graft occlusions were correctly localized by thallium scintigraphy in 61% of patients.

Exercise thallium imaging for localizing coronary artery disease

The location of coronary artery stenoses correlates with the location of perfusion defects on exercise thallium scintigraphy. Dunn and associates demonstrated a good correlation between septal, anteroseptal and anterior wall thallium defects and left anterior descending coronary artery disease [38]. Inferior, posteroinferior, and posterior segment defects correlated with either right or left circumflex coronary artery disease. Rigo and associates found that anterior and septal wall defects were specific for left anterior descending coronary artery disease [39]. Furthermore, inferior wall defects were specific for right coronary artery disease, and lateral wall defects were specific for circumflex artery disease. Apical defects have been shown to be nonspecific.

Quantitative techniques for interpreting exercise thallium images

Several computer techniques for analyzing exercise thallium images have been described. Most of the techniques generate circumferential profiles of peak myocardial activity. Such techniques require the assumption of a manually defined or computer defined geometric center point of reference. Furthermore, attempt to derive transmural count activities using radii originating from this center point lead to position-dependent errors, especially in the anterior projection where the ventricle is elongated. We have recently described a new computer technique which has several advantages over previously described methods. First, the program uses an ellipse rather than a circle to plot activity. Second, transmural rather than peak pixel activity is determined. Third, a comprehensive interpolative background correction approach is employed. Fourth, a registration technique using rotational and translational repositioning is used to align serial images. Fifth, functional color-coded images are generated which depict regions of redistribution. Sixth, regional myocardial thallium clearance can be calculated. Figure 10 demonstrates the computer display for one patient with left anterior coronary artery disease. Time activity curves were consistent with an initial septal defect with redistribution on delayed images.

We have used this new program to quantitate regional differences in thallium uptake before and after percutaneous transluminal coronary angioplasty [40]. After angioplasty, mean thalllium uptake in the left anterior descending coronary artery territory increased from 61% to 74% (p<.005). There was a reduction in the amount of redistribution from $13 \pm 23\%$ (1 S.D.) to $-1 \pm 15\%$ (p<.001). The color-coded subtraction image demonstrating redistribution showed similar improvement after angioplasty. Thus, the computer technique is not only clinically useful for quantitating and interpreting diagnostic exercise thallium images, but is also useful for comparing perfusion differences between exercise thallium scans obtained before and after interventions.

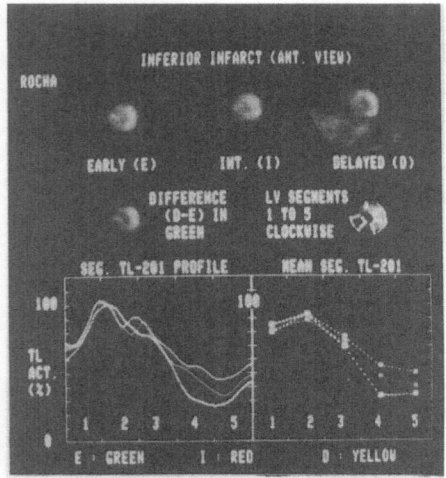

Figure 10. Immediate (Early), intermediate (Inter.), and delayed (Delayed) post-exercise thallium images obtained in the left anterior oblique projection in a patient with left anterior descending coronary artery disease. Time-activity curves (green = early, red = intermediate, yellow = delayed) demonstrated a septal defect (segment 4) with redistribution.

DIPYRIDAMOLE PROTOCOL

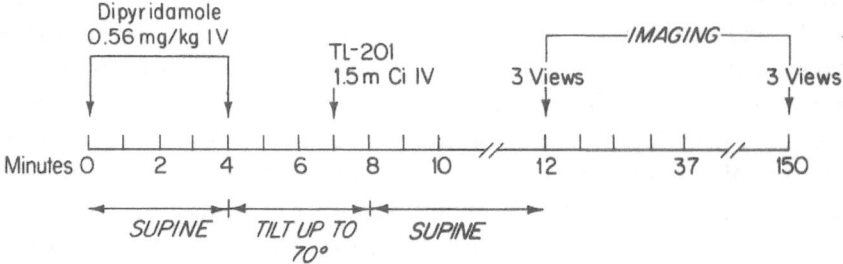

Figure 11. Dipyridamole protocol used for patient studies. The total dose of dipyridamole is 0.56 mg/kg over four minutes. Reprinted from Circulation 66; 650, 1982 with permission of the American Heart Association.

Dipyridamole thallium imaging

Background

Thallium imaging during dipyridamole-induced coronary hyperemia is based on the finding that normal coronary arteries dilate in response to dipyridamole, a potent vasodilator, and thereby greatly increase myocardial blood flow. However, the hyperemic response to dipyridamole is blunted or absent in myocardial regions supplied by stenotic coronary arteries. Such a technique is theoretically safer than exercise since myocardial work is not significantly increased, and ischemia is not used as an endpoint. Strauss and Pitt used ethyl adenosine to induce hyperemia and demonstrated thallium defects in dogs with experimental coronary artery stenoses [41]. Gould and associates used myocardial perfusion imaging during dipyridamole-induced coronary vasodilation to detect experimental coronary stenoses in dogs [42]. These same investigators subsequently were the first to describe a clinical protocol for studying patients with thallium and dipyridamole [43].

Protocol

Figure 11 demonstrates a clinical protocol for studying patients with dipyridamole and thallium. The patient is placed supine on a tilt table. A 20-gauge plastic cannula is placed in a large antecubital vein. Twelve-lead ECGs and blood pressure measurements are obtained at baseline and at one minute intervals during the first 15 minutes of the study. With the patient supine, intravenous dipyridamole is infused at a rate of 0.14 mg/kg/min for four minutes. After the infusion, the patient is tilted upright to 70 degrees, and 3 minutes later 1.5 to 2.0 mCi of intravenous thallium is injected. The patient is returned to the supine position one minute after the thallium injection, and myocardial images are collected immediately and again several hours later. Parenteral aminophylline (250 mg) is available to reverse significant side effects of the dipyridamole infusion. Images are collected and interpreted in a manner similar to that described above for exercise thallium images. Examples of dipyridamole thallium images are shown in Figure 12.

Diagnostic accuracy of dipyridamole thallium imaging

In a series of patients studied at our hospital, sensitivity was 93% and specificity 80% for coronary artery disease. The sensitivity and specificity were not affected by the extent of coronary artery disease, the presence of Q waves, or propranolol therapy. Most patients with initial thallium defects had complete thallium redistribution of one or more defects. Transient and persistent defects predicted abnormal resting wall motion by angiography better than ECG Q waves. Propranolol therapy and collaterals did not significantly affect the thallium redistribution results. Other investigators have found that the diagnostic accuracy of thallium imaging with dipyridamole is comparable to that following exercise [44].

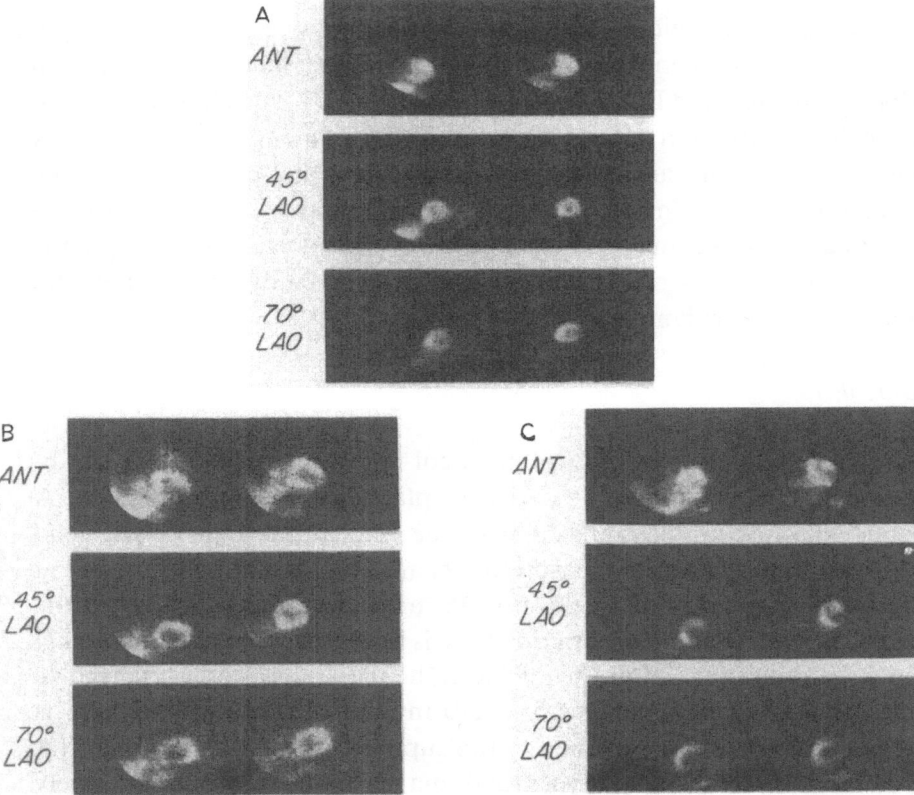

Figure 12. Initial postdipyridamole (left) and delayed (right) thallium scans in an anterior (ANT) and two left anterior oblique (LAO) views from three patients. (A) A 95% stenosis of the right coronary artery and a normal left ventriculogram. A transient defect is present in inferior and apical inferior segments. (B) Severe three-vessel disease and small region of apical akinesis on ventriculography. Transient defects are present in the inferior, anterior, septal, inferoposterior and apical inferior segments, but the apex in the ANT and 70 degree LAO views has a persistent defect. (C) A 90% stenosis of a dominant circumflex artery and posterolateral akinesis on ventriculography. A transient defect is present in the apical inferior and lateral as well as inferoposterior segments, but the posterior segment has a persistent defect. Reprinted from Circulation 66; 654, 1982 with permission of the American Heart Association.

As with exercise thallium imaging, initial and delayed right ventricular thallium imaging following dipyridamole has been shown to correlate with right coronary artery anatomy [45]. A transient right ventricular defect has been shown to correlate with the presence of proximal right coronary artery stenosis whereas normal right ventricular thallium uptake suggests the absence of proximal right coronary artery disease. Nonvisualization of the right ventricular activity was nondiagnostic. In a recent study, Bendersky and associates performed dipyridamole thallium imaging and exercise gated blood pool imaging in the same patients [46]. The dipyridamole thallium study had a sensitivity of 93% and a specificity of 72% for coronary artery disease. These values were not significantly different from the sensitivity of 94% and specificity of 64% for exercise gated blood pool imaging. Thus, dipyridamole thallium imaging is an acceptable alternative in patients unable to exercise.

Thallium imaging at rest

Rest thallium imaging in patients with stable or unstable angina pectoris

Defects on thallium images obtained with the patient at rest were initially described in patients with known prior myocardial infarction and scar. The location and size of the defect was found to correlate with the location and extent of myocardial scar [47]. Defects were more prominent in patients with transmural compared to nontransmural infarctions. Gewirtz and associates subsequently reported that rest thallium defects could be demonstrated in patients with severe coronary artery disease without myocardial scar [48]. Such transient defects were found in patients with severe but stable angina pectoris and were found to correlate with normal or minimally abnormal left ventricular wall motion. Transient thallium defects on rest images were also described in patients with variant angina during an episode of coronary artery spasm [49]. Finally, resting thallium defects have been described in patients with unstable angina during pain-free intervals. Wackers and associates reported that 63% of such patients have rest thallium defects [50]. Brown and associates studied 31 patients with unstable angina, 12 of whom had rest angina alone without exertional symptoms [51]. Only 25% of the 12 patients with rest angina alone had transient thallium defects. However, all of the remaining 19 patients with exertional unstable angina had transient thallium defects. Most of the zones demonstrating transient thallium defects in the latter group of 19 patients were associated with hypokinesis on the corresponding left ventriculogram segment. It was concluded that regional resting hypoperfusion of viable myocardium is far more common in patients with exertional unstable angina symptoms than in patients with rest angina alone. The authors postulated that patients with rapidly worsening exertional angina may be developing new critical stenoses or occlusions without adequate collateralization. However, unstable angina patients with rest symptoms alone may have angina as a result of a dynamic component to their coronary artery disease such as superimposed spasm or platelet aggregation producing transient occlusion.

Rest thallium imaging has also been used to differentiate patients with ischemic cardiomyopathy from those with idiopathic congestive cardiomyopathy. Bulkley and associates found that rest thallium images from patients with ischemic cardiomyopathy demonstrate defects of greater than 40% of the image circumference [52]. Studies from patients with idiopathic congestive cardiomyopathy demonstrate defects of less than 20% of the image circumference.

Rest thallium imaging in the setting of acuty myocardial infarction

Wackers and associates have shown that rest thallium imaging is 100% sensitive for acute myocardial infarction when performed within the first six hours after the onset of the pain [53, 54]. These investigators reported that thallium imaging detected myocardial infarction in 44 of 44 patients studied within 6 hours, in 90 of 96 (94%) patients studied within 24 hours, and in 75 of 104 (72%) patients studied more than 24 hours after the chest pain onset. Most of the false negative results occurred in patients with small or nontransmural myocardial infarcts. These same investigators studied the potential value of thallium imaging for selecting patients for admission to the coronary care unit. All patients had an atypical history of infarction and a nondiagnostic electrocardiogram [55]. Patients were imaged with thallium within 10 hours of the onset of chest pain. Thirty-four patients were found to have acute myocardial infarctions by enzyme determinations. Thirty of the 34 patients had an abnormal thallium study. Of the remaining 169 patients without acute infarction, only 14 had positive thallium images yielding a specificity of 92%. The same investigators have found a good correlation between the size of the myocardial scar post-mortem and the size determined by quantitative thallium scan analysis just before death [56]. The ability of the thallium scan to localize the site of infarction has been demonstrated in studies using electrocardiograms, ventriculography, and post-mortem examination [57].

A major disadvantage of rest thallium imaging in the setting of suspected acute myocardial infarction is the inability to differentiate acute infarction, severe ischemia and chronic scar on initial images. The possibility that serial imaging after thallium administration might distinguish ischemic from infarcted myocardium is under investigation. Preliminary data is available in 20 patients with acute myocardial infarctions studied within 12 hours of the onset of chest pain. All patients had initial thallium defects; however, only one third demonstrated redistribution of delayed images. Gated blood pool studies demonstrated akinetic or dyskinetic regional wall motion in zones corresponding to persistent thallium defects. However, transient thallium defects were associated with only hypokinetic regional wall motion [58].

Rest thallium imaging in patients admitted to the coronary care unit has also been used to predict hospital course [59]. One hundred and twenty-two patients were studied on admission to the coronary care unit. An eventful course was defined as either acute myocardial infarction or further ischemic episodes. Among 38 patients with previous myocardial infarction, 97% had abnormal scans and the presence or number of transient and/or persistent defects did not separate eventful from uneventful patients. Of the remaining 84 patients without prior myocardial infarction, 32% had an eventful course. In these patients, persistent defects were more predictive of subsequent hospital course than transient defects. The presence and number of persistent defects allowed identification of patients at high risk; 17 of 28 patients with 2 or more persistent defects and 15 of 20 patients with 3 or more persistent defects had an eventful course.

Thallium imaging at rest early after coronary artery reperfusion with streptokinase has been used as an indicator of myocardial salvage. Marcus and associates studied nine patients with acute myocardial infarction, all of whom had pre-streptokinase defects on thallium images [60]. After streptokinase, a second large dose of thallium was administered and images obtained. In all patients, the defects had resolved. However, preliminary canine studies have shown that thallium might be taken up initially by irreversibly ischemic myocardium [61]. Using a canine model of coronary occlusion followed by reperfusion, thallium images acquired immediately after and one hour after reperfusion often demonstrated normal thallium activity in regions subsequently undergoing infarction. Thus, further studies will be required before the initial distribution of thallium after coronary artery reperfusion can be used as a marker of myocardial salvage. Other investigators have described a thallium redistribution technique for assessing the effects of myocardial reperfusion. Simoons and associates administered intravenous thallium prior to myocardial reperfusion with streptokinase. Redistribution images were acquired four hours later. Significant thallium redistribution was found into the areas with initial defects after successful thrombolysis [62]. However, similar changes in thallium distribution were observed in a control group of patients without thrombolysis.

Myocardial imaging with gamma emitting fatty acids

Radiolabeled long-chain fatty acids could theoretically be important myo-cardial imaging agents since such fatty acids are a major substrate for myocardial energy production under anaerobic conditions. Furthermore the high utilization by the heart, minimal concentration in the lungs, and rapid fall in blood levels make fatty acids attractive potential imaging agents. Serial imaging with such agents to determine their clearance from the myocardium might also be a tool for studying myocardial metabolism. Sobel and associates have used carbon-11-labeled palmitic acid to image the heart and study myocardial metabolism [63, 64, 65, 66]. Palmitic acid uptake and clearance have been studied in normal, ischemic, and in-farcted human and canine myocardium [67, 68]. However, such tech-niques have not gained widespread clinical applicability for several rea-sons. First, an on-site cyclotron is required because of the short physical half-life of C-11 (20 minutes). Second, further expense is incurred by the necessity for a positron camera. Third, rapid decay of the C-11 makes static imaging difficult. Consequently, investigators have synthesized fatty acids labeled with gamma emitting radioisotopes.

Several long chain fatty acids terminally labeled with I-123 have been described [69, 70, 71, 72, 73, 74, 75]. Most investigators have reported a delayed myocardial clearance from ischemic regions. Feinendegen and associates reported a delayed myocardial clearance from ischemic zones using I-123-labeled-17-heptadecanoic acid [69, 70, 71, 75]. The mean myocardial half time was 25 minutes in normal subjects. However the mean half time was 35–50 minutes in patients with coronary artery dis-ease. Van der Wall and associates reported a monoexponential clearance of I-123-labeled-16-hexadecenoic acid from normal and infarcted zones, however the clearance was faster in infarcted zones [73, 76]. Huckell and associates also used I-123-labeled-16-hexadecenoic acid and found that normal regions and regions of old myocardial infarction had fast clear-ances, that ischemic regions had a slower clearance, and that acutely infarcted myocardium had no significant clearance. All of these studies utilized external gamma camera imaging with resultant problems with region of interest location, and foreground and background correction. In addition, correction for free I-123 in the blood was made using a second injection of NaI-123, as described in Chapter 5.

One study has examined the myocardial kinetics of I-123-labeled-16-hexadecenoic acid (I-123-HDA) in a canine model using implantable miniature radiation detectors [77]. In six anesthetized dogs with partial

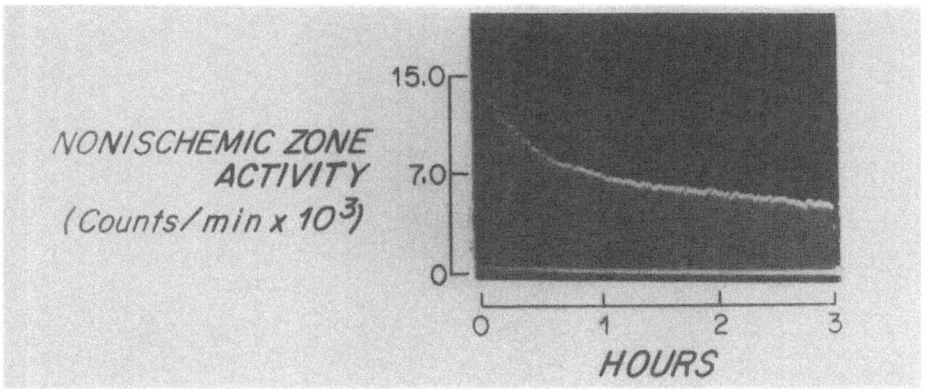

Figure 13. Nonischemic zone I-123 time-activity curve obtained with miniature radiation detectors. Reprinted from European Journal of Nuclear Medicine (in press).

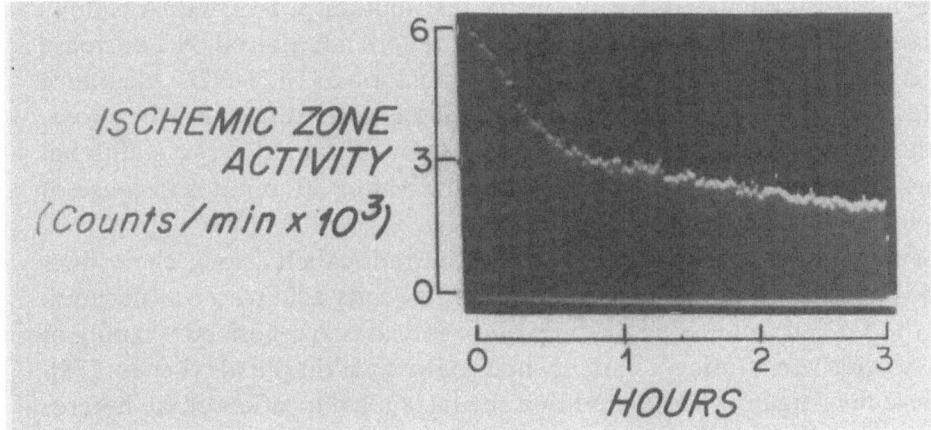

Figure 14. Ischemic zone I-123 time-activity curve obtained with miniature radiation detectors. Reprinted from European Journal of Nuclear Medicine (in press).

occlusion of the left anterior descending coronary artery, I-123-HDA was injected into the left atrium. Regional I-123 activities were monitored continuously using miniature cadmium telluride radiation detectors positioned over the normal and ischemic regions. In both zones, myocardial I-123 activity peaked within one minute of administration and then cleared bi-exponentially (Figures 13 and 14). There was a linear correlation between I-123 activity initially and microsphere-determined regional myocardial blood flow. There was no significant difference in myocardial clearance rates for normal and ischemic regions over a three-hour period.

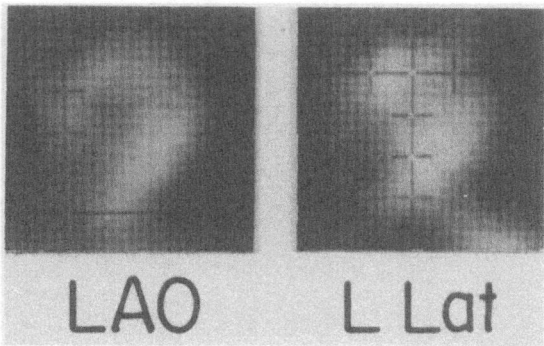

LAO   L Lat

Figure 15. Te-123m cardiac images obtained from a dog with a left anterior descending coronary artery occlusion. Reprinted from Circulation 65; 309, 1982 with permission of the American Heart Association.

The authors concluded that the initial distribution of I-123-HDA is flow-related and that I-123-HDA clearance rates are not altered by a decrease in myocardial perfusion. Thus, the extrapolation of I-123-HDA clearance rates to myocardial metabolism must be done with caution. Furthermore, although good quality myocardial images were obtained in two additional dogs, image quality decreased significantly after 30 minutes because of rapid myocardial tracer clearance.

The rapid myocardial clearance of the radiolabeled long chain fatty acids appears to be due to metabolism of the fatty acid with translocation of the I-123 to other sites. Knapp and associates synthesized a family of fatty acids substituting a metallic heteroatom within the alkyl chain [78]. These investigators postulated that the inter-alkyl location of the hetero-atom would protect it from translocation. One such radiopharmaceutical, tellurium-123m-labeled-9-telluraheptadecanoic acid (Te-123-THDA), has been shown to have a high myocardial uptake [79]. Biodistribution studies in the rat have shown the highest organ uptake in the heart [80]. Furthermore, threefold higher Te-123 activities were found in normal myocardium compared with infarcted myocardium. In canine studies using miniature implanted radiation detectors, there was minimal clearance of Te-123-THDA from normal and ischemic myocardium [81]. Good quality myocardial images were obtained using a gamma camera (Figure 15). Although this class of radiopharmaceuticals is promising as a myocardial perfusion imaging agent in man, further toxicology studies need to be performed. Furthermore, such agents may be unable to differentiate scar from ischemic myocardium.

References

1. Master AM: Two-step exercise electrocardiogram: Test for coronary insufficiency. Ann Intern Med 32: 842–63, 1950.
2. Rifkin RD, Hood WB: Bayesian analysis of electrocardiographic exercise stress testing. N Engl J Med 297: 681–6, 1977.
3. Kawana M, Drisek H, Porter J, Lathrop KA, Charleston D, Harper PV: The use of thallium-199 as a potassium analogue in scanning. J Nucl Med 11: 333, 1970.
4. Ritchie JL, Trobaugh GB, Williams DL, Hamilton GW: Myocardial imaging with thallium-201 at rest and exercise: Correlation with coronary anatomy and exercise electrocardiography (abstr). Circulation 53, 54; Suppl 11: 11–216, 1978.
5. Pohost GM, Zir LM, Moore RH, McKusick KA, Guiney TE, Beller GA: Differentiation of transiently ischemic from infarcted myocardium by serial imaging after a single dose of thallium-201. Circulation 55: 294–302, 1977.
6. Bradley-Moore PR, Lebowitz E, Greene MW, Atkins HL, Ansari AN: Thallium-201 for medical use. II. Biological behavior. J Nucl Med 16: 156–60, 1975.
7. Weich HF, Strauss HW, Pitt B: Myocardial extraction fraction of thallium-201 (abstr). Circulation 54; Suppl II: II–218, 1976.
8. Okada RD, Leppo JA, Strauss HW, Boucher CA, Pohost GM: Mechanisms and time course for the disappearance of thallium-201 defects at rest in dogs: Relationship of time to peak activity of myocardial blood flow. Am J Cardiol 49: 699–706, 1982.
9. Vogel RA, Kirch DL, LeFree MT, Rainwater JO, Jensen DP, Steele PP: Thallium-201 myocardial perfusion scintigraphy: results of standard and multipinhole tomographic technique. Am J Cardiol 43: 787–793, 1979.
10. Boucher CA, Zir LM, Beller GA, Okada RD, McKusick KA, Strauss HW, Pohost GM: Increased pulmonary uptake of thallium-201 during exercise myocardial imaging: Clinical, hemodynamic and angiographic implications in patients with coronary artery disease. Am J Cardiol 46: 189–96, 1980.
11. Kushner FG, Okada RD, Kirshenbaum HD, Boucher CA, Strauss HW, Pohost GM: Pulmonary thallium-201 after stress in patients with coronary artery disease (abstr). Clin Res 27: 182, 1979.
12. Okada RD, Boucher CA, Strauss HW, Pohost GM: Exercise radionuclide imaging approaches to coronary artery disease. Am J Cardiol 46: 1188–1204, 1980.
13. Okada RD, Raessler KL, Woolfenden JM, Groves BM, Patton D, Goldman S, Hager WD: Sensitivity and specificity in the detection of coronary artery disease: Clinical value of the thallium-201 stress tests. Int J Nucl Med Biol 5: 211–21, 1978.
14. Bailey IK, Griffith LSC, Rouleau J, Strauss HW, Pitt B: Thallium-201 myocardial perfusion imaging at rest and during exercise. Circulation 55: 79–87, 1977.
15. Wasserman L, Iskandrian AS, Segal BL, Bemis CE, Kimbiris D, Mintz GS, Croll MN: Merits of stress thallium-201 myocardial scans in patients with inconclusive exercise ECG. Clin Res 27: 213, 1979.
16. Amsterdam EA, Joye J, Glass E, Berman D, DeNardo G, Mason DT: Accuracy of thallium-201 myocardial exercise scintigraphy to detect coronary artery disease in patients with abnormal resting electrocardiograms (abstr). Clin Res 27: 147, 1979.
17. McCarthy DM, Blood DK, Sciacca RR, Cannon PJ: Single dose myocardial perfusion imaging with thallium-201: application in patients with nondiagnostic electrocardiographic stress tests. Am J Cardiol 43: 899–905, 1979.
18. Pohost GM, Boucher CA, Zir LM, McKusick KA, Beller GA, Strauss HW: The thallium stress test: the qualitative approach revisited (abstr). Circulation 59,60: Suppl II: II–49, 1979.
19. Dash H, Massie BM, Botvinick EH, Brundage BH: The noninvasive identification of left main and three-vessel coronary artery disease by myocardial stress perfusion scintigraphy and treadmill exercise electrocardiography. Circulation 60: 276–83, 1979.

20. Massie BM, Botvinick EH, Brundage BH: Correlation of thallium-201 scintigrams with coronary anatomy: factors affecting region by region sensitivity. Am J Cardiol 44: 616–22, 1979.

21. Leppo J, Yipintsoi T, Blankstein R, Bontemps R, Freeman LM, Zohman L, Scheuer J: Thallium-201 myocardial scintigraphy in patients with triple-vessel disease and ischemic exercise stress tests. Circulation 59: 714–21, 1979.

22. Rigo P, Becker LC, Griffith LSL, et al: Influence of coronary collateral vessels on the results of thallium-201 myocardial stress imaging. Am J Cardiol 44: 452–8, 1979.

23. Guiney TE, Pohost GM, Beller GA, McKusick KA: Differentiating false positive stress tests by single dose thallium-201 stress-scanning (abstr). Am J Cardiol 39: 321, 1977.

24. Mews GC, Zir LM, Strauss HW, Guiney TE, Dinsmore RE, Pohost GM: A critical look at "subcritical" coronary stenosis with Tl-201 (abstr). Circulation 58: Suppl II: II–181, 1978.

25. Cannon PJ, Schmidt DH, Weiss MB, Fowler DL, Sciacca RR, Ellis K, Casarella WJ: The relationship between regional myocardial perfusion at rest and arteriographic lesions in patients with coronary atherosclerosis. J Clin Invest 56: 1442–54, 1975.

26. Cannon PJ, Dell RB, Dwyer EM Jr: Regional myocardial perfusion ratio in patients with coronary artery disease. J Clin Invest 51: 978–94, 1972.

27. Bailey IK, Come PC, Kelly DT, Burrow RD, Griffith LSC, Strauss HW, Pitt B: Thallium-201 myocardial perfusion imaging in aortic valve stenosis. Am J Cardiol 40: 889–99, 1977.

28. Huckell VF, Staniloff HM, Feiglin DH, MacKenzie GW, Wald RW, Wigle ED, Morch JD, McLaughlin PR: The demonstration of segmental perfusion defects in hypertrophic cardiomyopathy imitating coronary artery disease (abstr). Am J Cardiol 41: 438, 1978.

29. Gaffney FA, Wohl AJ, Blomqvist CG, Parkley RW, Willerson JT: Thallium-201 myocardial perfusion studies in patients with the mitral valve prolapse syndrome. Am J Med 64: 21–26, 1978.

30. Ahmad M, Merry SL, Haibach H: Evidence of impaired myocardial perfusion in abnormal left ventricular function during exercise in patients with isolated systolic narrowing of the left anterior descending coronary artery. Am J Cardiol 48: 832–   , 1981.

31. Girod DA, Faris J, Hurwitz RA, Caldwell R, Burt RW, Siddiqui A: Thallium-201 assessment of myocardial perfusion in coronary artery anomalies in children (abstr). Am J Cardiol 43: 402,. 1979.

32. Okada RD, Boucher CA, Kirshenbaum HK, Kushner FG, Strauss HW, Block PC, McKusick KA, Pohost GM: Improved diagnostic accuracy of thallium-201 stress test using multiple observers and criteria derived from interobserver analysis of variance. Am J Cardiol 46: 619–24, 1980.

33. Kirshenbaum HE, Okada RD, Boucher CA, Kushner FG, Strauss HW, Pohost GM: Relationship of thallium-201 myocardial perfusion pattern to regional and global left ventricular function with exercise. Am Heart J 101: 734–41, 1981.

34. Brown KA, Boucher CA, Okada RD, Strauss HW, McKusick KA, Pohost GM: Serial right ventricular thallium-201 imaging after exercise: Relation to anatomy of the right coronary artery. Am J Cardiol 50: 1217–22, 1982.

35. Hirzel HO, Nuesch K, Gruentzig AR, et al.: Short and long term changes in myocardial perfusion after percutaneous transluminal coronary angioplasty assessed by thallium-201 exercise scintigraphy. Circulation 63: 1001–1007, 1981.

36. Greenberg BH, Hart R, Botvinick EH, Werner JA, Brundage BH, Shames DM, Chatterjee K, Parmley WW: Thallium-201 myocardial perfusion scintigraphy to evaluate patients after coronary bypass surgery. Am J Cardiol 42: 167–76, 1978.

37. Ritchie JL, Narahara KA, Trobaugh GB, Williams DL, Hamilton GW: Thallium-201 myocardial imaging before and after coronary revascularization. Assessment of regional myocardial blood flow and graft patency. Circulation 56: 830–6, 1977.

38. Dunn RF, Freedman B, Bailey IK, Uren RF, Kelly DT: Exercise thallium imaging: Location of perfusion abnormalities in single-vessel coronary disease. J Nucl Med 21: 717–22, 1980.

39. Rigo P, Bailey IK, Griffith SC, Pitt B, Burow RD, Wagner HN, Becker LC: Value and limitations of segmental analysis of stress thallium myocardial imaging for localization of coro-

nary artery disease. Circulation 61: 973–81, 1980.

40. Lim YL, Chesler DA, Boucher CA, Okada RD, Block PC, Pohost GM: A new computer analysis to quantitate and display regional thallium uptake following coronary angioplasty. Clin Res 30: 201,1982.

41. Strauss HW, Pitt B: Noninvasive detection of subcritical coronary arterial narrowings with a coronary vasodilator and myocardial perfusion imaging. Am J Cardiol 39: 403–6, 1977.

42. Gould KL: Noninvasive assessment of coronary stenosis by myocardial perfusion imaging during pharmacologic coronary vasodilatation: I. Physiologic basis and experimental validation. Am J Cardiol 41: 267–78, 1978.

43. Albro PC, Gould KL, Westcott RJ, Hamilton GW, Ritchie JL, Williams DL: Noninvasive assessment of coronary stenoses by myocardial imaging during pharmacologic coronary vasodilatation. III. Clinical trial. Am J Cardiol 42: 751–60, 1978.

44. Josephson MA, Brown BG, Hecht HS, et al.: Noninvasive detection and localization of coronary stenoses in patients: Comparison of resting dipyridamole and exercise thallium-201 myocardial perfusion imaging. Am Heart J 103: 1008–1018, 1982.

45. Brown KA, Boucher CA, Okada RD, Strauss HW, McKusick KA, Pohost GM: Right ventricular thallium-201 distribution following dipyridamole-induced coronary vasodilatation. Am Heart J 103: 1019–24, 1982.

46. Bendersky R, Okada RD, Boucher CA, Strauss HW, Pohost GM: Comparison of intravenous dipyridamole thallium imaging with exercise radionuclide angiography. Am J Cardiol (in press).

47. Niess GS, Logic JR, Russell RO, Rackley CE, Rogers WJ: Usefulness and limitations of thallium-201 myocardial scintigraphy in delineating location and size of prior myocardial infarction. Circulation 59: 1010–19, 1979.

48. Gewirtz H, Beller GA, Strauss HW, Dinsmore RE, Zir LM, McKusick KA, Pohost GM: Transient defects of resting thallium scans in patients with coronary artery disease. Circulation 59: 707–13, 1979.

49. Maseri A, Parodi O, Severi S, Pesola A: Transient transmural reduction of myocardial blood flow demonstrated by thallium-201 scintigraphy as a cause of variant angina. Circulation 54: 280–8, 1976.

50. Wackers FJ, Lie KI, Liem KL, Sokole EB, Samson G, Schoot JB, Durrer D: Thallium-201 scintigraphy in unstable angina pectoris. Circulation 57: 738–42, 1978.

51. Brown KA, Okada RD, Boucher CA, Phillips HR, Strauss HW, Pohost GM: Serial thallium-201 imaging at rest in patients with unstable and stable angina pectoris: Relationship of myocardial perfusion at rest to presenting clinical syndrome. Am Heart J (in press).

52. Bulkley BH, Hutchins GM, Bailey I, Strauss HW, Pitt B: Thallium-201 imaging and gated cardiac blood pool scans in patients with ischemic and idiopathic congestive cardiomyopathy. Circulation 55: 753–60, 1977.

53. Wackers FJT, Van Der Schoot JB, Sokole EB, et al.: Noninvasive visualization of acute myocardial infarction in man with thallium-201. Br Heart J 37: 741–4, 1975.

54. Wackers FJT, Sokole EB, Samson G, Van Der Schoot JB, Lie KI, Liem KL, Wellens HJJ: Value and limitations of thallium-201 scintigraphy in the acute phase of myocardial infarction. N Engl J Med 295: 1–5, 1976.

55. Wackers FJT, Lie KI, Liem KL, et al.: Potential value of thallium-201 scintigraphy as a means of selecting patients for the coronary care unit. Br Heart J 41: 111–7, 1979.

56. Wackers FJT, Becker AE, Samson G, Sokole EB, Van Der Schoot JB, Vet AJT, Lie KI, Durrer D, Wellens H: Location and size of acute transmural myocardial infarction estimated from thallium-201 scintiscans. Circulation 56: 72–8, 1977.

57. Niess GS, Logic JR, Russell RO, Rackley CE, Rogers WJ: Usefulness and limitations of thallium-201 myocardial scintigraphy in delineating location and size of prior myocardial infarction. Circulation 59: 1010–9, 1979.

58. Zir LM, Strauss HW, Gewirtz H, Shea WH, Forwand SA, Voukydis PC, Pohost GM: Tl-201

redistribution in patients with acute myocardial infarction (abstr). J Nucl Med 20: 649, 1979.

59. Boucher CA, Mulley AG, Okada RD, Thibault GE, Strauss HW, Green AM, Pohost GM: Serial thallium imaging at rest on admission to the coronary care unit: An analysis of transient and persistent defects and increased lung uptake in patients with suspected acute myocardial infarction (abstr). J Nucl Med 22: 55, 1981.

60. Markis JE, Malagold M, Parker JA, et al.: Myocardial salvage after intracoronary thrombolysis with streptokinase in acute myocardial infarction. Assessment by intracoronary thallium-201. N Engl J Med 305: 777–782, 1981.

61. Okada RD, Lim YL, Boucher CA, Pohost GM: Split-dose thallium imaging: A new technique for obtaining thallium images before and immediately after intervention (abstr). Circulation 66: 200, 1982.

62. Simoons ML, Wijns W, Balakumaran K, Serruys PW, Brand M van den, Fioretti P, Reiber JHC, Lie P, Hugenholtz PG: The effect of intracoronary thrombolysis with streptokinase on myocardial thallium distribution and left ventricular function assessed by blood-pool scintigraphy. Eur Heart J 3: 433–440, 1982.

63. Sobel BE, Weiss ES, Welch MJ, Siegel BA, Ter-Pogossian MM: Detection of remote myocardial infarction in patients with positron emission transaxial tomography with C-11-labeled palmitate. Circulation 55: 853–857, 1977.

64. Ter-Pogossian MM, Klein MS, Markham J, Roberts R, Sobel BE: Regional assessment of myocardial metabolic integrity in vivo by positron-emission tomography with 11-C-labeled palmitate. Circulation 61: 242–55, 1980.

65. Weiss ES, Hoffman EJ, Phelps ME, Welch MJ, Henry PD, Ter-Pogossian MM, Sobel BE: External detection and visualization of myocardial ischemia with 11-C-substrates in vitro and in vivo. Circulation Res 39: 24–32, 1976.

66. Hoffman EJ, Phelps ME, Weiss ES, Welch MJ, Coleman RE, Sobel BE, Ter-Pogossian MM: Transaxial tomographic imaging of canine myocardium with 11-C-palmitic acid. J Nucl Med 18: 57–61, 1977.

67. Klein MS, Goldstein RA, Welch MJ, Sobel BE: External assessment of myocardial metabolism with 11-C-palmitate in rabbit hearts. Am J Physiol 237: H51, 1979.

68. Goldstein RA, Klein MS, Welch MJ, Sobel BE: External assessment of myocardial metabolism with C-11-palmitate in vivo. J Nucl Med 21: 342, 1980.

69. Feinendegen LE, Vyska K, Freundlieb C, Hock A: Noninvasive analysis of metabolic reactions in body tissue; the case of myocardial fatty acids. Europ J Nucl Med (in press).

70. Freundlieb C, Hock A, Vyska K, Feinendegen LE, Machulla H-J, Stocklin G: Myocardial imaging and metabolic studies with [17-123-I]-iodoheptadecanoic acid. J Nucl Med 21: 1043–50, 1980.

71. Freundlieb C, Hock A, Vyska K, Feinendegen LE, Machulla H-J, Stocklin G: Elimination rate of labelled fatty acids from ischemic myocardium measuring ω-123-I-heptadecanoic acid. Nuklearmedizin: 338–940, 1980.

72. Freundlieb C, Hock A, Vyska K, Profant M, Feinendegen LE, Machulla HJ, Stocklin G: Noninvasive left ventricular imaging and assessment of myocardial fatty acid metabolism using ω-123-I-heptadecanoic acid. Nuklearmedizin: 439–42, 1979.

73. Wall EE van der, Heidendal GAK, Hollander W den, Westera G, Majid PA, Roos JP: Metabolic myocardial imaging with I-123 labeled free fatty acids (abstr.) Circulation Suppl III, 62: 8, 1980.

74. Huckell VF, Lyster DM, Morrison RT: The potential role of 123-Iodine-hexadecenoic acid in assessing normal and abnormal myocardial metabolism (abstr.) J Nucl Med 21: P57, 1980.

75. Vyska K, Hock A, Freundlieb C, Profant M, Feinendegen LE, Machulla HJ, Stocklin G: Myocardial imaging and measurement of myocardial fatty acid metabolism using ω-I-123-heptadecanoic acid (abstr.) J Nucl Med 20: 650, 1979.

76. Wall EE van der, Westera G, Hollander W den, Visser FC External detection of regional myocardial metabolism with radioiodinated hexadecenoic acid in the dog heart. Eur J Nucl Med 6: 147–51, 1981.

77. Okada Rd, Elmaleh D, Werre GS, Strauss HW: Myocardial kinetics of I-123-labeled-16-hexadecanoic acid. Europ J Nucl Med (in press).
78. Knapp FF Jr: Selenium and tellurium as carbon substitutes. In: International Symposium on Radiopharmaceuticals: Structure-Activity Relationships, edited by Spencer R. New York, Grune & Stratton, pp 101–8, 1980.
79. Knapp FF Jr, Ambrose KR, Callahan AP, Grigsby RA, Irgolic KJ: Tellurium-123m-labeled isosteres of palmitoleic and oleic acids show high myocardial uptake (abstr.) Proc 2nd Symposium on Radiopharmaceuticals, p 101, 1979.
80. Elmaleh DR, Knapp FF Jr, Yasuda T, Coffey JL, Kopiwoda S, Okada RD, Strauss HW: Myocardial imaging with Te-123m-9-telluraheptadecanoic acid. J Nucl Med (in press).
81. Okada RD, Knapp FF, Elmaleh DR, Yasuda T, Boucher CA, Strauss HW: Tellurium-123m-labeled-9-telluraheptadecanoic acid. A possible cardiac imaging agent. Circulation 65: 305–10, 1982.

5. Myocardial imaging with radiolabeled free fatty acids

E.E. van der Wall

Introduction

The regional, non-invasive assessment of myocardial functional integrity with the aim of identifying normal, ischemic and necrotic zones is highly desirable in patients with coronary artery disease (CAD). Therefore attempts have been made to determine the metabolic integrity of the myocardium quantitatively with radioactively labeled metabolic substrates. Since free fatty acids (FFA) are primary substrates of the normally perfused myocardium, it appears likely that radiolabeled FFA are suitable for the study of myocardial FFA metabolism.

Generally the following requirements for metabolic isotope tracers have to be met:

1. they should be highly specific indicators of a given metabolic pathway;
2. they must not alter the physiological behaviour of metabolic substrates;
3. they have to provide an adequate external detection by current imaging devices (gamma- or positron camera);
4. they must be clinically applicable.

These conditions are best fulfilled by radionuclides with chemical identities akin to physiological substrates such as carbon (C), nitrogen (N) and oxygen (O). C-11, N-13, and O-15 are the isotopes of the constituents of most living matter and of most molecules involved in the majority of metabolic processes. Moreover they are positron-emitting radionuclides (Table 1) and the combined use with positron emission tomography (PET) offers potential advantages for the assessment of myocardial integrity. An added advantage of these radionuclides is their short half-lives, allowing repeated measurements at short intervals which can be of much importance in intervention procedures.

In spite of the advantages of C-11, N-13 and O-15, their use in the assessment of myocardial integrity has been documented only in a limited number of studies. This is due to several factors. Because of the short half-lives, the production of these nuclides requires the availability of a

Table 1. Positron- and gamma-emitting radionuclides potentially used for evaluation of cardiac metabolism

Radionuclide	emission	half-life	production
O-15	positron (511 keV)	2.03 min	requires in-house cyclotron
N-13	positron (511 keV)	9.98 min	requires in-house cyclotron
C-11	positron (511 keV)	20.4 min	requires in-house cyclotron
I-123	gamma (159 keV)	13.3 h	cyclotron-produced
I-131	gamma (364 keV)	8.06 days	reactor-produced
Te-123m	gamma (159 keV)	120 days	cyclotron-produced

cyclotron (or other particle accelerator) in the laboratory where they are to be used. Furthermore, the rapid incorporation of these nuclides into useful molecules is difficult, and the tomographic devices (special positron cameras) necessary for the imaging of these nuclides are complex and expensive. In the recent past, however, the usefulness of this approach has become generally accepted, and the scientific literature contains an increasing number of reports of the use of PET and physiological indicators in the study of the myocardium. Regarding FFA, it would be very convenient to use the isotopes of the natural elements of FFA, which are C, O and hydrogen (H), but only C-11 has proven to be adequate as a label to FFA. Besides metabolic studies with PET, attention has been focused on gamma-emitting radionuclides labeled to FFA, because of potentially wider applicability and lower cost. Moreover, since most suitable gamma-emitting radionuclides have physical half-lives of more than several hours, no in-house cyclotron is required. For instance, iodine-123 (I-123, half-life 13.3 h) may be very well tagged to FFA and can easily be detected with any commercially available gamma-camera.

Although many different labeled fatty acids have been studied, this review will mainly call attention to the most important investigations in this field, i.e., the study of FFA labeled with the physiological tracer C-11 and with I-123 (Figure 1). We will first describe the myocardial FFA metabolism, then consider the metabolism and kinetics of radiolabeled FFA and finally discuss the potential clinical value of radiolabeled FFA.

Myocardial fatty acid metabolism

FFA are preferred myocardial substrates and fatty acid oxidation normally accounts for 60 to 80% of energy production by the heart. Even

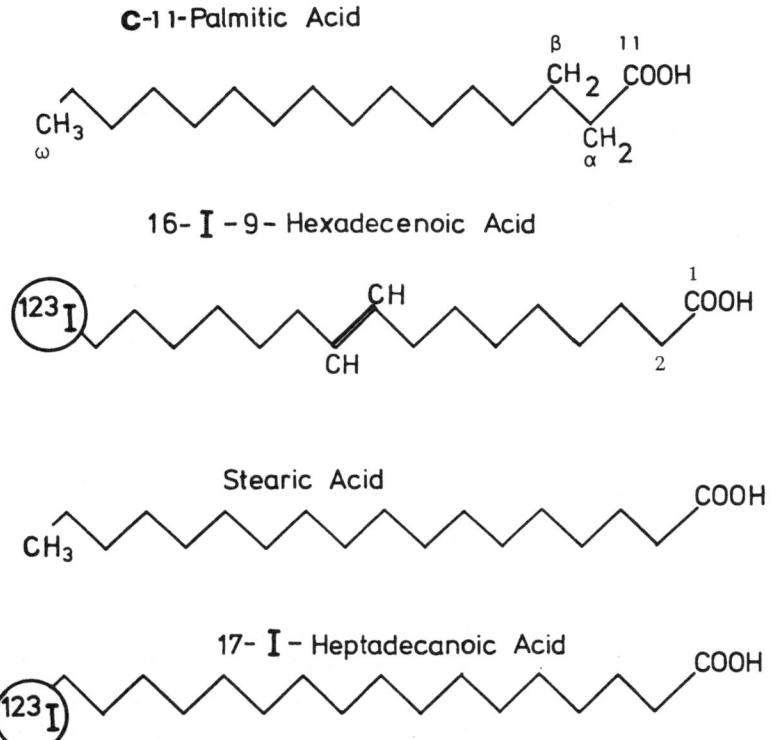

Figure 1. General structure of C-11-palmitate, stearic acid and the most currently used iodinated free fatty acids.

when moderate ischemia supervenes, FFA liberated from triglycerides are metabolized in preference to glucose. However, under conditions of marked ischemia or severe hypoxia (oxygen delivery less than 20% of normal), anaerobic metabolism provides a substantial proportion of energy via glycolytic mechanisms. The metabolic pathway of fatty acid has been well clarified (Figure 2). Long chain fatty acids are synthesized in the liver and adipose tissue, transported in blood bound primarily to albumin, and extracted by myocardium as a function of several factors including: chain length, molarity of both albumin and fatty acid, metabolic integrity of the cell, perfusion (since regional coronary flow determines residence time), and myocardial energy requirements. Both ischemia and hypoxia lead to decreased extraction.

Fatty acids in interstitial or intracellular fluid are bound to soluble proteins, and uptake of fatty acids into the cell appears to depend on competition between cellular binding sites and binding sites on albumin.

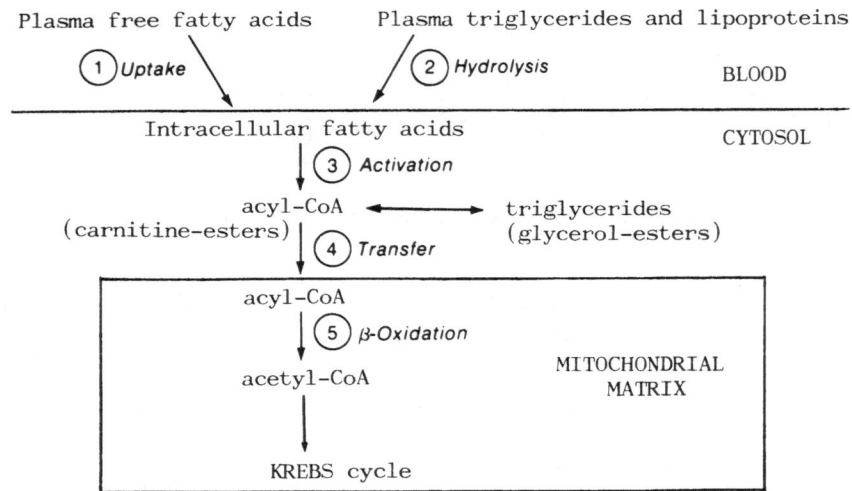

Figure 2. Overall scheme of fatty acid metabolism.

Intracellular fatty acids are activated and converted to thioester derivatives in the cytosol in reactions requiring both coenzyme A (CoA) and ATP. Esterified fatty acids may undergo oxidation or incorporation into triglycerides. Activated fatty acids in the cytosol cannot be oxidized directly. They are first transported across the mitochondrial membrane by acyl CoA carnitine transferases specific for chain length and intimately associated with mitochondrial membranes. Carnitine-dependent translocation facilitates ingress of acyl CoA into the mitochondrial matrix where beta oxidation occurs. Acyl CoA is oxidized to produce acetyl CoA which is oxidized via the Krebs cycle with liberation of CO_2 and synthesis of intracellular ATP. The knowledge of altered fatty acid metabolism in myocardial ischemia stimulated labeling procedures with FFA for the detection of CAD.

Metabolism and pharmacokinetic behaviour of labeled FFA

The first efforts with radiolabeled FFA were mainly pointed at the search for myocardial imaging agents. It was only recently that the non-invasive study of regional metabolic turnover rates in the myocardium has become a potential issue. For quantification of metabolic rates, the pharmacokinetics of these tracers in the myocardium in terms of uptake and clearance and their relationship to the biochemical process must be known.

Previous experimental studies [1, 2] have revealed a similar type of pharmacokinetics in the heart both for C-11-palmitic acid and for iodinated fatty acids (Figure 3.). The kinetics exhibit a fast uptake which represents the extraction from blood (phase I). This first phase simply reflects perfusion as has been demonstrated by studies [3] comparing N-13-H$_3$ and C-11-palmitic acid. Then, two elimination phases follow, a fast and a slow one. The fast elimination phase (phase II) is considered to represent beta-oxidation and is clinically the most relevant phase. The third phase can be attributed to release of fatty acids which has been stored before as triglycerides and phospholipids. Turnover rates of the labeled FFA can be expressed in terms of half-time values (minutes) calculated from the best-fit mono- or bi-exponential function of the different phases of the time-activity curve. For I-123 terminally labeled to

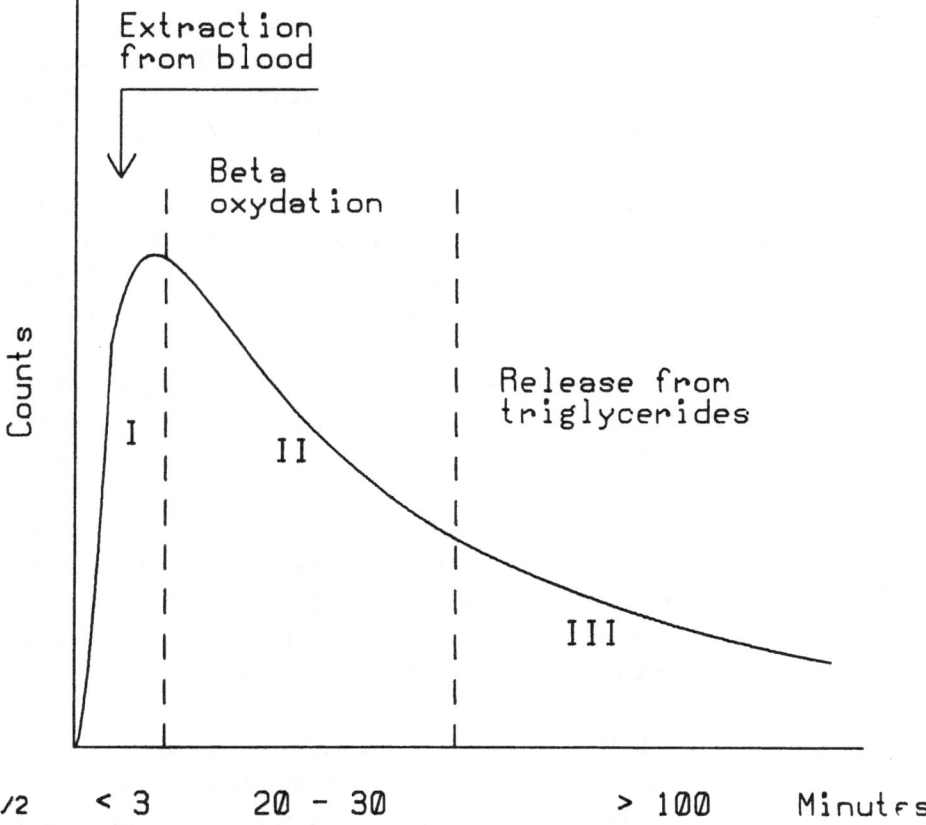

Figure 3. Schematic illustration of the characteristic time-activity curve of clinically used radiolabeled FFA in the myocardium. Three different phases are recognized.

heptadecanoic acid, the fast elimination phase has a half-time of about 25 min in man. Regarding C-11-palmitate, about similar half-time values have been clinically demonstrated [4]. The slow elimination (phase III) can hardly be seen in man and imaging is generally stopped 30 to 60 min after injection because the activity levels become too low for appropriate measurements.

The resemblance of the clearance curves of I-123-FFA and of C-11-palmitate suggests that clearance of I-123 reflects natural metabolism of FFA. Small differences in clearance pattern may still be expected since the C-11 label is removed from the fatty acid in the first step of beta-oxidation with subsequent degrading in the Krebs cycle and exhalation as $C-11-O_2$, while the radioiodine label at the terminal carbon atom is probably removed in the last step of beta-oxidation and released into the circulation before or in the Krebs cycle.

Accordingly, the kinetics of I-123-FFA may parallel metabolism of FFA in uptake of FFA and beta-oxidation pathway. Since the Krebs cycle is a relatively fast process (half-time about 4 min measured with C-11-acetate) [5], it will not considerably disturb the I-123-FFA turnover rates. From this point of view, clearance of I-123-FFA has been regarded to reflect metabolic turnover of FFA in the myocardium.

Considerable debate has nowadays arisen about the proper explanation for the elimination half-times in the second phase. It has been postulated that the measured half-times of iodinated FFA do not correlate with beta-oxidation but are due to the rate of diffusion of free iodide from the mitochondria into the coronary circulation [6].

On the other hand, with respect to C-11-palmitate, it remains to be proven that clearance of tracer is really due to oxidative metabolism with resultant formation of $C-11-O_2$ and not to washout of oxidation products, such as short-chain intermediates via the coronary circulation [7]. These factors become of crucial importance during reduced oxidative metabolism induced either by the decreased coronary flow (ischemia) or diminished oxygen delivery (hypoxia). Lerch et al. [8] demonstrated that clearance of C-11-palmitate was constantly depressed in regions with restricted oxygen supply regardless of concomitant reduction of flow, and they concluded that metabolism itself is the major determinant of reduced regional clearance. Schelbert et al. [9] suggested that results would be distorted because of altered residence time (i.e. duration of myocardial exposure to labeled substrates) or that altered washout would mask detection of impaired metabolism caused by ischemia or hypoxia. Later studies by his group indicated that measuring FFA oxidation rates is still possible in ischemia but probably with a lower accuracy than in normal myocardium [10].

The exact mechanism can only be clarified by experimentally studying the content of free I-123 or free $C-11-O_2$ per unit myocardial weight when measured acutely after injection and under different pathofysiological circumstances.

Recent results of dog hearts from our laboratory, in which a high percentage of free iodide was found a few minutes after injection of I-123-heptadecanoic acid (I-123-HDA), suggest that the diffusion-rate theory may be the most likely explanation for the elimination half-times of I-123-HDA. Further studies are therefore needed to unravel the intimate relationship between uptake and clearance of labeled FFA.

C-11-palmitate

C-11 provides a particularly suitable label for FFA imaging because of its property as a positron emitting radionuclide. C-11 labeled to palmitate was first used for the visualization of the myocardium by PET in 1976 [12]. C-11-palmitate was found to accumulate substantially in isolated perfused hearts under aerobic conditions, and since reduction of coronary flow is accompanied by decreased FFA extraction, C-11-palmitate was utilized to image normal, transiently ischemic, and irreversibly injured myocardium in intact dogs.

In later studies, Weiss et al. [13] determined the distribution of the tracer in the dog heart by positron emission transaxial tomography (PETT) and demonstrated that significant reversal of depressed C-11-palmitate accumulation in the ischemic zone occurred when coronary artery occlusion was maintained for less than 20 min, but that an irreversibly reduced uptake pattern was observed when reperfusion was delayed for 60 min or more. In a clinical study, Sobel et al. [14] demonstrated with PETT that the distribution of C-11-palmitate in patients with remote myocardial infarction was analogous to the distribution observed in animals with experimentally-induced infarction. Subsequent studies in man have shown that infarct size determined by PETT correlated with infarct size assessed by creatine kinase (MB) blood curves [15].

All these studies suggested a promising and practical application for C-11-palmitate, especially since the evaluation of the effectiveness of therapeutic intervention for the protection of ischemic myocardium requires the quantitative assessment of the distribution and extent of jeopardized and irreversibly injured myocardium. Bergman et al. [16] experimentally demonstrated in 1982 (by measuring uptake of C-11-palmitate) that successful streptokinase treatment, when initiated within 4 h after occlusion, showed preservation of cardiac metabolism while later treatment did not result in significant salutary metabolic effects.

Other recent studies [4, 7, 8, 17, 18] have delineated the myocardial kinetics under normal and ischemic conditions, and the rate of clearance of C-11 activity from the myocardium was proposed as an index of the oxidation rate of C-11-palmitate. It was shown in dogs and also in patients with exercise-induced ischemia that clearance of C-11-palmitate from ischemic regions was decreased compared to normal regions.

Table 2 shows the clearance rates of the most currently used labeled FFA expressed in min half-time.

Table 2. Metabolic clearance rates of various labeled FFA from normal and ischemic myocardial regions

FFA	Species	Clearance rates (Phase II) (minutes half-time)		Reference number
		normal	ischemia (1)	
C-11-palmitate	dog	8.8 ± 3.5	14.9 ± 7.0	[45]
	dog	11.6	≫12*	[7]
	man	22.6 ± 5.6	≫23*	[4]
I-131-HA	dog	20.0 ± 2.3	**	[2]
	dog	14.2 ± 1.4	22.6 ± 1.8	[29]
I-123-HA	dog	14.0 ± 6.7	**	[46]
	man	25	>48*	[23]
	man	34.0 ± 8.4	(18.5 ± 2.5, AMI)	[26]
I-123-HDA	man	25.0 ± 5.0	31.8 ± 19.6***	[24]
	man	24	46	[27]
	man	20-30	35-50	[47]
	man	27.5 ± 3.0	46.4 ± 7.1 (16.8 ± 3.5, AMI)	[26, 28]
I-123-PPA	man	50-60	80-150	[40]
	man	46	61	[48]
	man	≫60*	**	[49]

I-131-HA	I-131-hexadecenoic acid
I-123-HA	I-123-hexadecenoic acid
I-123-HDA	I-123-heptadecanoic acid
I-123-PPA	I-123-phenyl-pentadecanoic acid
AMI	acute myocardial infarction
(1)	transient ischemia, unless otherwise noted
*	no exact values mentioned
**	not studied
***	obtained from the entire myocardium

Radioiodinated FFA

One of the earliest attempts at cardiac imaging was performed with FFA labeled with iodine (I-131), half-life 8.06 days. In 1965, Evans et al. [19] iodinated oleic acid across the double bond and demonstrated that it could be used to visualize the myocardium and to detect myocardial infarction. This substance never became clinically useful because of its low specific activity, poor imaging quality and limitations in administered activity, dictated by radiation dosimetry. Moreover, iodination of FFA at the double bond strongly influenced extraction and elimination of the labeled compound.

In 1975, Robinson et al. [20] made considerable progress by introducing radioiodine into the terminal (omega) position of a fatty acid (hexa-decenoic acid) without altering its extraction efficiency compared to the naturally occurring compound. Poe et al. [21] postulated that the iodine atom in the terminal position maintains a configuration similar to a methyl group (both with an atomic radius of 2 Angstrom) and that the resultant molecule behaves as though it possesses an extra carbon atom. In this context 16-iodo-hexadecenoic acid would behave like heptadecanoic acid. Furthermore, it was shown that a chain length of 15 to 21 carbon atoms had the most optimal myocardial extraction [22], indicating that for metabolic studies a chain length of 16 or 17 carbon atoms appears to be very suitable.

Terminally labeled hexadecenoic acid demonstrated an initial myocar-dial distribution proportional to blood flow and, when labeled with I-123, its myocardial extraction of 78% and blood clearance half-time of 1.7 min closely resembled K-43 and Tl-201 distribution [2,50]. From these studies it was inferred that I-123-FFA are distributed according to myocardial blood flow and subsequently metabolized by known metabolic pathways. Compared to I-123, Tl-201 has a low photon-energy of 80 keV resulting in important tissue absorption, and moreover a rather long physical (72 h) and myocardial half-life (7 h) which gives a total body exposure of 210

Table 3. Radiophysical properties of Tl-201 and of I-123-FFA

		Tl-201	I-123-FFA
Gamma camera detection efficiency	keV	80	159
Myocardial extraction	%	87	78
Physical half-life	h	72	13
Biological half-life (myocardial)	h	7	0.5
Body exposure	mrads/mCi	210	30

mrads/mCi and precludes rapid sequential imaging. I-123 is a gamma-emitter with suitable photon-energy (159 keV) for the currently available gamma-cameras, it has a favourable physical half-life of 13.3 h and offers a relatively low whole body radiation dose to the patient (30 mrads/mCi). Table 3 shows the most important radiophysical properties of Tl-201 and I-123-FFA. In 1977, Poe *et al.* [23] injected 5 mCi I-123-HA intravenously in patients with CAD and images containing about one million net counts from the total myocardium could be obtained within 10 min. In 1978, Machulla *et al.* [1] experimentally used various radiolabeled FFA and showed that terminally labeled I-123-HDA had a myocardial uptake and elimination almost the same as that of C-11-palmitate. This study has been clinically extended in 1980 [24] and demonstrated reduced tracer uptake in ishemic myocardial zones using I-123-HDA. Not only high quality images were obtained, but also elimination of I-123 from the myocardium could be followed by calculating clearance half-times of I-123-HDA from distinct myocardial regions. All these investigative studies emphasized the potential value of I-123-FFA (hexadecenoic and heptadecanoic acid) for myocardial scintigraphy not only for myocardial imaging purposes, but also to evaluate myocardial metabolism in patients with CAD.

So far, clinical studies have been hampered by restricted commercial supply and the technical problem of a rapidly increasing background radioactivity due to release of free radioiodide into the circulation after administration of I-123-FFA. It has been shown that within 15 min after intravenous administration of I-123-HDA, about 50% of the radioactivity in the blood consists of free iodide, which implies that only within this time-limit (preferably within 10 min after administration) good analogoue images can be obtained [25]. Figure 4 shows a comparison in imaging quality between Tl-201 and I-123-FFA. A comparable imaging quality and a similar distribution pattern was noticed in controls and in patients with CAD.

The background problem has been met by a specially designed computer-aided correction procedure, thoroughly described by Van der Wall *et al.* [26]. The correction method must be used to correct the serial images for background activity from the I-123 in the blood pool, i.e., for iodide not bound to the myocardial cells. The procedure is based on the quantitative evaluation of the contribution of inorganic I-123 to the image. Its principle is schematically presented in Figure 5.

The correction procedure results in good quality scintigrams which provide a better contrast between myocardial and surrounding tissue (Figure 6), and this procedure enables the calculation of time-activity

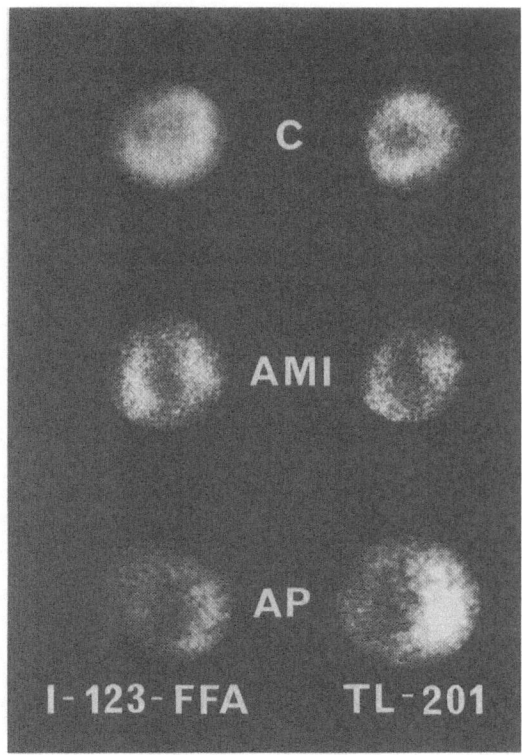

Figure 4. Comparison of imaging quality of I-123-FFA and Tl-201 scintigrams. Upper panel: control subject; middle panel: patient with inferior infarction; lower panel: patient with exercise-induced angina pectoris, showing anteroseptal defect. C = control, AMI = acute myocardial infarction, AP = angina pectoris.

curves which may serve as a parameter for the metabolic turnover of FFA in the myocardium. A drawback of turnover rate measurements is the long imaging period of 45 min and the acquisition of one single view per study which may underdiagnose the presence of CAD. The single view problem can of course be obviated by employment of a biplanar collimator [27].

We studied the kinetics of I-123-FFA in patients with stable and unstable angina pectoris, and patients with acute myocardial infarction (AMI) and we observed different turnover rates of normally perfused, transient ischemic and acutely infarcted areas [26, 28]. With reference to half-time values measured in apparently normal regions (20–30 min), we demonstrated increased values in ischemic zones and decreased values in infarcted zones, suggesting a slow and a fast metabolic turnover of I-123-

94

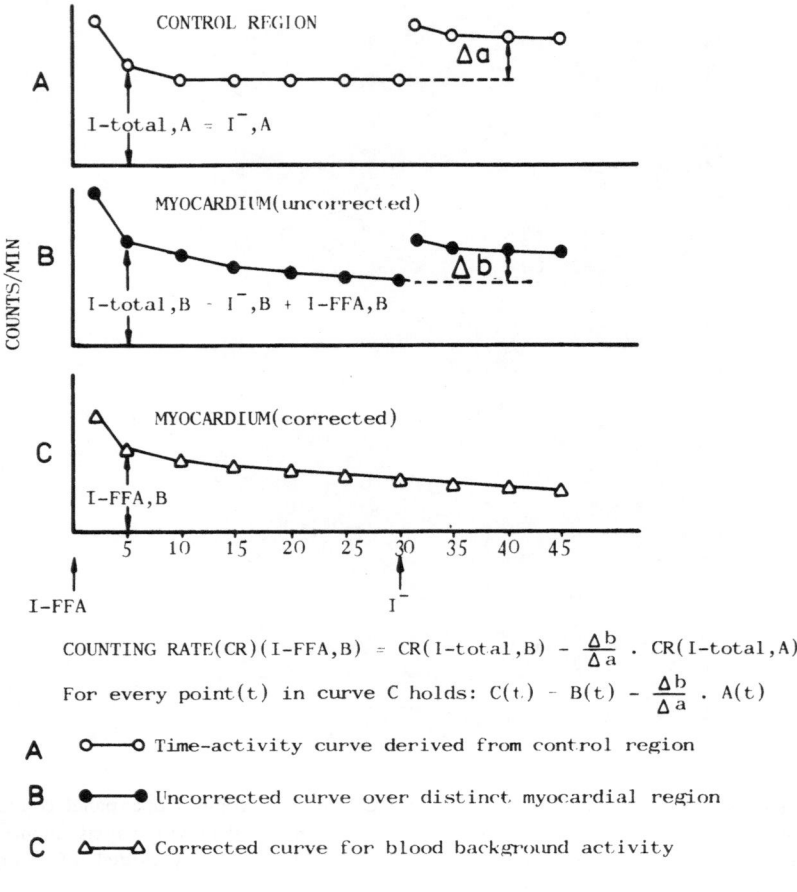

COUNTING RATE(CR)(I-FFA,B) $= CR(I\text{-total},B) - \dfrac{\Delta b}{\Delta a} \cdot CR(I\text{-total},A)$

For every point(t) in curve C holds: $C(t) - B(t) - \dfrac{\Delta b}{\Delta a} \cdot A(t)$

A ○——○ Time-activity curve derived from control region

B ●——● Uncorrected curve over distinct myocardial region

C △——△ Corrected curve for blood background activity

Regions if interest (ROI) are made over lung tissue and a distinct
part of the myocardium, resulting in curve A, resp. B.
After administration of 123-I-iodide, 30 min after injection of
123-I-FFA, in both regions an increase is found proportional to the
amount of circulating blood in the ROI(Δ a, resp.Δ b).
Consequently the count-rate (CR) in lung tissue is proportional to
the concentration of circulating iodide in the blood i.e. CR (I-total,A)=
CR(I⁻,A). Furthermore the CR in the myocardium will be proportional
to the amount of circulating blood iodide plus the amount of 'bound'
fatty acid, CR(I-FFA,B). Therefore the following equation is valid:

$$CR(I\text{-FFA},B = CR(I\text{-total},B) - \frac{\Delta b}{\Delta a} \cdot CR\ (I\text{-total},A).$$

If CR(I-FFA,B) is plotted versus time, the blood background **corrected**
curve is found, which represents the net turnover of 123-I-FFA in the
myocardium. So for every point (t)* in the corrected curve C holds:

$$C(t) = B(t) - \frac{\Delta b}{\Delta a} \cdot A(t). \qquad \text{* every fifth point plotted}$$

Figure 5. Schematic illustration of the correction method.

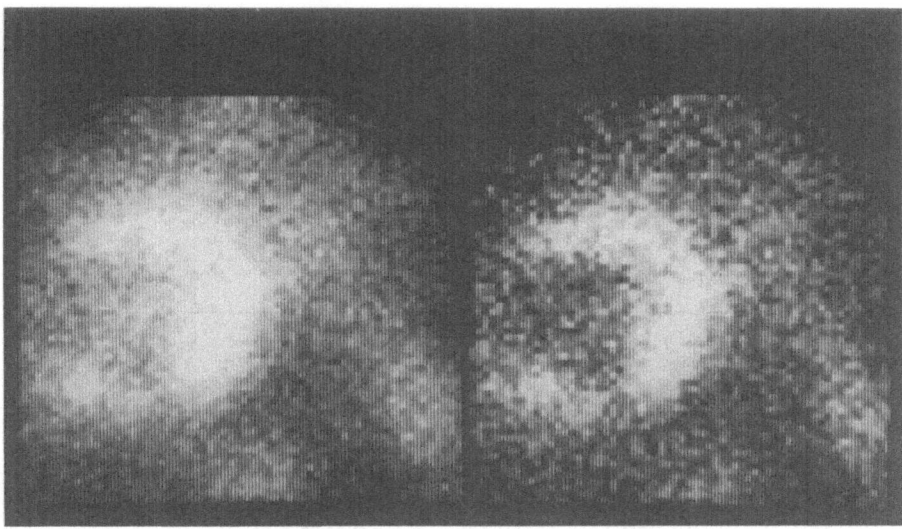

Figure 6. Myocardial I-123-heptadecanoic acid scintigram before (left) and after correction in a patient with anteroseptal infarction.

FFA respectively. Figure 7 gives schematically the observed turnover rates from different myocardial regions. Based on these results, it was postulated that I-123-FFA offer the diagnostic potential to distinguish reversible from irreversible ischemia. Although clinically interesting, and supported by animal experiments [29] and other clinical studies [30], these findings have to be confirmed by studies in much larger populations. Another application of I-123-HDA is its use in patients after successful trombolysis. Two clinical studies [31, 32] reported the value of I-123-HDA in assessing the metabolic integrity of reperfused myocardium within one week after AMI, based on the reduction of defect size and normalization of half-time values. In a recent study [33] it has also been shown that in patients with congestive cardomyopathy (COCM), the determination of clearance rates could be of significant value. All patients with COCM showed inhomogeneous tracer distribution and slow clearance rates of I-123-HDA, suggesting altered FFA metabolism in diseased myocardial regions. Classification of primary cardiomyopathies is currently based on anatomic and functional abnormalities regardless of the underlying etiology. Biochemical studies will not only enhance our understanding of these disorders as well as their detection and characterization but will also aid in the development of effective treatment. Also results of venous bypass surgery and the effect of cardiac rehabilitation have been assessed with

96

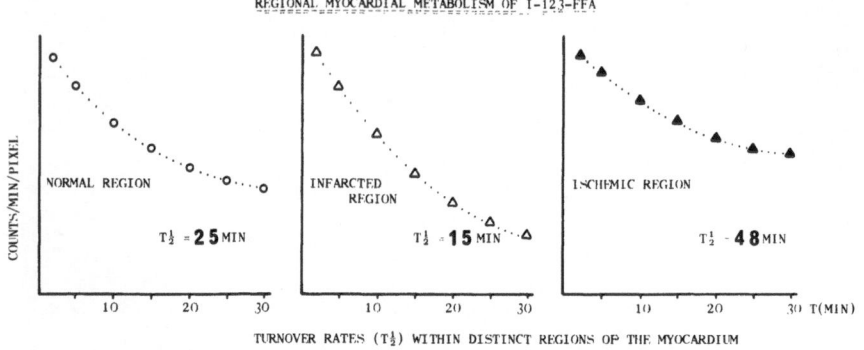

Figure 7. Time-activity curves derived from normal, ischemic and infarcted myocardial region.

I-123-HDA by the measurement of clearance rates [34, 35].

Other recent pharmacological studies [36, 37] evaluated the influence of beta-blocking agents (metoprolol and pindolol) on myocardial uptake of iodinated FFA in dog hearts. Both beta-blocking agents decreased uptake in the normal as well in the acutely ischemic heart, indicating a direct metabolic effect of beta-blockade. Since FFA are supposed to have dele- terious effects on the myocardium by increasing oxygen consumption, these data suggest an additional beneficial influence of beta-blockade. From the above mentioned studies, it will be clear that many different points of entry of myocardial metabolism can be observed with the use of radioiodinated FFA.

Future prospects

Recently, new biochemical concepts have been proposed to avoid the high background activity in imaging studies of the myocardium [38]. Attaching the iodine label to a benzene ring located in the terminal position of a fatty acid (I-123-phenyl-pentadecanoic acid; I-123-PPA) results in a radio- pharmaceutical which shows essentially no release of free radioiodide into the circulation (Figure 8). The final catabolite of I-123-PPA consists of benzoic acid, which is fastly detoxificated and so obviates background problems.

Although I-123-PPA can be employed for imaging purposes, no useful clearance rates have been determined. Since the breakdown products of phenyl-fatty acids will reside much longer in the cells, myocardial clearance will be considerably delayed, making proper metabolic studies virtually impossible [39]. In our institution, elimination half-times of much more than 60 min from normal human hearts have been calculated, which excludes measurement of oxidative metabolism and will only reflect turnover of triglycerides [40].

A next labeled fatty acid that recently [41] has been proposed is tellurium-123m-9-telluraheptadecanoic acid (Te-123m-THDA). This radiopharmaceutical gives a reasonable imaging quality in dog hearts. However, the physical and myocardial biological half-lives of Te-123m are respectively 120 and 7 days, which precludes metabolic clearance studies. In addition, and apart from high radiation doses, experimental studies [42] showed toxic effects in rats, and further toxicity studies are necessary before considering Te-123m-THDA as a myocardial imaging agent in man.

An other new metabolic tracer is C-11-beta-methylheptadecanoic acid (C-11-BMHDA) [43]. This compound is obtained by inserting a methyl radical in the beta-position and so inhibits beta-oxidation. It is therefore trapped in the myocardium and can not further be metabolized (nearly constant level of activity in the dog myocardium for 60 minutes). Needless to say, that C-11-BMHDA is not suitable for studying metabolic clearance

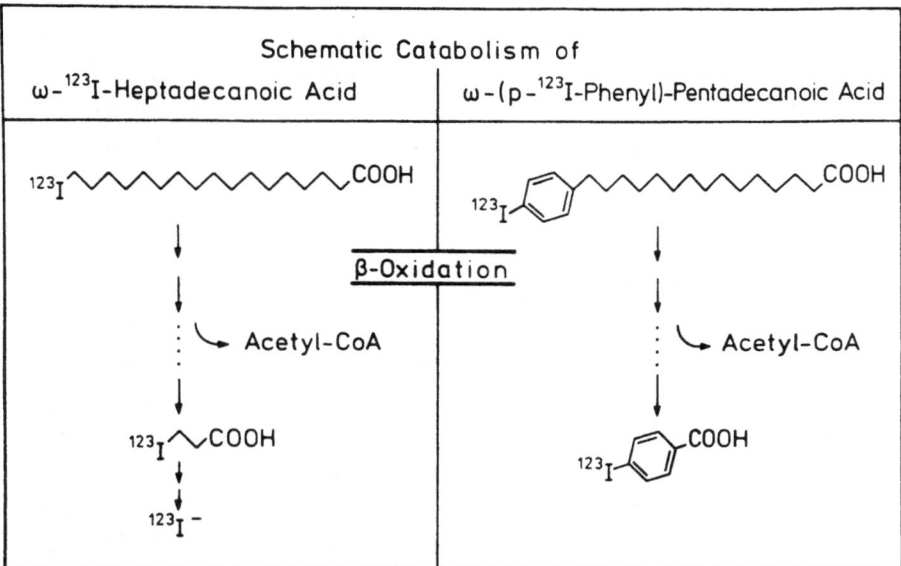

Figure 8. Final products from I-123-heptadecanoic acid (free radioiodide) and from I-123-phenyl-pentadecanoic acid (benzoic acid). (Reproduced from Machulla [38]).

rates, and can thus only be used as an imaging agent.

Other developments are concerned with different biochemical steps in the metabolism of FFA such as studies with C-11 labeled acetate and pyruvate [5, 44]. These labeled metabolic products may provide insight into the overall metabolism of the heart under various conditions. Moreover, enzyme deficiences (for instance lack of carnitine) can be detected with these labeled metabolic products and the therapeutic effectiveness can be evaluated.

Conclusion

Cardiac disease, in particular CAD, is at present most frequently diagnosed and treated in its final stage, i.e., when structural or anatomical derangements have already occurred.

However, disease begins at the biochemical level and therapies are designed to halt or reverse abnormal biochemical processes, restore delivery of biochemical nutrients, or supplement depleted ones. Any technique that provides biochemically specific information about the myocardium could play a vital role in the early diagnosis and effective management of human cardiac disease.

Although the interest for metabolism of the human heart dates from more than 15 years ago, it was only very recently that labeled fatty acids could be applied for non-invasive metabolic studies in the myocardium. Until now, clinical studies have been scarse mainly due to restricted availability of radiopharmaceuticals and to limited equipment facilities.

Positron emission tomography

The initial as well as the operational costs of positron emission tomography have been major limitations for widespread application and the number of positron cameras throughout the world is still very small (1982; North America 19, Europe 13, Asia 4). In addition, one might legitimately question the usefulnesss of an imaging technique limited to the small number of positron-emitting radionuclides as compared to the considerably greater number of gamma-emitters, particularly in light of the fact that positron emission tomographs are expensive and complex devices which cannot be used for the imaging of the more common gamma-ray emitters. However, dedicated and reliable medical minicyclotrons with less technical requirements and lower costs are currently being developed, combined with automated synthesis techniques. At present, clinical studies with C-11-palmitate are limited and its interest is of pure investigational value.

Radioiodinated FFA

Radioiodinated FFA have become commercially available since the beginning of 1983 in the Netherlands (CYGNE, Eindhoven; Magnapharma b.v., Laren) and can therefore be used on a routine basis in clinical practice. Regarding clinical use, we think it is wise to make a clear distinction between studies for imaging purposes and for metabolic investigations. As for imaging in patients with CAD, Tl-201 is still preferable because of lower cost, wider availability and better understanding of its uptake and kinetics in the myocardium. Particularly under exercise conditions Tl-201 will preserve its pivotal role, since redistribution of I-123-FFA can not be used for the evaluation of the exercise scintigrams. Because of the relatively short half-time in the myocardium a second injection of I-123-FFA will be necessary at rest. However, one could speculate that a different pattern of myocardial FFA turnover rates obtained during exercise from diseased myocardial regions (transiently ischemic versus infarcted) will circumvent the need for the performance of resting studies. The study of myocardial FFA metabolism by the noninvasive measurement of turnover rates is still in the experimental phase and its understanding needs the combined efforts of both nuclear medicine and myocardial biochemistry. An urgent problem that has to be solved is the understanding of the coupling of flow and metabolism, i.e., the relation between uptake and elimination of metabolic tracers especially under conditions of myocardial exercise and ischemia. Unless the exact mechanism of the metabolic kinetics has been elucidated, the clinical value of labeled FFA as metabolic tracers will only be superficial. Well-controlled experimental studies have to be carried out to make the labeled FFA clinically useful and to unlabel them from always being promising.

Acknowledgements

The author wishes to express his appreciation for the valuable discussions with Dr. G. Westera, for the critical reading of the manuscript by Ir. M. van Eenige and for excellent secretarial help by A.G. Scholtalbers.

References

1. Machulla HJ, Stoecklin G, Kupfernagel C, Freundlieb C, Hoeck A, Vyska K, Feinendegen LE: Comparative evaluation of fatty acids labeled with C-11, Cl-34m, Br-77 and I-123 for metabolic studies of the myocardium: concise communication. J Nucl Med 19: 298–302, 1978.
2. Poe ND, Robinson Jr GD, Graham LS, MacDonald NS: Experimental basis for myocardial imaging with I-123-labeled hexadecenoic acid. J Nucl Med 17: 1077–1082, 1976.
3. Schelbert HR, Henze E, Huang SC, Phelps ME: Relationship between myocardial blood flow and uptake and utilization of free fatty acids (FFA). J Nucl Med 22: P10, 1981.
4. Henze E, Guzy P, Schelbert H: Metabolic effects of cardiac work on normal and ischemic myocardium in man measured noninvasively with C-11 palmitate and positron emission tomography (PET). Eur Soc Cardiol; Working group on use of isotopes in Cardiology; Rotterdam: 26, 1983 (abstract).
5. Selwyn AP, MacArthur C, Allan R, Pike V, Jones T: Myocardial ischemia; metabolic studies using positron tomography. 8th Eur Congr Cardiol Paris: 194, 1980 (abstract).
6. Stoecklin G: Evaluation of radiohalogen labelled fatty acids for heart studies. Nuklearmedizin (supp 19): 1981.
7. Lerch RA, Ambos HD, Bergmann SR, Welch MJ, Ter-Pogossian MM, Sobal BE: Localization of viable, ischemic myocardium by positronemission tomography with C-11-palmitate. Circulation 64: 689–699, 1981.
8. Lerch RA, Bergmann SR, Ambos HD, Welch MJ, Ter-Pogossian MM, Sobel BE: Effect of flow-independent reduction of metabolism on regional myocardial clearance of C-11-palmitate. Circulation 65: 731–738, 1982.
9. Schelbert HR, Phelps ME, Hoffman E, Huang SC, Kuhl DE: Regional myocardial blood flow, metabolism and function assessed noninvasively with positron emission tomography. Am J Cardiol 46: 1269–1277, 1980.
10. Schoen HR, Schelbert HR, Najafi A, Hansen H, Huang H, Barrio J, Phelps ME: C-11 labeled palmitic acid for the noninvasive evaluation of regional myocardial fatty acid metabolism with positron-computed tomography. II. Kinetics of C-11 palmitic acid in acutely ischemic myocardium. Am Heart H 103: 548–561, 1982.
11. Scheuer J, Brachfeld N: Myocardial uptake and fractional distribution of palmitate-1-C-14 by the ischemic dog heart. Metabolism 15: 945–954, 1966.
12. Weiss ES, Hoffman EJ, Phelps ME, Welch MJ, Henry PD, Ter-Pogossian MM, Sobel BE: External detection and visualization of myocardial ischemia with C-11-substrates in vitro and in vivo. Circ Res 39: 24–32, 1976.
13. Weiss ES, Ahmed SA, Welch MJ, Williamson JR, Ter-Pogossian MM, Sobel BE: Quantification of infarction in cross sections of canine myocardium in vivo with positron emission transaxial tomography and C-11-palmitate. Circulation 55: 66–73, 1977.
14. Sobel BE, Weiss ES, Welch MJ, Siegel BA, Ter-Pogossian MM: Detection of remote myocardial infarction in patients with positron emission transaxial tomography and intravenous C-11-palmitate. Circulation 55: 853–857, 1977.
15. Ter-Pogossian MM, Klein MS, Markham J, Roberts R, Sobel BE: Regional assessment of myocardial metabolic integrity in vivo by positron-emission tomography with C-11-labeled palmitate. Circulation 61: 242–255, 1980.
16. Bergmann SR, Lerch RA, Fox KAA, Ludbrook PA, Welch MJ, Ter-Pogossian MM, Sobel BE: Temporal dependence of beneficial effects of coronary thrombolysis characterized by positron tomography. Am J Med 73: 573–581, 1982.
17. Goldstein RA, Klein MS, Welch MJ, Sobel BE: External assessment of myocardial metabolism with C-11 palmitate in vivo. J Nucl Med 21: 342–348, 1980.
18. Schoen HR, Schelbert HR, Robinson G, Najafi A, Huang SC, Hansen H, Barrio J, Kuhl DE, Phelps ME: C-11 labeled palmitic acid for the noninvasive evaluation of regional myocardial fatty

acid metabolism with positron-computed tomography. I. Kinetics of C-11 palmitic acid in normal myocardium. Am Heart J 103:532–547, 1982.

19. Evans JR, Phil D, Gunton RW, Phil D, Baker RG, Beanlands DS, Spears JC: Use of radioiodinated fatty acid for photoscans of the heart. Circ Res 16: 1–10, 1965.

20. Robinson Jr GD, Lee AW: Radioiodinated fatty acids for heart imaging: iodine monochloride addition compared with iodide replacement labeling. J Nucl Med 16: 17–21, 1975.

21. Poe ND, Robinson Jr GD, MacDonald NS: Myocardial extraction of labeled long-chain fatty acid analogs. Proc Soc Exp Biol and Med 148: 215–218, 1975.

22. Otto CA, Brown LE, Wieland DM, Beierwaltes WH: Radioiodinated fatty acids for myocardial imaging: Effects of chain length. J Nucl Med 22: 613–618, 1981.

23. Poe ND, Robinson Jr GD, Zielinski FW, Cabeen Jr WR, Smith JW, Gomes AS: Myocardial imaging with I-123-hexadecenoic acid. Radiology 124: 419–424, 1977.

24. Freundlieb C, Hoeck A, Vyska K, Feinendegen LE, Machulla HJ, Stoecklin G: Myocardial imaging and metabolic studies with [17-I-123]iodoheptadecanoic acid. J Nucl Med 21: 1043–1050, 1980.

25. Wall EE van der, Heidendal GAK, Hollander W den, Westera G, Roos JP: I-123 labeled hexadecenoic acid in comparison with Tl-201 for myocardial imaging in coronary heart disease. A preliminary study. Eur J Nucl Med 5: 401–405, 1980.

26. Wall EE van der, Hollander W den, Heidendal GAK, Westera G, Majid PA, Roos JP: Dynamic myocardial scintigraphy with I-123 labeled free fatty acids in patients with myocardial infarction. Eur J Nucl Med 6: 383–390, 1981a.

27. Aurich D, Reske SN, Biersack HJ, Schmidt H, Simon HJ, Knopp R, Winkler C: Biplanar sequential scintigraphy of the myocardium by means of 123-I-heptadecanoic acid. In: Nuclear Medicine and Biology. C. Raynaud (ed), Pergamon Press) Proc 3rd World Congr Nucl Med Biol Paris II, 1982, 1389–1391.

28. Wall EE van der, Heidendal GAK, Hollander W den, Westera G, Roos JP: Metabolic myocardial imaging with I-123 labeled heptadecanoic acid in patients with angina pectoris. Eur J Nucl Med 6: 391–396, 1981c.

29. Wall EE van der, Westera G, Hollander W den, Visser FC: External detection of regional myocardial metabolism with radioiodinated hexadecenoic acid in the dog heart. Eur J Nucl Med 6: 147–151, 1981b.

30. Huckell VF, Lyster DM, Morrison RT: The potential role of 123 iodine-hexadecenoic acid in assessing normal and abnormal myocardial metabolism. J Nucl Med 21: P57, 1980.

31. Pachinger O, Sochor H, Ogris E, Probst P, Klicpera M, Kaindl F: Salvage of ischemic myocardium by intracoronary streptokinase therapy. In: Non invasive methods in ischemic heart disease. Faivre G, Bertrand A, Cherrier F, Amor M, Neimann JL (eds). Specia, Nancy 1982: 410–414.

32. Visser FC, Westera G, Wall EE van der, Roos JP: Dynamic free fatty acid scintigraphy in patients with successful thrombolysis after acute myocardial infarction. Eur Soc Cardiol; Working group on use of isotopes in Cardiology; Rotterdam: 23, 1983 (abstract).

33. Hoeck A, Freundlieb C, Vyska K, Loesse B, Erbel R, Feinendegen LE: Myocardial imaging and metabolic studies with [17-I-123]iodoheptadecanoic acid in patients with idiopathic congestive cardiomyopathy. J Nucl Med 24: 22–28, 1983.

34. Freundlieb C, Hoeck A, Vyska K, Erbel R, Feinendegen LE: Fatty acid uptake and turnover rate in the ischemic heart before and after bypass surgery. In: Nuclear Medicine and Biology. C Raynaud (ed), Pergamon Press Proc 3rd World Congr Nucl Med Biol Paris II, 1982, 1392–1395.

35. Hoeck A, Freundlieb C, Vyska K, Feinendegen LE, Rost R, Schuerch PM, Hollmann W: The influence of rehabilitation training on fatty acid metabolism in patients with myocardial infarction. In: Non invasive methods in ischemic heart disease. G Faiver, A Bertrand, F Cherrier, M Amor, JL Neimann (eds). Specia, Nancy 1982: 300–303.

36. Wall EE van der, Westera G, Visser FC, Eenige MJ van, Hollander W den, Roos JP: Influence of metoprolol on myocardial uptake of free fatty acids in experimental myocardial ischemia. Curr Ther Res 32: 653–662, 1982.

37. Wall EE van der, Westera G, Hollander W den, Visser FC, Roos JP, Heidendal GAK: The effect of pindolol on myocardial uptake of free fatty acids in the dog. Curr Ther Res 33: 591–600, 1983.
38. Machulla HJ, Marsmann M, Dutschka K: Biochemical concept and synthesis of a radioiodinated phenylfatty acid for in vivo metabolic studies of the myocardium. Eur J Nucl Med 5: 171–173, 1980.
39. Coenen HH, Harmand MF, Kloster G, Stoecklin G: 15-(p-[Br-75]bromophenyl)-pentadecanoic acid: Pharmacokinetics and potential as heart agent. J Nucl Med 22: 891–896, 1981.
40. Reske SN, Machulla HJ, Biersack HJ, Simon H, Knopp R, Winkler C: Metabolic turnover of P-I-123 phenylpentadecanoic acid in the myocardium. In: Nuclear Medicine and Biology. C Raynaud (ed), Pergamon Press, Proc 3rd World Congr Nucl Med Biol Paris III, 1982, 2522–2525.
41. Okada RD, Knapp Jr FF, Elmaleh DR, Yasuda T, Boucher CA, Strauss HW: Tellurium-123m-labeled-9-telluraheptadecanoic acid: A possible cardiac imaging agent. Circulation 65: 305–310, 1982.
42. Elmaleh DR, Knapp Jr FF, Yasuda T, Coffey JL, Kopiwoda S, Okada R, Strauss HW: Myocardial imaging with 9-[Te-123m]telluraheptadecanoic acid. J Nucl Med 22: 994–999, 1981.
43. Livni E, Elmaleh DR, Levy S, Brownell GL, Strauss WH: Beta-methyl[1-C-11]heptadecanoic acid: A new myocardial metabolic tracer for positron emission tomography. J Nucl Med 23: 169–175, 1982.
44. Goldstein RA, Klein MS, Sobel BE: Detection of myocardial ischemia before infarction, based on accumulation of labeled pyruvate. J Nucl Med 21: 1101–1104, 1980.
45. Schelbert HR, Henze E, Keen R, Huang H, Barrio J, Phelps M: Regional fatty acid metabolism in acute myocardial ischemia demonstrated noninvasively by C-11 palmitate (CPA) and positron tomography (PET). Circulation 66 (supp II): 126, 1982 (abstract).
46. Comet M, Wolf JE, Pilichowski P, Mathieu JP, Dubois F, Riche F, Busquet G, Vidal M, Godart J, Pernin C, Gaudy M: Influence du propranolol sur l'activité myocardique après injection i.v. d'acide 16 I(123) hexadecene 9 oique. In: Non invasive methods in ischemic heart disease, G Faivre, A Bertrand, F Cherrier, M Amor, JL Neimann. (eds), Specia, Nancy 1982: 295–299.
47. Vyska K, Hoeck A, Freundlieb C, Profant M, Feinendegen LE, Machulla HJ, Stoecklin G: Myocardial imaging and measurement of myocardial fatty acid metabolism using omega-I-123-heptadecanoic acid. J Nucl Med 20: 650, 1979 (abstract).
48. Dudczak R, Schmoliner R, Angelberger P, Kletter K, Frischauf H: Myocardial studies with I-123 p-phenylpentadecanoic acid (PPA) in patients with coronary artery disease (CAD) and cardiomyopathy (CMP). J Nucl Med 23: P35, 1982.
49. Wall EE van der: Preliminary findings. 1983.
50. Westera G, Wall EE van der, Heidendal GAK, Bos GC van den: A comparison between terminally radioiodinated hexadecenoic acid (I-HA) and Tl-201-thallium chloride in the dog heart. Implications for the use of I-HA for myocardial imaging. Eur J Nucl Med 5: 339–343, 1980.

6. Quantitative analysis of the distribution and washout of thallium-201 in the myocardium: description of the method and its clinical applications

Jamshid Maddahi, Ernest V. Garcia and Daniel S. Berman

Introduction

Exercise thallium-201 (Tl-201) myocardial perfusion scintigraphy is a useful noninvasive method for detecting and evaluating patients with significant coronary artery disease (CAD). Visual interpretation of analogue Tl-201 images for evaluation of regional myocardial perfusion, even when performed by experienced readers, is subject to substantial observer variability [1]. This approach is further limited by dependence on the quality of the hard copy output and the inability to accurately compensate for background activity. Furthermore, although the visual method is highly specific for localization of CAD, it has major limitations in sensitivity for detection of individual coronary stenoses [2, 3], especially in patients with multiple vessel CAD [2–6] and when the degree of coronary stenosis is not severe [2, 3]. Finally, although the regional washout characteristics of the myocardium for Tl-201 contain important diagnostic information, washout abnormalities are difficult to detect by visual inspection.

Recently, several approaches have provided significant contributions to the quantitation of initial myocardial distribution [7–13] and washout of Tl-201 [10–13]. The purpose of this report is to discuss the steps involved in quantitation of stress-redistribution Tl-201 scintigrams and to compare the quantitative and visual interpretation method in their applications to the evaluation of patients with coronary artery disease.

The value of regional myocardial Tl-201 washout rate analysis

Interpretation of stress-redistribution Tl-201 myocardial scintigrams using analysis of perfusion defects fails to identify all hypoperfused myocardial segments resulting in frequent underestimation of the extent of disease in patients with multivessel coronary involvement [2–6, 14]. This limitation has been thought to be in part related to the fact that initial Tl-201 distribution reflects relative rather than absolute reduction in myocardial blood flow. Thus, areas with less hypoperfusion may appear relatively normal compared with the most severely hypoperfused segments. It is also likely that in an occasional patient with extensive coronary artery disease and rather uniform reduction in myocardial perfusion during stress, no perfusion defect will be apparent on the initial myocardial Tl-201 images.

Detection of relatively mildly ischemic regions may be possible by several approaches. Application of appropriate background subtraction or image processing and display [15] to planar Tl-201 images may enhance the differences between the normal and mildly hypoperfused areas, and result in the detection of the latter. Use of tomographic Tl-201 imaging may help detect small areas of hypoperfusion that are obscured by super-position of normal regions. Furthermore, a spatially nonrelative indicator of segmental myocardial hypoperfusion may demonstrate abnormality in a hypoperfused myocardial region that is otherwise undetected by spatially relative perfusion defect analysis. Recent investigations regarding the myocardial kinetics of Tl-201 suggest that not only initial uptake of Tl-201 is reduced in a hypoperfused myocardial region, but also subsequent washout rate of Tl-201 slower [16, 17]. Regional myocardial washout rate can be analyzed without interregional comparisons (i.e., in a spatially nonrelative fashion). This is accomplished by quantitating the percent regional loss of thallium from the immediate postinjection to four hour redistribution time and by comparing the calculated value to a previously established normal reference value [10]. Slower than normal regional washout rate will then identify regions with less than normal perfusion.

Figure 1 demonstrates the above hypothesis in a diagrammatic fashion. In the example of single-region ischemia, the hypoperfused segment (B) compared to the normally perfused area (A) demonstrates both lower relative initial uptake of Tl-201 and slower 4 hour % washout for Tl-201. In the example of double-region (imbalanced) ischemia, although regional blood flow is reduced to both segments (C) and (D), segment (C) is less hypoperfused and therefore is considered to be normal (without perfusion defect) relative to segment (D). Segment (C), however, demonstrates slower than normal washout rate for Tl-201 indicative of regional hypoperfusion.

Figure 2 diagrammatically demonstrates an example of double region balanced ischemia. In this example, neither of the hypoperfused regions show perfusion defect at the time of stress. Both regions, however, show slower than normal Tl-201 washout rate.

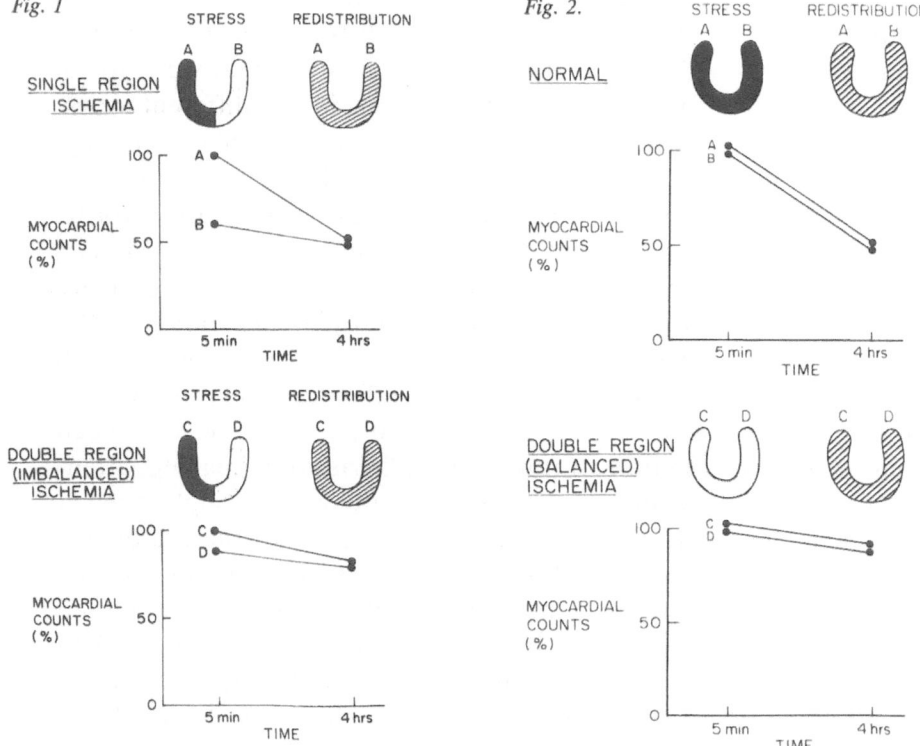

Figure 1. Diagrammatic representation of initial distribution and subsequent washout rate of myocardial Tl-201 in an example of single region ischemia and double region (imbalanced) ischemia. In the latter conditions, the less hypoperfused myocardial region (C) does not show an initial perfusion defect, but demonstrates a slower than normal washout rate for Tl-201.

Figure 2. Diagrammatic example of single region ischemia and double region balanced ischemia. Balanced ischemia is detected by slower than normal washout rate for Tl-201 rather than perfusion defects.

Description of the method

Exercise & imaging protocols

Patients are exercised using a multistage treadmill test according to the Bruce protocol or multi-stage bicycle test. Exercise is terminated only with exhaustion, development of severe angina, serious arrhythmia, or hypotension. A dose of 1.5–2 mCi of Tl-201 is injected at peak exercise, and exercise is continued for 45 to 90 seconds after injection. After termination of exercise, multiple-view myocardial scintigrams are obtained at approximately six minutes and three to five hours after injection of Tl-201. At each interval, imaging is performed in the anterior, 45-degree, and 75 to 85-degree left anterior oblique (LAO) views for 10 minutes per view. It has been shown that imaging in five different views, even when combined with gated acquisition, does not increase the diagnostic information obtained by the standard three view nongated imaging [12]. During the acquisition of the anterior view, the shape of the myocardium is evaluated. If significant heart rotation is noted, the view is repeated by changing the angulation of the camera. Subsequent images are compensated accordingly for heart rotation by the technologist. Patients are routinely instructed to discontinue propranolol for 24 to 48 hours and avoid nitrates, food and drinks for three hours before exercise testing, and to limit their activity and have only a small meal between imaging periods. At the time of four hour redistribution imaging, attention should be paid to identical reproduction of the viewing angles used at the earlier imaging period. This can be facilitated with the aid of two external markers (9.5 μCi Co-57 point sources), which are taped to the patient's chest during the early imaging [12]. The positions are marked with a felt pen, so that the same positions can be used at the time of late imaging. For imaging, a standard-field-of-view camera is used, equipped with 37 photomultiplier tubes, 1/4"-thick sodium iodide crystal, and a high-resolution, parallel-hole collimator. A 25% energy window centered on the 80 keV photopeak and a 15% window centered on the 167 keV photopeak are used. If the positioning point source is used, a third energy spectrum is set up for Cobalt-57. All images are stored by the computer on magnetic disc in a 64×64 or $128 \times 128 \times 8$ bit matrix.

Computer processing

The image processing steps vary from one method to another, however, the following principles apply to most of the available techniques:

a. Background subtraction.
Each image is compensated for tissue crosstalk by performing bilinear interpolative background subtraction as described by Goris *et al.* [18]. For this purpose, a rectangular boundary enclosing the heart is positioned by the computer operator approximately four pixels away from the myocardium (Figure 3). The background subtraction method may be modified by use of the proximity waiting function described by Watson *et al.* [19]. The effect of this modification is to produce more rapid falloff of the computed

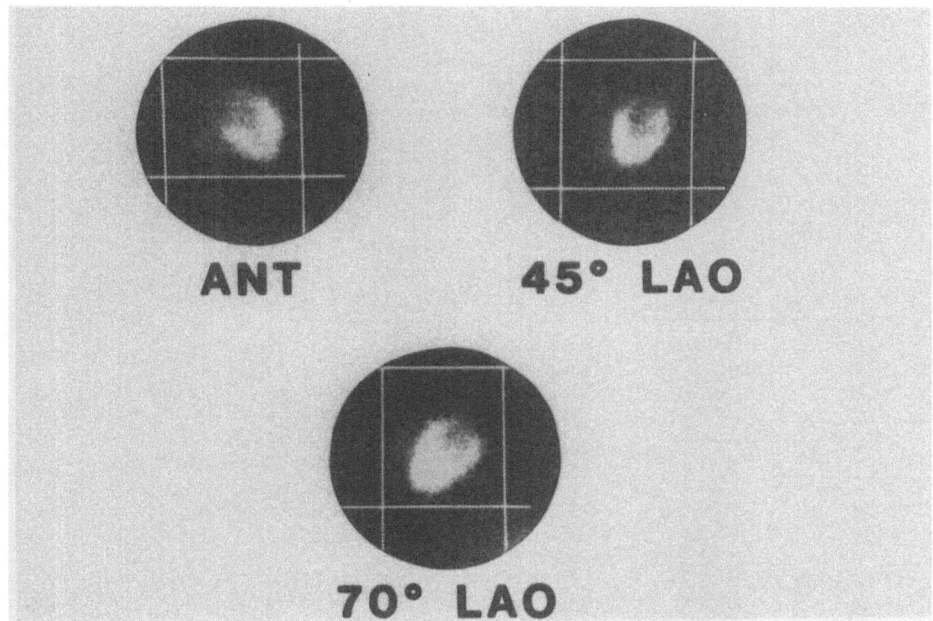

Figure 3. Placement of rectangular boundary relative to the heart used for performing bilinear interpolative background subtraction in the anterior (ANT), 45 degree and 70 degree LAO positions.

tissue crosstalk, this being particularly important where the rectangle surrounding the myocardium crosses areas of high uptake, such as the liver.

b. *Smoothing*
After background subtraction, the images are smoothed using a standard algorithm for nine-point weighted averaging [10]. Unweighted five-point smoothing has also been used [13].

c. *Generation of circumferential profiles*
From the smoothed images, circumferential maximum count profiles of the myocardial distribution of Tl-201 are obtained [9, 10, 13] (Figure 4). Each point in these profiles represents the maximum count per pixel along a radius traversing the myocardium. The profile is constructed by the computer from the values of 60 radii spaced at six-degree intervals plotted clockwise. These profiles quantitate the segmental activity as an angular function referenced from the center of the left ventricular cavity which is located visually or objectively. The latter may be accomplished by automated determination of its geometric center [13]. The operator also as-

ALGORITHM

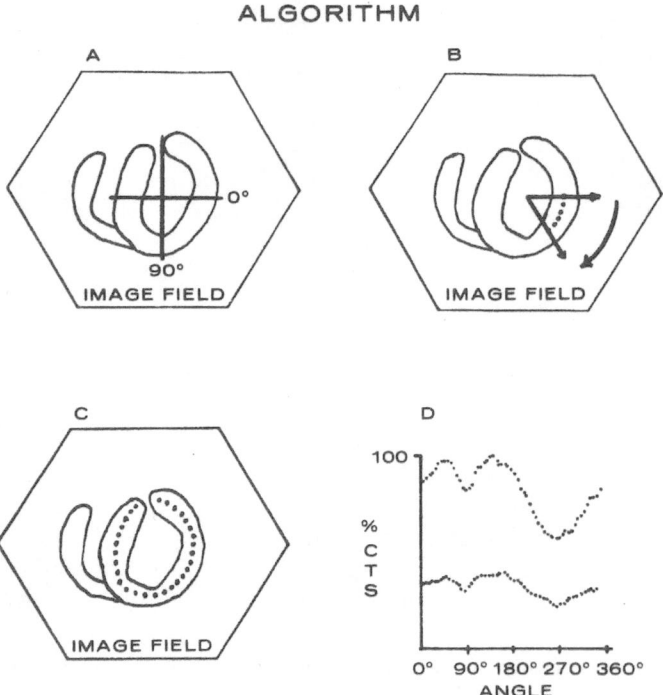

Figure 4. Diagrammatic representation of method for obtaining circumferential profiles of the myocardium. Coordinate reference axis is shown in (A). Image pixels for circumferential profile analysis are found by performing a radial search for maximum value at 6 degree intervals (B) throughout 360 degrees. Maximal values shown as black dots in (B) and (C) are then plotted in (D) for each angle as a percentage of the maximum value for the circumferential profile. Top curve in (D) represents circumferential profile from stress thallium-201 image; below, that from the four hour delayed image.

signs the maximum radius to which the computer will search. This is done to prevent the algorithm from searching outside the left ventricular myocardium into other structures, such as the right ventricle.

d. Profile alignment

These circumferential profiles are then aligned by visually identifying the location of the scintigraphic apex on the stress and redistribution profiles. The computer then automatically shifts that point in the circumferential profile to coincide with 90 degrees. These profiles are subsequently plotted for each view at each time interval. The curves are normalized to the maximum pixel value found in any of the profiles.

e. Generation of washout rate profiles

In addition to the distribution (stress and 4 hour) profiles, washout rate circumferential profiles are calculated as percent washout from stress to the approximately four-hour redistribution time. Figure 5 demonstrates the manner in which each point on washout rate profile is calculated. As shown, despite regional count variation at the time of stress and four-hour redistribution, percent regional washout rate of Tl-201 is fairly uniform from all myocardial regions.

Establishment of normal limits

Thirty-one normal patients undergoing stress-redistribution scintigraphy were used for establishment of normal limits [10]. The mean value and standard deviations were established from the pooled data of these patients for each of the 60 angular locations of the anterior, 45-degree LAO and steep (70–85-degree) LAO images for each time interval. The time between the stress and redistribution imaging, if other than four hours, was used to extrapolate the washout rate profiles to exactly four hours [10]. The lower limit of normal for the stress profile was established as the profile that was two standard deviations below the mean observed stress profile. The normal limits for washout rate at four hours was determined in an identical manner. Use of two standard deviations with one-tailed analysis established statistical criteria that included 97.5% of the normal population.

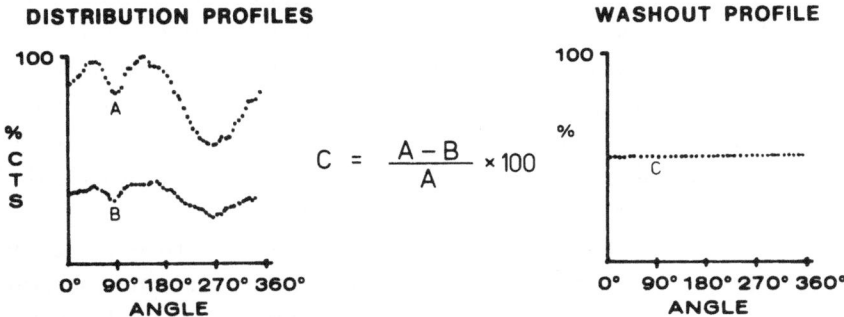

Figure 5. Generation of the washout rate circumferential profile (right) from initial and four hour redistribution circumferential profiles (left top and left bottom respectively). Note that despite interregional variations in thallium counts, Tl-201 washout rate is fairly uniform throughout the myocardium.

Development of quantitative criteria for abnormality

In a prospective group of 31 normal patients and 20 patients with angiographically documented coronary artery disease, stress and washout rate circumferential profiles were compared to the normal limits described above [10]. The computer was programmed to identify any arc of the profile that was outside the normal limits. Different quantitative criteria for type and magnitude of abnormality were assessed in all 51 patients for their ability to best discriminate normal subjects from patients with coronary artery disease. The following criteria best separated the two populations:

1. A "stress defect" was defined by any 18-degree segment (three contiguous radii) of the stress profile falling below the normal limit;

2. "Slow washout" was defined by any 18-degree segment (three contiguous radii) of the washout profile falling below the normal limit; and

3. To be considered abnormal, the patient needed at least two abnormal 18-degree arcs in the combined stress and washout rate profiles in three views.

Using the above criteria, quantitative analysis of Tl-201 images was normal in all 31 normal patients and was abnormal in 19 of the 20 CAD patients.

Computerized display of the results

Figure 6 demonstrates an example of the computerized display of the quantitative results which has recently been developed by Van Train *et al.* [21]. The stress and washout rate circumferential profiles in this patient with coronary disease were compared to the established normal limits. Using the above criteria, myocardial regions with stress perfusion defect or slow washout abnormality were identified. Findings were then displayed on concentric ellipses in the anterior, 45-degree LAO, and steep LAO views. In each view, the inner ellipse is the diagrammatic representation of the myocardium in that view, the border of different myocardial regions being shown as small break points on this ellipse. The missing portions of the middle ellipse demonstrate presence of stress perfusion defect. In this patient, stress defects are present in the anterolateral, apical and distal inferior region in the anterior view. Additionally, stress defects are present in the septal and inferoapical left ventricular regions in the 45 degree LAO view, and the anteroseptal, apical, and distal inferior walls in the steep LAO view. The missing portions of the outer ellipse

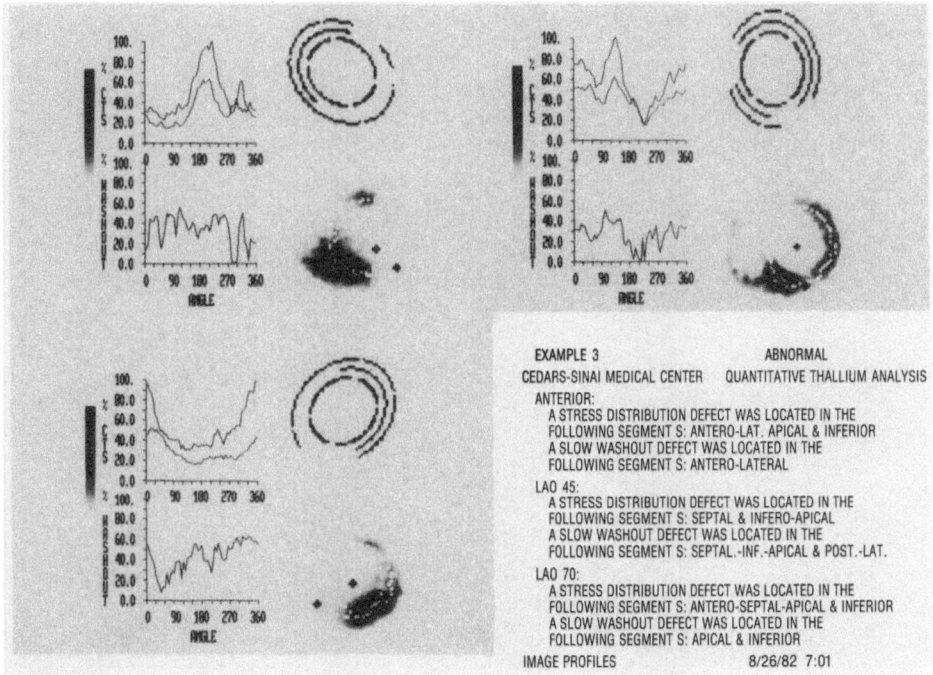

EXAMPLE 3   ABNORMAL
CEDARS-SINAI MEDICAL CENTER   QUANTITATIVE THALLIUM ANALYSIS
ANTERIOR:
     A STRESS DISTRIBUTION DEFECT WAS LOCATED IN THE
     FOLLOWING SEGMENT S: ANTERO-LAT. APICAL & INFERIOR
     A SLOW WASHOUT DEFECT WAS LOCATED IN THE
     FOLLOWING SEGMENT S: ANTERO-LATERAL

LAO 45:
     A STRESS DISTRIBUTION DEFECT WAS LOCATED IN THE
     FOLLOWING SEGMENT S: SEPTAL & INFERO-APICAL
     A SLOW WASHOUT DEFECT WAS LOCATED IN THE
     FOLLOWING SEGMENT S: SEPTAL.-INF.-APICAL & POST.-LAT.

LAO 70:
     A STRESS DISTRIBUTION DEFECT WAS LOCATED IN THE
     FOLLOWING SEGMENT S: ANTERO-SEPTAL-APICAL & INFERIOR
     A SLOW WASHOUT DEFECT WAS LOCATED IN THE
     FOLLOWING SEGMENT S: APICAL & INFERIOR

IMAGE PROFILES   8/26/82 7:01

Figure 6. Computerized display of the quantitative stress-redistribution Tl-201 interpretation in patient with coronary artery disease. Multiple regions with perfusion defects and slower than normal washout rate are identified.

indicate presence of slow washout abnormality. In this example, (Figure 6), slow washout abnormality is also present in the anterolateral, septal, inferoapical, distal posterolateral, apical, and distal inferior walls of the left ventricle. This concentric ellipse display system not only facilitates interpretation of a given case as normal or abnormal but also aids in assignment of abnormalities to specific myocardial regions. Figure 7 shows an example of computerized display of quantitative stress-re-distribution Tl-201 interpretation in a normal patient. Lack of any breaks in the middle and outer ellipses indicate absence of either perfusion defect or slow washout abnormality. Another method for display of quantitative results has been described by Reiber *et al.* [13]. With this method, the localization, extent and type of abnormalities are presented in different grey levels in a functional image (Figure 8). To this end, for each radial line it is determined whether the stress, redistribution and washout profile values are normal or abnormal. These outcomes are then compared with

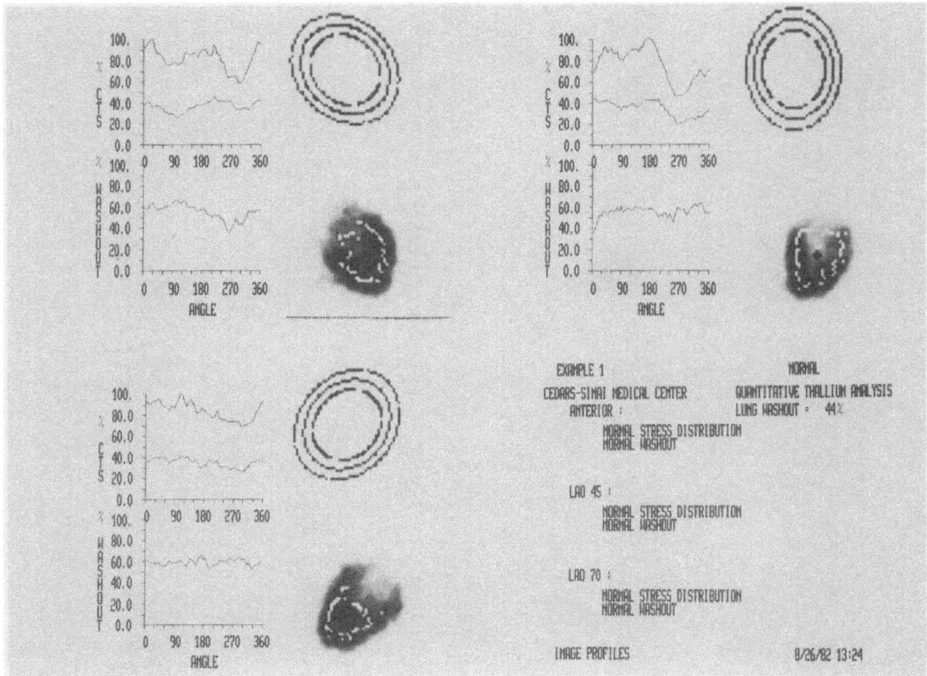

Figure 7. Computerized display of the quantitative stress-redistribution Tl-201 interpretation results in a normal patient.

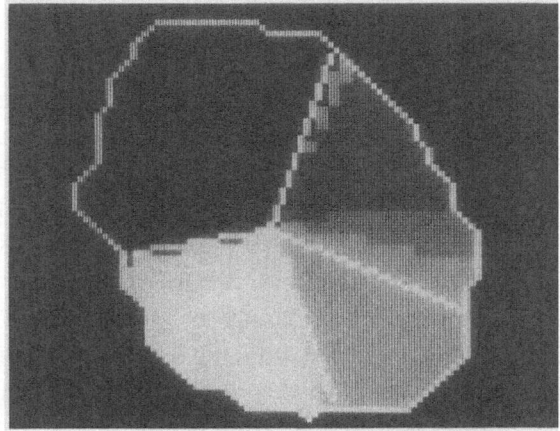

Figure 8. Functional image of quantitative analysis showing location, extent and type of abnormalities. (Used with permission of Reiber, JHC, *et al.* [13]).

the entries of a decision table to define the type of abnormality for that particular radial line [13].

Interobserver agreement of computerized quantitative Tl-201 analysis

In 14 patients used for assessment of reproducibility of computer analysis [10], each of the three views was divided into three segments, for a total of nine segments per patient. Each segment was analyzed by computer as to whether it was normal or abnormal. Concordant results were obtained by two independent observers in 115 of 126 segments (93% agreement). No patient was erroneously called normal or abnormal due to this variation. The main cause of discrepancy was variation in aligning the apex at 90 degrees in patients with large apical defects, which explained eight of the nine discordant results.

Clinical applications

Overall detection of coronary artery disease

We compared the quantitative method to consensus visual interpretation of analog Tl-201 images in a group of 67 patients undergoing stress-redistribution Tl-201 scintigraphy [20]. Forty-one of 45 patients with angiographically documented coronary artery disease were considered abnormal by visual assessment and 42 of 45 by the quantitative technique. Thus, the sensitivity of the visual and quantitative techniques were 91% and 93%. These were not significantly different from one another. Of the 22 normal subjects, 20 had normal circumferential profiles, yielding a 91% specificity for the quantitative method. Three of these 22 normal subjects were considered abnormal by visual assessment, yielding a specificity of 86%, which was not statistically different from that of the quantitative technique. The quantitative method therefore had a similar sensitivity and specificity for overall detection of coronary artery disease when compared with visual interpretation. Quantitative analysis, however, offered the advantage of objectivity over visual analysis in this specific application.

Detection of disease in individual coronary arteries

For detection of disease in individual coronary arteries, abnormality in each myocardial region was assigned to a specific coronary artery; three

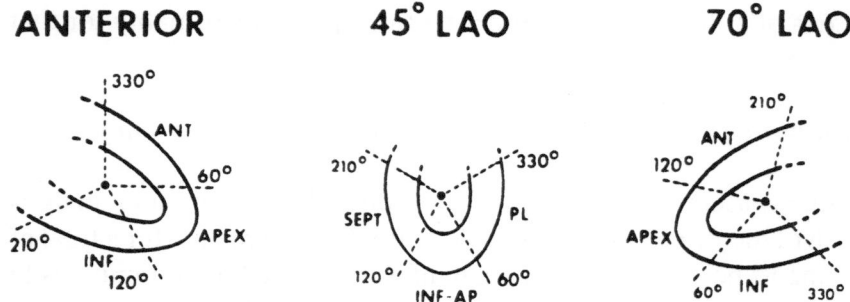

Figure 9. Myocardial regions assessed visually (A) and quantitatively (B) in each view. In quantitative analysis, the arc from 210–330 degrees in each view was considered to represent the outflow track and was not evaluated. See text for assignment of the different myocardial regions to specific coronary arteries. ANT = anterior; INF = inferior; SEPT = septum; INF-AP = inferoapical; PL = posterolateral.

regions in each view were individually assessed visually and quantitatively (Figure 9). In quantitative analysis, the profile in each view which corresponded to the arc from 210–330 degrees was considered to represent the outflow track. The arc from 60–120 degrees was designated as representing the apex in the anterior and 70 degree LAO views and to represent the inferoapical area in the 45 degree LAO view. For localization of anatomic disease, the anterior wall (anterior and 70 degree LAO views) and the intraventricular septum (45 degree LAO view) were considered to represent the distribution of left anterior descending coronary artery, the inferior wall (anterior and 70 degree LAO view), the distribution of the right coronary artery and the posterolateral wall (45 degree LAO view), left circumflex distribution [20]. An apical or inferoapical abnormality alone was interpreted as indicating coronary artery disease but was not used to localize disease to a specific coronary artery.

The sensitivity of visual and quantitative Tl-201 interpretation for detection of disease in each of the three major coronary arteries is shown in Figure 10. The sensitivity of the visual method for detection of individual coronary stenoses was low, 56%, 34%, and 65% for the LAD, LCX, and RCA respectively. Thus, of 110 diseased vessels, only 57 were detected by the visual method (52% sensitivity). The quantitative technique, however, had significantly higher sensitivity for detection of disease in individual coronary arteries (80% for LAD, 63% for LCX, and 94% for RCA). The overall sensitivity for detection of disease in any vessel was 79%.

The specificity of the visual and quantitative technique for identification of absence of disease in individual coronary arteries is shown in Figure 11.

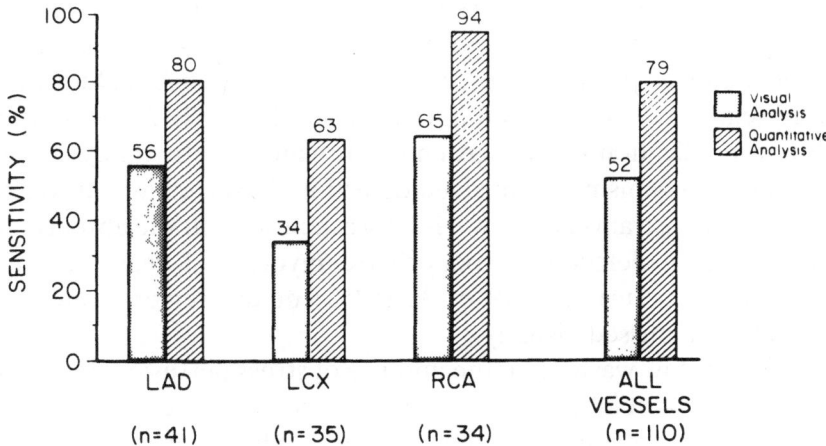

Figure 10. Comparative sensitivities of the visual and quantitative techniques for detection of disease in individual coronary arteries.

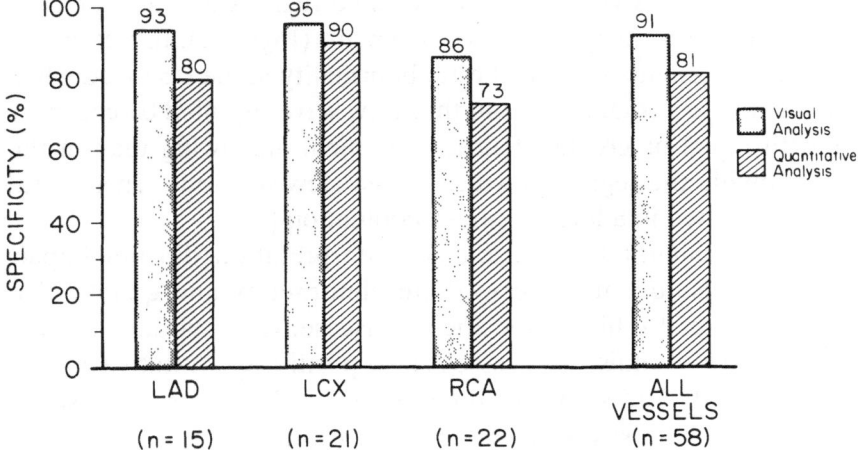

Figure 11. Comparative specificity of the visual and quantitative techniques for identification of absence of disease in individual coronary arteries.

The specificity of the visual and the quantitative techniques was 92% and 85% for the LAD, 97% and 94% for the LCX, 91% and 82% for the RCA, and 93% and 87% for any normal vessel. None of the specificity values were significantly different between the two methods of analysis.

The improvement by the quantitative analysis in sensitivity for detection of individual coronary stenoses was due to correct detection of an additional 35 hypoperfused regions that were missed visually. None of these 35 regions had prior infarction. Sixteen of 35 (46%) of these diseased segments showed perfusion defect by quantitative analysis. Detection of these 16 segments with reduced initial distribution of Tl-201 was most likely due to application of background subtraction to the images. The most frequent mechanism of improved detection, however, was through quantitative demonstration of slow Tl-201 washout rate in the absence of apparent perfusion defect in hypoperfused myocardial regions. This mechanism alone occurred in 19 of 35 (54%) of the regions detected quantitatively and missed visually.

The finding of slow washout in the absence of stress perfusion defect in hypoperfused myocardial segments may superficially appear contradictory to animal experiments which have shown that hypoperfused regions demonstrate both reduced initial uptake as well as slow Tl-201 washout rate. However, these experiments and findings were obtained in a model with single region ischemia in which uptake and washout of Tl-201 were compared with those of absolutely normal segments. Stress-redistribution scintigrams in patients with multiple ischemic regions may not demonstrate stress defects in all hypoperfused segments (Figure 1). In fact, in our study, 16 of 19 segments with washout abnormality alone occurred when the remaining myocardial regions in that view were supplied by coronary arteries with equal or greater degree of luminal narrowing than in the arteries supplying the segments with isolated slow washout. These findings were confirmed in a larger patient population [22].

Use of these quantitative criteria for interpretation did not impair specificity, because quantitative washout abnormality and quantitative stress defects were also highly specific for disease. Of 85 visually normal regions supplied by nondiseased vessels, false positive quantitative finding was present in only 7 (2 showed slow washout, 2 showed isolated stress defect, and 3 had both stress defect and slow washout).

Detection of moderate coronary artery narrowing

Figure 12 shows the sensitivity of the visual and the quantitative Tl-201 analyses in relation to severity of coronary stenosis. Seventy vessels demonstrated greater than 75% luminal diameter narrowing on coronary arteriography. Of these, 43 (61%) were detected visually and 59 (84%) quantitatively. An even greater difference between the two techniques was observed when the sensitivity for detection of 50–75% coronary narrowing (moderate coronary stenosis) was examined. Only 14 of 40

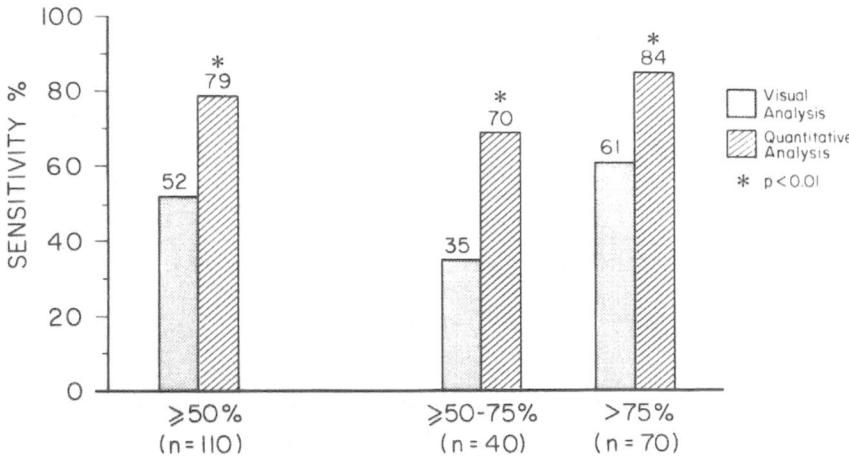

Figure 12. Sensitivity of the visual and the quantitative Tl-201 analyses in relation to severity of coronary stenosis.

(35%) coronary arteries with 50–75% narrowing were detected visually, compared with 28 of 40 (70%) by the quantitative method.

Correct identification of patients with triple vessel and/or left main coronary disease

We compared the value of quantitative analysis of perfusion defect and washout rate of myocardial Tl-201 to that of visual thallium interpretation, stress electrocardiography, and exertional hypotension for correct identification of patients with left main and/or triple vessel coronary artery disease [23]. One hundred and eight consecutive patients were studied who underwent coronary arteriography, exercise electrocardiography, and stress redistribution Tl-201 myocardial scintigraphy. Sixty-one patients demonstrated triple vessel and/or left main disease and were designated as angiographic high risk group (Group I). The remaining 47 patients had less extensive coronary disease and were considered as angiographic non-high risk patients (Group II). The Group II patients included 15 patients with normal coronary arteries, 16 with single vessel, and 16 with double vessel disease.

Table 1 demonstrates the sensitivity and specificity of different testing modalities alone or in combination for correct identification of high risk angiographic patients. Exercise electrocardiogram was considered positive for high risk angiographic disease if greater than or equal to 2 mm ST

Table 1. ·Sensitivity and specificity of different noninvasive testing modalities for correct identification of patients with high risk angiographic (triple vessel and/or left main) disease

	EX-Hypo-tension	EX-ECG	VTL	QTL	EX-ECG +VTL	EX-ECG +QTL
Sensitivity	20%	36%	16%	64%*	48%*	79%*
Specificity	98%	96%	94%	89%	89%	85%

EX = exercise, ECG = electrocardiography, VTL = visual Tl-201 analysis, and QTL = quantitative Tl-201 analysis.
* = p<.01 versus Ex-hypotension, EX-ECG, VTL, and EX-ECG + VTL.

segment depression developed with onset of 1 mm depression within the first six minutes of exercise. Scintigraphic evidence for angiographic high risk disease was considered to be present if images were abnormal in either combined anterior, septal, and posterolateral left ventricular myocardial regions or in the regions representing distribution of all three major coronary arteries. Using individual testing modalities, of 61 patients with high risk disease, 12 had exertional hypotension and 22 demonstrated high risk pattern stress electrocardiograms leading to sensitivities of 20% and 36% respectively. With Tl-201 scintigraphy, visual interpretation correctly identified 10 and quantitative analysis 40 of these 61 patients resulting in sensitivity values of 16% and 64% respectively. The sensitivity of the quantitative method was significantly (p<.01) higher than other tests individually. Absence of high risk angiographic pattern was correctly identified (specificity) in 46/47 (98%) by stress blood pressure response, in 45/47 (96%) by stress ECG, in 44/47 (94%) by visual Tl-201 analysis, and in 42/47 (89%) by quantitative Tl-201 interpretation. These specificities were not significantly different from one another.

Using combination testing approach, a high risk pattern stress electrocardiogram and/or visually interpreted Tl-201 scintigram was present in 29 of 62 Group I patients (sensitivity 48%), and 5 of 47 in Group II patients (specificity 89%). A high risk pattern of stress electrocardiogram and/or quantitatively interpreted Tl-201 scintigram was present in 48 of 61 Group I patients (sensitivity 79%) and 7 of 47 Group II patients (specificity 85%). This combination offered the highest overall accuracy for identification of high risk disease patients than the other combination or other individual testing modalities.

In order to investigate what feature of quantitative Tl-201 analysis helped diagnosis of additional high risk patients, the contribution of different quantitative criteria to the detection of additional ischemic myocardial regions were analyzed in 28 angiographic high risk patients who were identified as high risk by the quantitative method but were designated non-high risk by visual analysis. Additional analysis of washout rate of Tl-201 led to correct identification of 18/28 (64%) of misclassified high risk disease patients.

Detection of unsuspected high risk CAD patients by diffuse slow washout of myocardium Tl-201

When coronary artery disease is uniformly severe and extensive, regional myocardial hypoperfusion may be balanced during stress precluding development of spatially relative perfusion defects. Extensive coronary disease may then be shown only by a diffuse slow washout pattern (DSWP) of thallium from all the myocardial regions (Figure 2). In 1265 consecutive patients [24] having undergone quantitatively analyzed stress-redistribution Tl-201 scintigraphy, 62 patients were identified who had no or a maximum of one perfusion defect and thus not suspected of having extensive coronary disease by perfusion defect analysis. All of these patients have undergone clinically indicated coronary arteriography. Of these 62 patients, 32 had associated DSWP (Group A) who were compared to the remaining 30 who did not have DSWP (Group B). The prevalence of triple vessel and left main disease was 72% (23/32) in Group A and only 17% (5/30) in Group B. An independent relationship between DSWP and extensive coronary disease was demonstrated by a Mantel-Ahaentzel chi-square analysis of a wide variety of other indices of extensive disease. The positive and negative predictive value of DSWP for high-risk angiographic disease was 72% and 83% respectively. This high predictive accuracy was demonstrated even in the absence of other scintigraphic, clinical, or electrocardiographic indicators of high-risk angiographic disease. The predictive value was as strong in patients who exercised submaximally. Discrimination between Groups A and B was not possible by age, sex, symptoms, exercise duration, exertional hypotension, or marked exercise ST depression.

Figure 13 demonstrates stress-redistribution scintigrams of a patient referred to our stress test laboratories because of a nonanginal chest pain. No perfusion defects are present. Because he exercised for 13 minutes and to 92% of predicted maximal heart rate, developed no chest pain, no exertional hypotension, and had an equivocal stress electrocardiogram (1 mm upsloping ST segment depression at peak exercise), combined test results predicted a low likelihood for significant coronary disease. Quan-

120

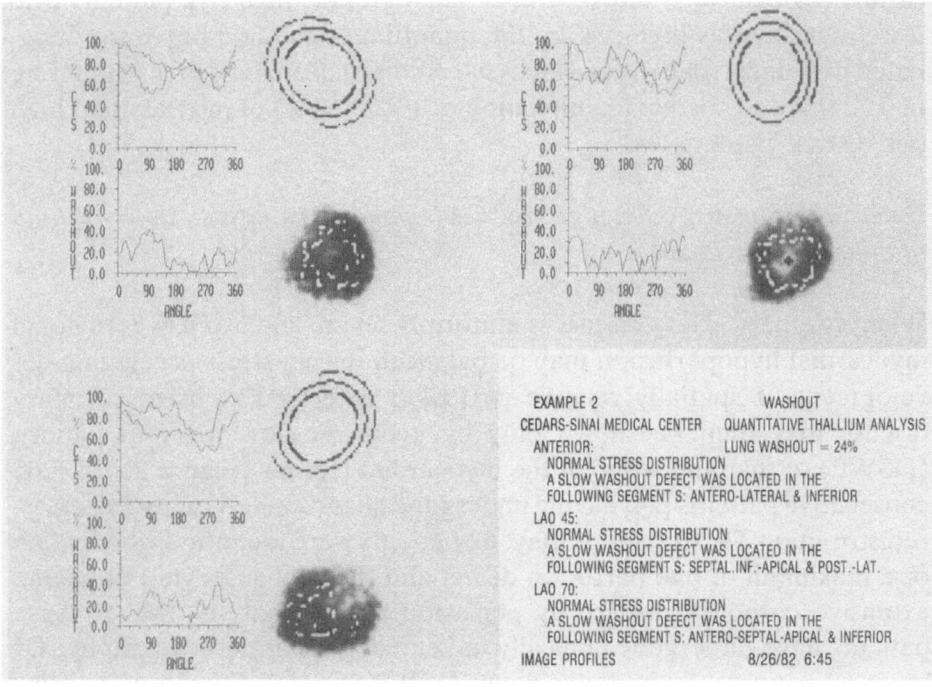

EXAMPLE 2   WASHOUT
CEDARS-SINAI MEDICAL CENTER   QUANTITATIVE THALLIUM ANALYSIS
ANTERIOR: LUNG WASHOUT = 24%
   NORMAL STRESS DISTRIBUTION
   A SLOW WASHOUT DEFECT WAS LOCATED IN THE
   FOLLOWING SEGMENT S: ANTERO-LATERAL & INFERIOR
LAO 45:
   NORMAL STRESS DISTRIBUTION
   A SLOW WASHOUT DEFECT WAS LOCATED IN THE
   FOLLOWING SEGMENT S: SEPTAL.INF.-APICAL & POST.-LAT.
LAO 70:
   NORMAL STRESS DISTRIBUTION
   A SLOW WASHOUT DEFECT WAS LOCATED IN THE
   FOLLOWING SEGMENT S: ANTERO-SEPTAL-APICAL & INFERIOR
IMAGE PROFILES   8/26/82 6:45

Figure 13. Diffuse myocardial slow washout pattern in the absence of perfusion defect in a patient with triple vessel coronary artery disease.

titative scintigraphic analysis, however, while confirming the visual impression of no perfusion defects, revealed washout abnormalities of the anterior, inferior, and posterolateral walls suggesting presence of extensive coronary disease. Angiography, done on the specific request of the patient, confirmed the presence of triple vessel coronary artery disease as predicted by diffuse slow washout pattern of myocardial Tl-201.

Possible mechanisms for slow myocardial Tl-201 washout rate in the absence of coronary disease

(1) Low exercise heart rate
Following intravenous injection of Tl-201, the initial myocardial uptake and subsequent washout is directly related to coronary blood flow; i.e., myocardial regions with higher coronary blood flow demonstrate a higher initial uptake and a faster subsequent washout rate for Tl-201 compared to regions with lower coronary blood flow. During exercise, increase in myocardial blood flow is related to exercise heart rate. It is conceivable,

therefore, that in the absence of coronary disease, intravenous injection of Tl-201 at a very low exercise heart rate may result in slower myocardial washout rate of Tl-201 compared to that expected when the tracer is injected at higher exercise heart rates. Massie *et al.* have shown that in normal patients myocardial washout of Tl-201 is slower when the tracer is injected during submaximal exercise compared to maximum exercise [25]. Myocardial washout rate for Tl-201 is even slower when the tracer is injected at rest [26]. These observations have led to the concern that in a patient who undergoes stress-redistribution Tl-201 scintigraphy and achieves a submaximal heart rate, slower than normal myocardial wash-out rate for Tl-201 may occur in myocardial regions subtended by normal coronary arteries resulting in lower specificity of washout rate analysis for detection of regional disease. We undertook a study [27] to determine the effect of exercise heart rate on the sensitivity and specificity of quantitative Tl-201 analysis in 226 consecutive patients with stress-redistribution Tl-201 scintigraphy and coronary arteriography. There were a total of 438 diseased and 240 normal vessels in these 226 patients. Patients were divided into three groups according to percent maximal predicted heart rate achieved; 59 patients in Group A achieved <75% predicted maximum heart rate, 56 patients in Group B achieved 75–84% predicted maximum heart rate, and 111 patients in Group C achieved ≥85% predicted maximum heart rate. Table 2 demonstrates the sensitivity and specificity of the quantitative analysis of perfusion defect alone or in combination with washout rate analysis in the three groups. Sensitivity and specificity of perfusion defect analysis alone was not affected by the achieved exercise heart rate. The addition of washout rate analysis significantly increased the sensitivities of segmental disease detection over perfusion defect analysis alone in all three groups. The specificities, however, were not significantly decreased except in Group A where a

Table 2. Comparative sensitivity and specificity of quantitative Tl-201 analysis in patients achieving different maximum heart rates

	PD + SW			PD only		
Group	A	B	C	A	B	C
Sensitivity	.74*	.86*	.69*	.57	.64	.58
Specificity	.44*	.60	.68	.76	.72	.74

* p<0.05
PD = perfusion defect abnormality, SW = slow washout abnormality. For description of group A, B and C, please refer to the text.

high false positive slow washout was noted. Appearance of higher false positive rate in this group was independent of whether the clinical or electrocardiographic response to exercise was ischemic or nonischemic. This study suggested that the specificity of washout rate analysis for detection of regional myocardial hypoperfusion is only impaired in patients who achieve less than 75% maximal predicted heart rate.

(2) Subcutaneous infiltration of thallium dose at the site of injection
We and others have made anecdotal observations that in patients in whom Tl-201 injectate infiltrated subcutaneously, the initial myocardial uptake of Tl-201 was delayed, had a lower peak, and slower subsequent washout, compared to patients in whom the dose was delivered intravenously as a bolus. It is important, therefore, that subcutaneous infiltration of Tl-201 be avoided during injection by inserting an intravenous line prior to exercise and checking the free flow prior to and after injection of the dose.

(3) Unusually slow blood disappearance rate of Tl-201
Since myocardial washout rate of Tl-201 ultimately depends on plasma disappearance rate of Tl-201, it is possible that in patients with unusually slow plasma disappearance rate for Tl-201, myocardial washout rate would also be slow in the absence of coronary artery disease. This conceptual problem requires further investigation.

(4) Inappropriate data acquisition
As indicated above, for reliable washout rate analysis, the scintigraphic data should be acquired for an identical duration at each time interval (e.g., 10 minutes per view). Inappropriate acquisition of data by changing the imaging duration between early poststress and 4 hour delayed study invalidates washout rate calculations. For example, if the early poststress images are acquired for 10 minutes per view but the 4 hour delay study for 20 minutes per view the calculated washout rates will be falsely slower than normally expected.

Conclusion

Comprehensive computerized quantitative approaches to analysis of the regional stress myocardial distribution and washout rate of thallium-201 have been developed. These methods minimizes many of the problems associated with subjectivity of visual analysis of Tl-201 scintigrams. Additionally, the quantitative technique is more accurate than visual image interpretation for detection of disease in individual coronary arteries, especially in patients with multiple vessel coronary artery disease and those with moderate coronary artery stenosis. Importantly, the quantitative technique significantly enhances the potential of stress-redistribution scintigraphy for correct identification of patients with triple vessel and/or left main coronary artery disease. These improvements have been primarily due to additional analysis of regional myocardial washout rate for Tl-201 which is a spatially nonrelative index of myocardial hypoperfusion. These improvements may expand the diagnostic capability of Tl-201 scintigraphy in the noninvasive evaluation of patients with coronary artery disease.

Acknowledgements

The authors gratefully acknowledge the research assistance of Ana Becerra, Paciano Tapnio, David Brown and Ken Van Train and the secretarial assistance of Judy Smith.

References

1. Trobaugh GB, Wackers FJTh, Sokole EB, DeRouen TA, Ritchie JL, Hamilton GW: Thallium-201 myocardial imaging: an interinstitutional study of observer variability. J Nucl Med 19: 359, 1978.
2. Massie BM, Botinick EH, Brundage BH: Correlation of thallium-201 scintigrams with coronary anatomy: factors affecting region by region sensitivity. Am J Cardiol 44: 616, 1979.
3. Rigo P, Bailey IK, Griffith LSC, Pitt B, Burow RD, Wagner HN, Becker LC: Value and limitations of segmental analysis of stress thallium myocardial imaging for localization of coronary artery disease. Circulation 61: 973, 1970.
4. Dash H, Massie BM, Botvinick EH, Brundage BH: The oninvasive identification of left main and three-vessel coronary artery disease by myocardial stress perfusion scintigraphy and treadmill exercise electrocardiography. Circulation 60: 276, 1979.
5. McKillop JH, Murray RG, Turner JG, Bessent BG, Lorimer AR, Greig WR: Can the extent of coronary artery disease by predicted from thallium-201 myocardial images? J Nucl Med 20: 715, 1979.
6. Lenaers A, Block P, Thiel EV, Lebedelle M, Becquevort P, Erbsmann F, Ermans AM: Segmental analysis of Tl-201 stress myocardial scintigraphy. J Nucl Med 18: 509, 1977.
7. Meade RC, Bamrah VS, Horgan JD et al: Quantitative methods in the evaluation of thallium-201 myocardial perfusion images. J Nucl Med 19: 1175, 1978.
8. Vogel RA, Kirch DL, LeFree MT, et al: Thallium-201 myocardial perfusion scintigraphy: results of standard and multi-pinhole tomographic techniques. Am J Cardiol 43: 787, 1979.
9. Burow RD, Pond M, Schafer AW, et al: "Circumferential profiles:" a new method for computer analysis of thallium-201 myocardial perfusion images. J Nucl Med 20: 771, 1979.

124

10. Garcia E, Maddahi J, Berman D, Waxman A: Space-time quantitation of 201 Tl myocardial scintigraphy. J Nucl Med 22: 309, 1981.
11. Berger BC, Watson DD, Burwell LR, et al: Redistribution of thallium at rest in patients with stable and unstable angina and the effects of coronary artery bypass surgery. Circulation 60: 1114, 1979.
12. Reiber JHC, Simoons ML, Lie SP, Balakumaran K, Withagen AJA: Improved sensitivity of thallium-201 scintigrams by computer analysis. In: Noninvasive Methods in Ischemic Heart Disease. Faivre G, Bertrand, A, Cherrier F, Amor M, Neimann J-L (eds). Specia Nancy 1982: 163–172.
13. Reiber JHC, Lie SP, Simoons ML, Wijns W, Gerbrands JJ: Computer quantitation location, extent and type of thallium-201 myocardial perfusion abnormalities. Proc. 1st International Symposium on Medical Imaging and Image Interpretation ISMIII, IEEE Cat. No. CH 1804-4/82: 123–128, 1982.
14. Berman DS, Garcia EV, Maddahi J: Role of thallium-201 imaging in the diagnosis of myocardial ischemia and infarction. In: Nuclear Medicine Annual, edited by Freeman L, Weissman H, New York, Raven Press, 1980.
15. Watson DD, Leidholtz E, Beller GA, Teates CD: Defect perception in myocardial perfusion images. J Nucl Med 21: P61, 1980.
16. Pohost GM, O'Keefe DD, Gewirtz H, Strauss HW, Beller GA, Newell JB, Chaffin JS, Daggett WM: Thallium redistribution in the presence of severe fixed coronary stenosis. (abstr) Clin Res 26: 260A, 1978.
17. Beller GA, Pohost GM: Time course and mechanism of resolution of thallium-201 defects after transient myocardial ischemia (abstr) Am J Cardiol 41: 379, 1978.
18. Goris ML, Daspit SG, McLaughlin P, Kriss JP: Interpolative background subtraction. J Nucl Med 17: 744, 1976.
19. Watson DD, Beller GA, Berger BC, Teates CD: Notes on the quantitation of sequential Tl-201 images. Software 6: 4, 1979.
20. Maddahi J, Garcia EV, Berman DS, Waxman A, Swan HJC, Forrester J: Improved noninvasive assessment of coronary artery disease by quantitative analysis of regional stress myocardial distribution and washout of thallium-201. Circulation 64(5): 924, 1981.
21. Van Train K, Garcia E, Maddahi J, Brown D, Hulse S, Waxman A, Berman D: Improved space-time quantitation of segmental thallium-201 myocardial scintigrams. Clin Nucl Med 6: 449, 1981.
22. Abdulla A, Maddahi J, Garcia E, Rozanski A, Gutman J, Swan HJC, Berman D: Myocardial Tl-201 isolated washout abnormality: Mechanism for its occurrence and its contribution to enhanced detection of ischemic myocardial segments. Circulation 64: IV–105, 1981.
23. Maddahi J, Abdulla A, Berman D, Garcia E, Rozanski A, Waxman A, Forrester J, Swan HJC: Quantitative analysis of Tl-201 myocardial stress distribution and washout improves the identification of left main and triple vessel coronary artery disease. J Nucl Med 22(6): P25, 1981.
24. Bateman TM, Maddahi J, Gray RJ, Murphy FL, Raymond M, Stewart ME, Swan HJC, Berman DS: Diffuse slow washout of myocardial thallium-201: Predictive value in the detection of unsuspected extensive coronary disease. Circulation 66: II–62, 1982.
25. Massie BM, Wisneski J, Kramer B, Hollenberg M, Gertz E, Stern D: Comparison of myocardial thallium-201 clearance after maximal and submaximal exercise: Implications for diagnosis of coronary disease: Concise communication. J Nucl Med 23(5): 381, 1982.
26. Murphy FL, Maddahi J, Van Train K, Garcia E, Brown D, Swan HJC, Berman D: Thallium-201 uptake and washout at rest vs exercise in patients without coronary artery disease – Implications for quantitation. Am J Cardiol (in press), 1983.
27. Murphy FL, Maddahi J, Bateman T, Becerra A, Steuer M, Reisman SA, Kimchi A, Rozanski A, Garcia E, Swan HJC, Berman D: Effect of submaximal exercise heart rate on the results of quantiative thallium-201 stress testing. Clin Nucl Med 7(9S): P33, 1982.

7. First-pass and equilibrium radionuclide angiocardiography for evaluating ventricular performance

Barry L. Zaret and Harvey J. Berger

Introduction

In 1971, gated equilibrium radionuclide angiocardiography was developed [1, 2] and in the following year, an alternative technique, first-pass radionuclide angiocardiography was described [3]. Since their introduction ten years ago, these two radionuclide techniques for assessment of cardiac function have undergone substantial technical development and have progressed from the investigational stage to that of clinical application. Both techniques have advantages and limitations. In many instances, the approaches are complementary, and both can and should be performed in an individual patient. The decision as to which technique to utilize and when to combine them should be based upon available instrumentation, clinical setting, and type of patient being studied. In general, these nuclear studies provide important physiologic insights into both right and left ventricular function. They require only intravenous injection of minimal amounts of radioactive tracers, which do not perturb hemodynamics or other aspects of human physiology. Indices of global and regional left and right ventricular performance have been developed, providing a means of characterizing cardiac pump function under a number of conditions [4].

First-pass radionuclide angiocardiography

With this technique analysis is limited to the initial transit of radioactivity through the central circulation, following rapid intravenous injection of an intact bolus. Evaluation is based upon indicator-dilution principles. The major assumption is that there is homogeneous mixing of the radioactive tracer with blood prior to its arrival in the chamber being evaluated. Because there is temporal and anatomic segregation of radioactivity within each of the cardiac chambers, both right and left ventricular performance can be evaluated from the same study [5].

Technetium-99m radiopharmaceuticals of high specific activity generally have been employed. Since each study requires a separate injection, technetium-99m radiopharmaceuticals other than pertechnetate often may be preferable. For example, when serial studies are performed, such as at rest and exercise or after interventions, the first injection can be made with either technetium-99m sulfur colloid, which is cleared from the blood pool by the reticuloendothelial system, or with technetium-99m diethylenetriamine-pentaacetic acid (DTPA), which is cleared by the kidneys. First-pass studies also can be performed in combination with subsequent equilibrium blood pool imaging. In fact, this is relatively commonly performed, especially when analysis of right ventricular function is needed.

The medial right antecubital or external jugular vein are the preferable sites for injection. Careful bolus administration and injection technique are essential for the validity of first-pass data. The appropriateness of the bolus technique can be monitored by following a region of interest over the superior vena cava during the early phase of the study. If the bolus injection is inadequate, the study should be repeated.

The need for separate repeat injections for each first-pass study is a limitation of this approach. In addition, because of background considerations, the time interval between technetium-99m studies may be longer than desired. An ideal intravascular tracer for first-pass studies would have a short half-life, allowing multiple sequential studies with both high count rates and reduced radiation exposure. Several short-lived tracers have been developed and appear to be potential alternatives for the first-pass technique. These include gold-195m (half-life of 30.5 seconds) [6], tantalum-178 (half-life of 9.3 minutes) [7], and iridium-191m (half-life of 4.9 seconds) [8]. All three are obtained from shielded table top generators, and are derived from longer lived parents. Of these three, the results with gold-195m have been the most encouraging. In fact, this radiotracer is presently undergoing clinical trials and is commercially available in Europe. It is likely that this tracer will be employed extensively in the future with the first-pass approach. We have had experience with this agent in both animals and man. Because of the very short half-life of gold-195m, studies of ventricular function may be combined with Tl-201 perfusion imaging using a single exercise study [9].

Instrumentation

The choice of scintillation camera and computer for first-pass studies is a critical issue. Systems must provide adequate temporal and spatial resolution with acceptable counting statistics. Because data are derived from only several cardiac cycles during the initial transit of the radionuclide bolus, the limiting factor of the first-pass approach is the relatively low count rates of the raw data compared to the equilibrium approach. When studies are performed on conventional Anger cameras, the maximal count rates are limited by the system's dead time. These instruments generally have linear response rates up to approximately 60,000 counts per second.

There are two distinct instrumentation alternatives: the computerized multi-crystal scintillation camera and the computerized digital single crystal camera. Both systems allow accumulation of high count rates, up to approximately 450,000 counts per second for the multicrystal camera. The multicrystal camera is composed of a mosaic of 294 individual crystals that are coupled through a complex light-pipe array to 35 photomultiplier tubes. The dead time of the system is primarily a function of the speed at which the electronics can process an event. With a high sensitivity parallel hole collimator, a 25 mCi dose of technetium-99m results in over 400,000 counts per second in the overall image frame and a count density of approximately 500 counts/cm^2 in the left ventricle during a first-pass study. The newly-developed digital cameras also permit rapid data acquisition and processing using high speed buffer memories. These instruments, which are undergoing further development and testing, have the advantage of employing the routine complement of 37 photomultiplier tubes and a spectrum of routine collimators, ranging from the high sensitivity to the high resolution versions. This potentially gives the added flexibility of performing high quality static imaging and equilibrium studies on the same system as high count rate first-pass studies. To date, such flexibility has generally not been available with the multicrystal camera.

Although the entire first-pass study is acquired on the computer usually in frame mode, data are analyzed only when the bolus is in the chamber of interest, either the right or left ventricle. While the first-pass study can be obtained in any position relative to the imaging device, we prefer the anterior position for assessment of both right and left ventricular function [10, 11, 12, 13, 14]. In the gated first-pass technique, an alternative which is applicable to the analysis of right ventricular function on a routine Anger camera, data are stored directly in a series of equal frames starting immediately after the R wave. The picture file that is formed is identical to that obtained in equilibrium blood pool imaging, except that only a few beats are used. When the gated first-pass technique is used for analysis of the right ventricle, the 15 to 30° right anterior oblique position is prefera-

128

ble, because the right atrium and right ventricle can be separated.

The first step in analysis of the first-pass radionuclide angiocardiogram involves visual evaluation of the series of images at 1 to 2 frames/second. The morphology of the cardiac blood pool and of the great vessels is used to determine the overall flow pattern. For calculation of left ventricular ejection fraction, the steps used in analysis involve definition of the region of interest, summation of beats, and background correction [5]. However, in this case meaningful quantitative analysis of global ventricular function can be generated from data obtained in any position. Radioactivity is analyzed only at the time when it is in the chamber being assessed (Figure 1). Although the relative background correction for first-pass studies is substantially lower than that for gated equilibrium imaging, it still must be taken into account. Based upon counts detected in the left ventricular region of interest at end-diastole, background contributes approximately 25 to 30% using the first-pass technique, as compared to 50 to 55% in the equilibrium imaging approach.

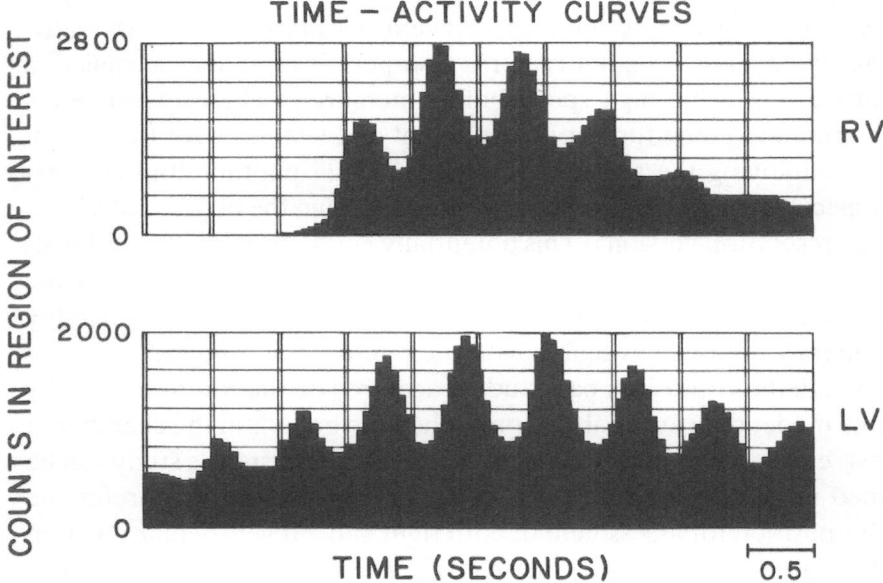

Figure 1. Regional time-activity curves for the right and left ventricles obtained with a first-pass radionuclide angiocardiogram using a computerized multi-crystal camera. The peaks of each curve correspond to end-diastole, and the valleys to end-systole. Note the extremely high count rates in both curves. Data from several consecutive beats are summed to produce a representative cardiac cycle. RV = right ventricle, LV = left ventricle. Reproduced with permission from Berger HJ, Matthay RA, Pytlik LM, Gottschalk A, Zaret BL: First-pass radionuclide assessment of right and left ventricular performance in patients with cardiac and pulmonary disease. Semin Nucl Med 9: 275–295, 1979.

With the first-pass approach, a fixed region of interest corresponding to the end-diastolic image usually is employed. Over- or under-estimation of the region will result in inaccurate determinations [12, 14]. The most important factor is exclusion of the proximal aorta from the left ventricular region. Three approaches to left ventricular background correction have been employed. In the method used in our laboratory, a series of frames is chosen immediately prior to the first discernible left ventricular beat on the time-activity curve [12]. This constant background image represents overlying and scattered radiation from the left atrium and lungs. An alternative approach involves placement of a horseshoe-shaped region of interest around the apex of the left ventricle and generation of a low frequency time-activity curve through this region in a manner similar to that employed for the equilibrium technique. Others have suggested either subtracting a constant percentage from all studies or suppressing background activity with constant isocount contour subtraction. Irrespective of the technique employed, correct choice of the background is essential.

Left ventricular ejection fraction is determined either as an average of several individual beats or from a summed cardiac cycle (representative cardiac cycle) formed by adding several beats frame by frame. In patients with occasional premature beats, the premature contraction and the post-premature beat should be excluded from analysis. This poses potential problems, since only a limited number of beats are available for analysis. The major limiting factor of the first-pass technique when acquired on a routine Anger camera is the inadequacy of count rates. In a left ventricular region of interest, at a temporal resolution of 20 frames per second, it is common to have less than 200 counts per frame when the study is obtained on a single crystal camera, compared with greater than 1,000 counts per frame when the study is obtained on the multicrystal camera.

Using techniques analogous to those employed for assessment of the left ventricle, a high frequency time-activity curve can be generated from a right ventricular region of interest. We believe this is the optimal manner of determining right ventricular ejection fraction under varying physiologic conditions such as exercise, and in the presence of varying degrees of anatomic distortion or right ventricular dysfunction. There is now extensive experience in applying this approach in coronary and congenital heart disease as well as chronic obstructive pulmonary disease [11].

Although regional left ventricular function can be derived from the first-pass study, statistical considerations play a predominant role in determining the adequacy of first-pass data for assessment of wall motion.

Although the count density of first-pass images is substantially lower than that from equilibrium blood pool imaging, data are acquired over a far shorter period of time, minimizing patient motion, and the target-to-background ratio for the first-pass studies is higher, potentially improving edge definition.

Several approaches have been proposed for analysis of first-pass data. First, the end-diastolic perimeter can be superimposed upon the end-systolic image or perimeter, and regional wall motion can be evaluated from the difference between these two images [12, 15, 16]. The approach that has been found to be the most advantageous with the first-pass method is use of functional images, especially the regional ejection fraction image [17, 18]. Such images must be displayed using at least 64 shades of grey or 16 discrete colors. A regional ejection fraction approach based upon changes in counts in sectors of the left ventricle also has been described. Although each of these radionuclide approaches has been shown to agree with contrast angiographic assessment of wall motion, for detailed evaluation of wall motion in patients with coronary artery disease, studies must be performed in more than one position. If a single position study is obtained, the anterior view probably is preferable. In this view, particular care must be taken when analyzing the anterobasal and inferoposterior regions of the ventricle because of overlap with the left atrium and descending aorta, respectively.

The end-diastolic perimeter also can be used to calculate end-diastolic volume [18]. This can be accomplished using conventional area-length approximations. Even in patients with regional dysfunction, the end-diastolic perimeter resembles an ellipsoid quite closely. From this measurement, as well as the count-based ejection fraction and the heart rate, end-systolic volume, stroke volume, cardiac output, and pulmonary blood volume can be derived. The major sources of error in this technique are accurate determination of the left ventricular edges and delineation of the aortic valve plane.

Equilibrium radionuclide angiocardiography

This technique provides a means of cardiac blood pool imaging throughout the cardiac cycle by synchronizing collection of scintillation data with electrocardiographic events [1, 19, 20]. Several requirements must be met to assure high quality valid data: (1) cardiac performance should be relatively stable during data acquisition; (2) patient motion relative to the detector must be minimized; (3) radioactivity must remain intravascular at relatively constant concentration during data acquisition; (4) framing intervals chosen must be sufficiently short to allow for a temporal resolution that is adequate for the given heart rate; and (5) the duration of data acquisition must be sufficiently long for adequate count density and resultant spatial resolution.

The entire intravascular blood pool is labeled. Thus, an optimal blood pool label is essential for an adequate study. Currently, labeled autologous red blood cells are used almost exclusively. Red blood cells can be labeled with technetium-99m using either *in vivo* or *in vitro* techniques. With *in vivo* labeling, unlabeled stannous pyrophosphate (usually 1 to 3 mg reconstituted in normal saline) is injected intravenously approximately 15 minutes prior to injection of 15 to 30 mCi of technetium-99m pertechnetate [21]. The direct labeling occurs within the intravascular space. In the *in vitro* technique, which is not employed commonly, the labeling process is performed in a sterile vial. Recently, a modified *in vivo* technique also has been adopted [22]. With this approach, stannous pyrophosphate is injected into the patient as in the conventional *in vivo* technique. However, the labeling then is performed in a closed heparinized syringe-extension tube system attached directly by needle to the patient's vein. The labeling efficiency of this approach appears to be substantially higher than that of the *in vivo* technique, and there is almost no free pertechnetate in the patient. This technique definitely improves the quality of the gated blood pool study and now is performed routinely in our laboratory. In order to maximize the count density of a study, 30 mCi of technetium-99m pertechnetate is recommended as the most appropriate dose in adults. The dominant factor determining blood pool activity is the physical half-life of the radionuclide (6 hours). Serial imaging can be performed following a single injection for periods up to 12 hours.

Instrumentation

In most instances, gated blood pool imaging is performed with a single crystal scintillation camera, equipped with a parallel hole collimator. The uniformity of the detector is important for quantitative studies, and if possible, there should be less than a five percent variation in uniformity with a field flood across the detector. The choice of collimator to be used is based upon anticipated count rate and acceptable imaging time. When determination of regional wall motion is an important consideration, a general all-purpose collimator or high-resolution collimator should be employed. However, imaging time increases as the collimator's resolution increases and there is a trade-off between sensitivity and resolution. Under certain circumstances the potential benefits gained by using a collimator with a higher intrinsic resolution may be offset by more prolonged imaging time and resultant patient motion. For these reasons, in exercise or multiple interventional studies, a high sensitivity collimator often is used. However, resolution with this collimator is relatively poor, making analysis of regional function more difficult.

All scintillation data are collected temporally in synchrony with the electrocardiographic trigger. Depending upon the heart rate and mode of data acquisition, the R-R interval usually is divided into equal framing interval subdivisions (Figure 2). Generally, a framing interval of 30 to 50 milliseconds is employed at rest and 20 to 30 milliseconds at exercise. To obtain data concerning ventricular filling and emptying characteristics, higher temporal resolution at 10 to 20 millisecond intervals is required [23, 24, 25]. Data occurring during consecutive cardiac cycles are sorted in a temporal sequence determined by their relationship to the onset of the R wave and summed. The end result is a single image sequence spanning the entire cardiac cycle, which is made up of data from several hundred individual cardiac beats.

Gating may be performed through either frame or list mode collections. In frame mode, scintillation data are sorted into the appropriate location of the picture file, added to the previous data in that memory, and then discarded. This is the approach used by most computer systems and

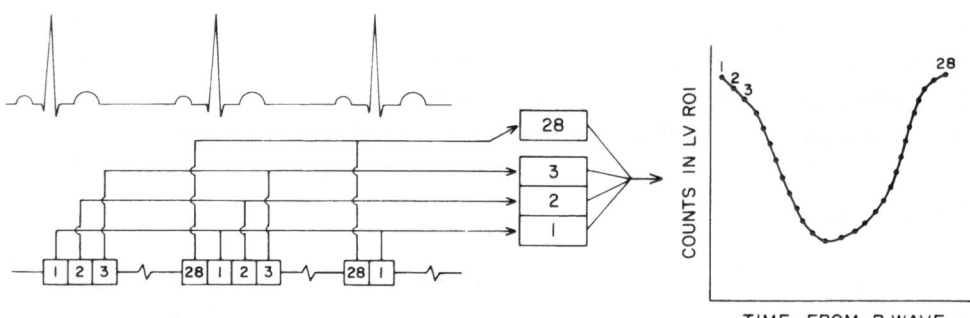

Figure 2. Diagram representing the method of multiple gated cardiac blood pool imaging. Each RR interval is subdivided into 28 equal frames. Data from consecutive beats are summed, resulting in a single representative cardiac cycle. This approach assumes that the time interval between R waves is constant. Each one of the 28 frames has a corresponding image. When analyzing the counts in the left ventricular region of interest (ROI), a relative left ventricular volume curve can be derived. Reproduced with permission from Zaret B, Berger H: Techniques of nuclear cardiology, in Hurst JW (ed.): The Heart. New York, McGraw-Hill, 1981, pp 1803–1843.

requires the least memory capability. In list mode, scintillation data are stored consecutively, word by word, in one of two buffer memories. This mode requires substantial computer memory in excess of that employed routinely. Use of list mode acquisition allows reformatting of data which can provide significant advantages. With the list mode method, the left ventricular time-activity curve can be constructed using forward/backward framing, improving the accuracy of the diastolic portion of the volume curve. In addition, data obtained from ectopic beats or those with varying R-R intervals can either be excluded or analyzed independently.

Gated blood pool data become interpretable approximately 30 seconds after acquisition. However, data with moderate spatial resolution generally require a minimum of two to three minutes, depending upon the collimation. At rest, studies usually are acquired until a preset left ventricular count density of at least 200–250 counts per picture element (pixel) is reached. This generally results in a total of 200–250,000 counts per frame and requires from seven to ten minutes. When imaging is performed during exercise, approximately 100–150,000 counts per frame are collected. With a high sensitivity collimator, this can be accomplished in approximately two minutes. It should be emphasized that the resolution of such exercise studies is degraded compared to routine resting data, making analysis of regional wall motion difficult.

For complete analysis of all cardiac chambers and the great vessels, imaging at rest should be performed in at least three, but preferably four, separate positions: antero-posterior, approximately 45° left anterior oblique (the obliquity which gives the best separation of the two ventricles), left lateral, and 30° left posterior oblique [26]. These latter two steep views are obtained with the patient in the right-side-down decubitus position. The right anterior oblique view is not recommended because it places the left ventricle furthest from the detector. The left anterior oblique view chosen for quantitative analysis of global left ventricular function must optimally separate the two ventricles. Although this is usually at an approximate 45° obliquity, dependent upon cardiac orientation this obliquity may vary substantially and should be individualized in each patient. Care must be taken to assure that the two ventricles are separated from base to apex. Furthermore, a 10° caudal tilt (with the detector pointed towards the feet) should be employed to minimize left atrial contributions within the left ventricular region of interest. An alternative technique involves the use of a 30° slant hole collimator [27, 28]. An advantage of the slant hole collimator is that it can be placed directly over the patient's chest, bringing the heart closer to the detector.

This may result in less distortion or foreshortening of the ventricle.

The gated blood pool study allows evaluation of the entire blood pool. Each cardiac chamber should be analyzed with respect to relative position, size, synchrony, and symmetry of contraction. This is best performed using a cine display. The size of the chambers should be assessed by comparing them to the known dimensions of the detector, as well as to placed radioactive markers or other standard dimension calibrations. An overall assessment of global function should be reached prior to approaching analysis of regional wall motion.

Regional wall motion is best assessed from the cine display. The left ventricle is subdivided anatomically into multiple segments according to standard definitions. While quantitative methods for analysis of regional wall motion do exist (see below), standardized visual analysis of the entire gated blood pool study also provides relevant semiquantitative data. The left ventricle as visualized in three or four views is divided into 11 anatomic segments. Each segment is graded on a five-point scale with 3 being normal, 2 mildly hypokinetic, 1 severely hypokinetic, 0 akinetic, and −1 dyskinetic. A total score for the left ventricle then is derived (normal score = 33). Various regional abnormalities may be detectable only in a single position as a result of overlap of segments or chambers. For example, inferior and posterior wall regional abnormalities, including aneurysms, only may be apparent in the left lateral or left posterior oblique images (Figure 3) [26]. Particularly for the inferior wall, the anterior position often may be misleading or incorrect because of overlap of margins of the right and left ventricular blood pools.

Many definitions for left ventricular aneurysms have been proposed in the literature based upon a combination of pathologic, angiographic, and direct surgical visual assessment. The functional definition of a left ventricular aneurysm used in our laboratory involves demonstration of a region of dyskinesis or akinesis with sharp margins adjacent to relatively well contracting myocardium with deformity of the left ventricular contour during both systole and diastole. It also may be helpful to describe the presence or absence of an aneurysm using a probability scale as devised for receiver operating characteristic (ROC) curves.

Because of the nature of the gated blood pool study, both sides of the interventricular septum are visualized. Evaluation of septal motion is perhaps the most difficult regional analysis to make on a pure visual basis with this technique. The best way to characterize septal wall motion is by systolic thickening, although edge motion towards the long axis of the left ventricle also does occur. The presence of paradoxical septal motion

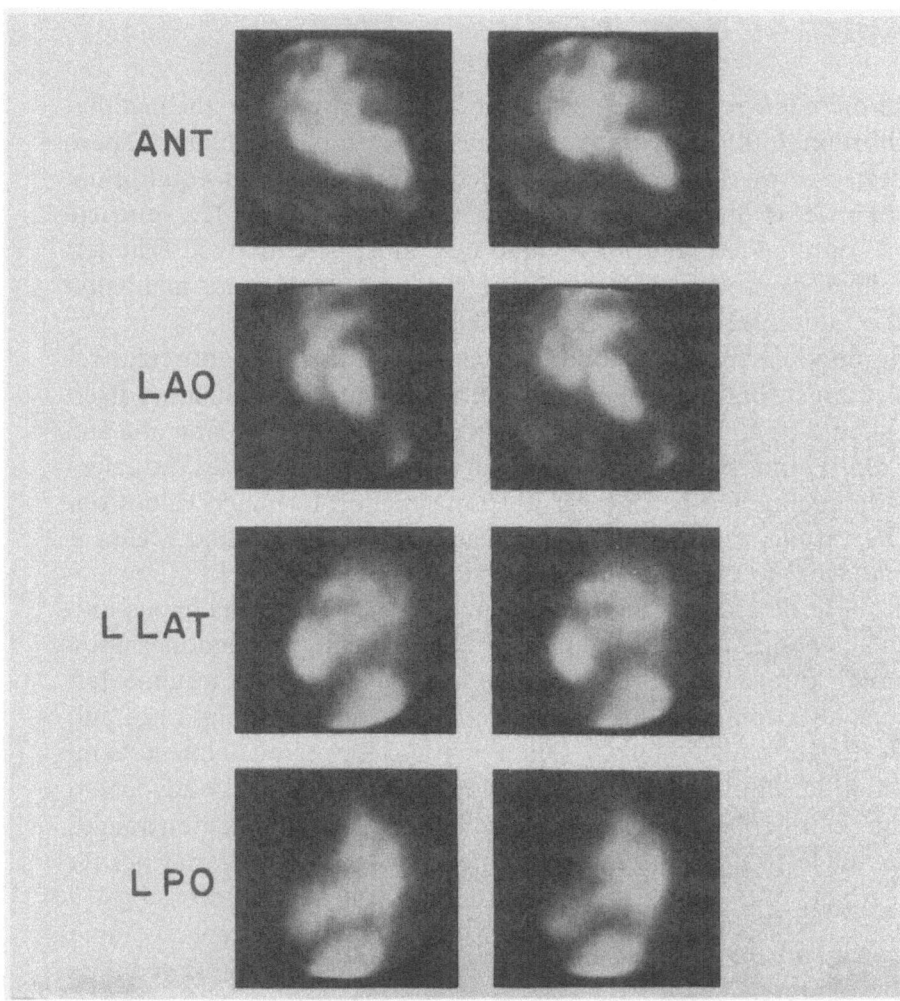

ANT

LAO

L LAT

LPO

Figure 3. Multiple gated cardiac blood pool imaging in a patient with previous anterior wall myocardial infarction and a large anteroapical left ventricular aneurysm. Note that the aneurysm only is appreciated on the left lateral and left posterior oblique studies, highlighting the need for acquiring studies in multiple obliquities. ANT = anterior, LAO = left anterior oblique, LLAT = left lateral, LPO = left posterior oblique. End-diastolic images are shown on the left, end-systolic images on the right.

should be evaluated. With this finding, the septum (basal, apical, or both segments) moves towards the right ventricle during systole. This is a common postoperative event after cardiac surgery and does not necessarily imply septal infarction or ischemia. Paradoxical septal motion also is seen in patients with conduction defects, right ventricular dilatation (especially volume overload), and anteroseptal infarction.

Left ventricular ejection fraction

Calculation of left ventricular ejection fraction is based upon the fact that at equilibrium, left ventricular counts are proportional to volume. There are a series of systematic steps involved in processing an equilibrium study. In order to limit analysis of count rate changes to the left ventricle alone, an optimal left anterior oblique view must be employed. The left ventricular region of interest can be determined using either manually-derived or automated approaches [29, 30, 31, 32, 33].

Background correction accounts for activity in the left ventricular region of interest, but not originating from the ventricular chamber itself [19]. It should be stressed that background correction is a systematic and standardized but arbitrary and emperical correction that raises the calculated radionuclide left ventricular ejection fraction to match values obtained by cardiac catheterization. In general, the background region is placed adjacent to the posterolateral wall of the left ventricle.

From these data, a left ventricular time-activity curve analogous to a ventricular volume curve, is generated automatically. Depending upon the framing rate employed, this curve can be used to determine left ventricular ejection fraction, peak ejection rate, peak filling rate, and relative left ventricular volumes. Other methods for region of interest and background selection are under evaluation. Some studies have advocated use of the Fourier phase images, stroke volume or ejection fraction images to define the left ventricular region of interest [34, 35]. These may permit more accurate automated definition of the left ventricular edges.

Several studies have demonstrated recently that left ventricular volume can be calculated from left ventricular counts. This technique requires determination of the total number of counts in the left ventricle, as well as the depth of the left ventricle relative to the detector. Using the linear attenuation coefficient for technetium-99m in soft tissue, absolute left ventricular volume can be derived directly after accounting for framing interval and blood concentration during the study [48, 49, 50].

Quantitative analysis of regional wall motion

Although the most widely used approach for analysis of regional wall motion involves visual interpretation, several quantitative techniques also have been proposed for determination of regional function. These include: 1. computer generated chords, hemiaxes, radii, and contours [36]; 2. regional count-based ejection fractions [37, 38]; 3. ejection fraction or

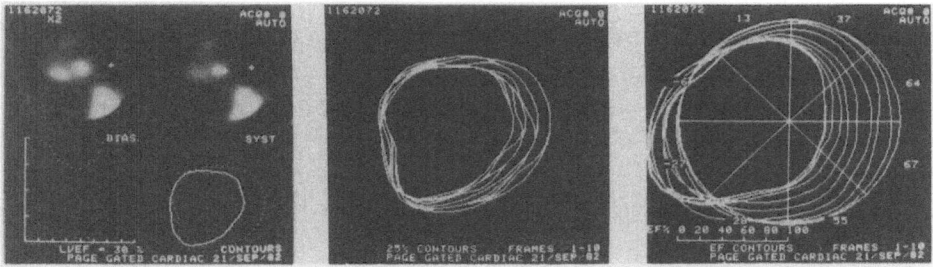

Figure 4. Automated methods for evaluation of regional wall motion. In the panel on the left, the end-diastolic (dashed) and end-systolic (solid) images and contours are shown. Note the severe regional dysfunction of the interventricular septum, but preserved posterolateral motion. In the center panel, a series of left ventricular contours is displayed. Note once again the markedly diminished septal motion. In the panel on the right, the left ventricle has been divided into 8 sectors. Regional count-based ejection fractions for each of the sectors are displayed. Note the disparity between regional ejection fractions in the septum and apex compared with the lateral wall. This patient had a documented anteroseptal myocardial infarction.

stroke volume functional image [34, 39]; and 4. Fourier phase and amplitude images and histograms [39, 40]. Except for the first method, the remainder only can be performed on the left anterior oblique position study. Although studies have demonstrated the utility of each approach, especially when quantifying the response of regional function to interventions, it is unclear which, if any, is optimal in most patients. In addition, those clinical or technical instances in which a specific technique will be unreliable remain to be defined.

An advantage of the radial shortening technique is that this can be applied to studies obtained in multiple obliquities. In the regional ejection fraction technique, time activity curves are derived from several regions of the left ventricle as seen in the left anterior oblique view. The left ventricle usually is divided into from three to eight regions (Figure 4). The regions at the base of the left ventricle in the area of the mitral valve plane are excluded because of overlap with the aortic root and left atrium. In functional imaging, a specific characteristic of volume change, such as the ejection fraction, stroke volume, or Fourier phase or amplitude is calculated for each pixel in the interpolated matrix. The range of values for this parameter then is displayed using grey shades or color. In this way, small regions of normal ejection can be differentiated from those with abnormal function.

The Fourier filtering technique also can be employed to visualize the temporal sequence of mechanical events [41, 42, 43, 44, 45]. By extracting pixel-by-pixel time-activity curves, the timing of mechanical systole can be displayed in a cinematic format. The phase histogram is scanned, and as each phase angle is passed, the corresponding pixels are identified. This newly developed technique allows characterization of the pattern of regional function in conduction disturbances.

Additional quantitative measurements

The proportionality between externally detected counts and intravascular volume allows changes in counts in regions corresponding to left ventricle, lung, or peripheral extremity to be used to assess relative changes in respective blood volumes [46, 47]. As long as the intravascular distribution of the radiotracer remains constant and the physical decay of technetium-99m is taken into consideration, the effects of interventions can be determined. Assessment of regional pulmonary blood volume is of interest as an indirect measure of pulmonary artery and left ventricular filling pressures both at rest and exercise. Assessment of peripheral blood volumes and capacity is of interest in evaluating distribution of cardiac output and physiologic effects of vasodilators and inotropic agents.

Assuming one can define the right ventricular and left ventricular regions of interest accurately, the ratio of right to left ventricular stroke counts can be used as a measure of the degree of valvular regurgitation [51, 52, 53]. In the absence of regurgitation or intracardiac shunting, the stroke volumes of the two ventricles should be equal. Moderate to severe degrees of valvular regurgitation can be identified. However, this method requires validation in each laboratory, and mild degrees of regurgitation may not be differentiated reliably from normal. Furthermore, errors are introduced in evaluating patients with substantial resting left ventricular dysfunction [54]. Further details are given in Chapter 8.

Right ventricle
Right ventricular size and contraction are best evaluated on the anterior or right anterior oblique views. During right ventricular systole, the tricuspid valve plane moves towards the left ventricle. The inferior diaphragmatic surface of the right ventricle and the right ventricular apex move upward. This movement often is not apparent at all on the left anterior oblique position study, even in the absence of any right ventricular dysfunction. In this view, there is substantial right atrial/right ventricular overlap, such that a major portion of the visualized blood pool is a combination of these two chambers. Therefore, motion of the right ventricular walls may not be defined properly. This issue also is of substantial

importance in quantifying right ventricular volume and ejection fraction. Furthermore, the tangential walls seen in this view do not reflect the areas of major contraction. In addition, because of the bellows shape of the right ventricle, an increase in right ventricular volume may be difficult to define in any single position. In the presence of right ventricular dilatation or cardiac rotation, overlap of the right ventricular blood pool may make analysis of the anteroapical and inferoapical portions of the left ventricle difficult. Several laboratories have reported on the efficacy of the equilibrium technique for evaluating right ventricular ejection fraction. Because of the geometric factors discussed above, we continue to favor the first-pass approach for this measurement.

Nonimaging nuclear probe

A modification of the equilibrium blood pool imaging technique involves the use of a specially collimated nonimaging nuclear probe and dedicated microprocessor instead of the conventional scintillation gamma camera and computer [55, 56, 57]. This instrument has the advantages of extensive portability, decreased cost, and augmented detector sensitivity. It is used only for assessing global left ventricular function and hence its disadvantages involve an inability to assess regional left ventricular function, right ventricular function or myocardial perfusion. The computerized nuclear probe consists of a two inch in diameter by one and one-half inch thick crystal and a single bore three and one-half inch converging collimator. The isosensitivity response contours of this collimator are such that radioactivity emanating from the left ventricle can be identified clearly and separated from surrounding structures. The analog scintillation data and electrocardiogram are input simultaneously and sampled in real time at 10 millisecond intervals by a dedicated microprocessor. The beat-to-beat left ventricular time-activity curve is displayed and can be analyzed directly. A gated cardiac cycle from the same data also can be obtained. Data are summed for any length of time, usually ranging from 30 seconds through two minutes. This generates a high temporal resolution volume curve analogous to that obtained with multiple gated cardiac blood pool imaging.

Studies are performed after labeling of the intravascular blood pool with technetium-99m as noted previously for blood pool imaging. Especially for serial studies over several hours or beat-to-beat analysis, a comparable dose as is used for imaging studies should be employed. However, accurate studies can be obtained with doses as low as 5 mCi or less.

Positioning of the nonimaging probe requires appropriate orientation of the detector relative to the left ventricular blood pool based upon a logically-derived series of algorithms. Detector positions are based upon both the stroke counts and average counts as recorded by the probe. The left ventricular region of interest is chosen as the position with the maximal ratio of stroke counts to average counts.

We have had substantial experience with this instrument over the past three years. The ability to assess beat-by-beat changes in left ventricular function is of value in a number of clinical and investigative areas, including assessment of the hemodynamic consequences of rhythm disturbances [58] and rapidly changing reflex events [59], and the assessment of pressure-volume relations [60]. In addition, its small size and portability allow dispersion of technology to areas such as the operating room that would not be routinely accessible to larger scintillation cameras.

Factors associated with errors in left ventricular ejection fraction

Although both first-pass and equilibrium radionuclide angiocardiography are accurate means of determining left ventricular ejection fraction, there are a number of technical factors which may introduce errors. These generally relate to problems in definition of the left ventricular region of interest and background. These errors can be encountered with either technique [12, 14, 19].

Overestimation

With the equilibrium technique, the major cause for an overestimation of left ventricular ejection fraction is an inappropriately high background correction. This may result from placement of the background region of interest either over or too close to the spleen or descending aorta or positioning over another more poorly defined anatomic region with markedly increased radionuclide activity. Such regions would not be representative of the activity behind and scattering into the left ventricular region of interest. If the end-diastolic region of interest is too large (but not including the left atrium), the ejection fraction also will be overestimated. With the computerized nuclear probe, there is a potential for mispositioning of the detector primarily over a relatively normal region of myocardium, and thereby potentially minimizing the contribution of dyssynergic segments to global performance.

In the first-pass study, the major cause of overestimation of the ejection fraction also is overestimation of the background. If background is determined temporally from the time-activity curve, choice of background frames too late in the time-activity curve will increase the background. Similarly, any factor resulting in poor temporal separation of the right and left ventricular phases of the first-pass study can result in an overestimation of background.

Underestimation

In the equilibrium technique, inclusion of the left atrium in the left ventricular region of interest during ventricular systole will lower the ejection fraction. Although predominantly a problem in patients with enlarged left atria, this may occur in other patients as well. This problem can be minimized by use of increased caudal tilt or a slant hole collimator. Poor separation of the left and right ventricles, particularly in the region of the lower septum, and inclusion of the ascending aorta in the region of interest also can artifactually decrease left ventricular ejection fraction. Use of a fixed (nonvariable) region of interest for calculation of left ventricular ejection fraction results in underestimation of ejection fraction.

In a patient with a large or loculated pleural or pericardial effusion, as well as marked left ventricular hypertrophy, the background region of interest may be placed over a photopenic area. This may not be an accurate representation of the true left ventricular background, resulting in too low a background correction.

Problems in electrocardiographic gating also will affect the ejection fraction determination. If the gate is working only variably, or if the temporal resolution is too slow, there may be a substantial underestimation of ejection fraction.

Count detection is physically dependent upon distance from the collimator. In a patient with an anteroapical aneurysm, where the akinetic or dyskinetic segment is closest to the detector, there may be an underestimation of global left ventricular ejection fraction, since contribution of the well-contracting basal segments to the change in counts may be obscured or attenuated by the aneurysm. In a similar fashion, in a markedly enlarged left ventricle or posterobasal aneurysm, the assumption that counts are proportional to volume may not hold, because of self attenuation.

Comparison between the first-pass and equilibrium techniques

Each technique has limitations and attributes. With the gated equilibrium technique, following a *single* radionuclide injection, multiple studies can be performed over several hours or regional wall motion can be assessed in multiple views. This allows sequential evaluation of a variety of physiologic and pharmacologic interventions. This ability to obtain multiple studies from a single radionuclide injection presents a potential advantage over the first-pass technique. On the other hand, especially with newer imaging systems, the development and availability of new short half-lived tracers may impact substantially upon this difference. It is possible that in the near future gold-195m could replace technetium-99m for first-transit studies [6, 9]. The high count density of the equilibrium study represents a major advantage in terms of evaluating regional wall motion. However, because the entire intravascular blood pool is labeled, there is a somewhat lower target-to-background ratio with the equilibrium technique than with the first-pass study. The equilibrium method allows simultaneous assessment of all cardiac structures and great vessels; however, at times this also may detract from assessment of any individual chamber. In contrast, direct assessment of *each* ventricle can be accomplished with the first-pass technique without superimposed activity or '"noise" from other cardiac and extra-cardiac structures.

A major advantage of the first-pass technique is that it can be performed rapidly. At resting heart rates, the period of data acquisition is less than 30 seconds. This characteristic permits accurate definition of rapidly changing physiologic states. In contrast, a disadvantage of the equilibrium technique is the duration of the examination. Equilibrium radionuclide angiocardiography requires two to ten minutes for data acquisition. This is not optimal for the study of acutely ill patients or those on ventilators, or those who cannot remain in a stable position for a prolonged period of time. If analysis of regional wall motion is important in a particular clinical setting and the period of data acquisition must be limited (such as during exercise), the first-pass technique using a multicrystal or digital camera may provide preferable results. Exercise ventricular performance can be evaluated with either technique. However, patient motion will degrade image quality. For equilibrium exercise studies, it appears easier to immobilize the patient in the supine or minimally erect position. With the first-pass approach, where patient motion is not a problem, upright exercise is employed almost exclusively; while equilibrium studies, because of patient motion, usually are performed in the supine position. This problem has been circumvented to some extent by using more extensive restraining devices. In terms of patient comfort, upright exercise is generally preferred, especially in those with heart failure or respiratory impairment. Furthermore, these two types of exercise result in different preload and afterload stresses, a factor which may result in different ventricular performance responses in the two positions. This may be particularly relevant in certain disease states such as aortic regurgitation [61].

In our opinion, the first-pass technique appears to be a better way of evaluating right ventricular function and is preferred for assessing and quantifying intracardiac shunts. Using right and left ventricular regions of interest, the equilibrium technique allows determination of valvular regurgitation. Although the methods are different, both equilibrium blood pool imaging and first-pass radionuclide angiocardiography provide a means of measuring left ventricular volumes.

Major problems with the first-pass technique are encountered when the bolus injection technique is poor, when there are arrhythmias during the period of data acquisition, and when there is marked pulmonary artery hypertension resulting in delayed clearance from the right heart. Excellent venous access and standardized bolus injection technique are critical and at times limiting requirements of the first-pass method.

Exercise studies

Ventricular performance is evaluated during exercise using either equilibrium gated or first-pass techniques [13, 62, 63, 64]. Although the exercise protocols for these two approaches are similar, some differences do exist. The protocol for exercise equilibrium blood pool imaging involves serial acquisition of two-minute left anterior oblique blood pool studies. When performing supine exercise, it is preferable to adjust the ergometer component of the stress table so that the patient's legs are outstretched and at the same level as the body torso. Following control acquisitions, exercise is begun at a workload of 150 to 200 kilopond meters per minute, or approximately 25 to 30 Watts. The workload is increased every three minutes by 150 to 200 kilopond meters per minute or 25 to 30 Watts until symptom-limited. Imaging is performed during the last two minutes of each three-minute exercise stage. The major changes in heart rate that occur are noted during the initial minute of exercise. Thereafter, the heart rate generally is relatively constant. In order to improve image resolution, some laboratories have elected to exercise patients for four minutes per load, with three minutes of data acquisition. Many laboratories obtain an additional study during the immediate post-exercise period [65]. This may be of particular value in the assessment of the reversibility of regional dysfunction present at rest.

When performing an exercise equilibrium blood pool study, it is essential that the left anterior oblique view is optimized. While separation of the right and left ventricles may be adequate at rest, with the poorer resolution and motion associated with bicycle exercise, separation no longer may be adequate. Unfortunately, the left anterior oblique position image, which is required for calculation of left ventricular ejection fraction, is a suboptimal view for visual evaluation of left ventricular regional wall motion. Definition of septal wall motion abnormalities is difficult and the reproducibility of defining septal wall motion abnormalities is poor [66]. The significance of an inferoapical wall motion abnormality often is difficult to assess in the left anterior oblique position, because this region may represent either the inferior wall, the apex, or a combination of the two. The left ventricular apex may be tipped superiorly and anteriorly, making it difficult to delineate the actual anatomic region involved. Thus, only the inferolateral and posterolateral segments can be evaluated well visually on this view. Because of these problems, some laboratories now perform equilibrium exercise imaging in two positions. This requires repeating the entire study from rest to exercise in the anterior position. Nevertheless, independent of the number of views acquired, regional wall motion is difficult to evaluate from a two-minute acquisition with a high sensitivity collimator and superimposed patient motion.

Exercise ventricular performance studies also can be obtained with first-pass radionuclide angiocardiography. In the future with further development in new instrumentation and radionuclides, this may well evolve into the preferred method of evaluating ventricular performance during exercise. When using technetium-99m as the radiotracer, the resting study frequently is performed with technetium-99m di-ethylene-triamine-penta-acetic acid (DTPA). The peak exercise study then can be performed with technetium-99m pertechnetate following renal clearance of the initially injected tracer. The resting study is performed initially, with the patient fully positioned in front of the detector and his feet in the bicycle ergometry pedals. A similar exercise protocol as described earlier for equilibrium blood pool imaging is employed. The exercise radionuclide angiocardiogram is obtained at the peak of exercise with the patient still pedaling maximally. When studies are performed with the computerized multicrystal camera, it often is helpful to hold the patient directly against the vertical detector. The bolus injection should be made while the thorax is stabilized, but while the patient is still exercising. If studies are performed only in the immediate post-exercise period, non-diagnostic information may be obtained.

Careful definition of the normal left ventricular response to exercise is mandatory. There have been differences in various reports in the literature concerning the normal left ventricular response. Some of the differences may reside in the definition of the normal population selected for study. The so-called "normal" standard may be based upon data acquired in relatively young presumably normal volunteers without evidence of cardiopulmonary disease such as laboratory personnel, trainees or investigators, patients with chest pain but normal coronary angiograms, and patients with a very low pre-test likelihood of disease based upon sequential Bayesian analysis [62, 66]. It should be noted that those with chest pain and normal coronary arteriograms may not always behave normally [67]. Most laboratories define the normal left ventricular response to exercise as an *absolute* increment in ejection fraction of at least 5% (ejection fraction units) without development of regional wall motion abnormalities [62, 68]. This may be associated with a small increase in left ventricular end-diastolic volume. A similar definition of normal exercise left ventricular reserve involves a *relative* 10% increase in left ventricular ejection fraction from rest to exercise [65]. However, within the normal range of left ventricular ejection fractions (greater than 50%), this definition is almost identical to the one previously described. In the uncommon cases when left ventricular ejection fraction is markedly elevated at rest (greater than 75%), usually due to exaggerated resting sympathetic tone, a normal response has been defined as no fall in ejection fraction with stress. The definition of normal exercise left ventricular reserve has been based upon studies involving both submaximal and maximal exercise workloads. Other have defined the normal response only by the absolute level of ejection fraction reached during exercise. This presents several problems and we do not advocate this definition. First, within the spectrum of normal, there can be a wide range of resting values. Of more importance, in the presence of an abnormal baseline, an individual may augment substantially but fail to reach a prescribed level derived from experience with patients with higher baseline levels. Clearly, increasing ejection fraction from 30% to 50% is substantial and indicates excellent reserve, irrespective of the absolute value obtained with exercise.

It is critical to recognize that inadequate stress due to physical limitations may result in apparently normal responses in spite of severe coronary artery disease. In the presence of an inadequate exercise end-point, the sensitivity for detecting coronary disease by virtue of an abnormal left ventricular response may fall from approximately 90% to 60% (Figure 5) [62]. In addition, when performed for diagnostic reasons, exercise radionuclide angiocardiography should not be performed when patients are receiving beta-adrenergic blocking agents or other antianginals. Several studies have indicated that beta blockers in particular can totally convert an abnormal response to normal [69]. The same may hold for other therapeutic modalities [70]. If this is not clinically feasible, the

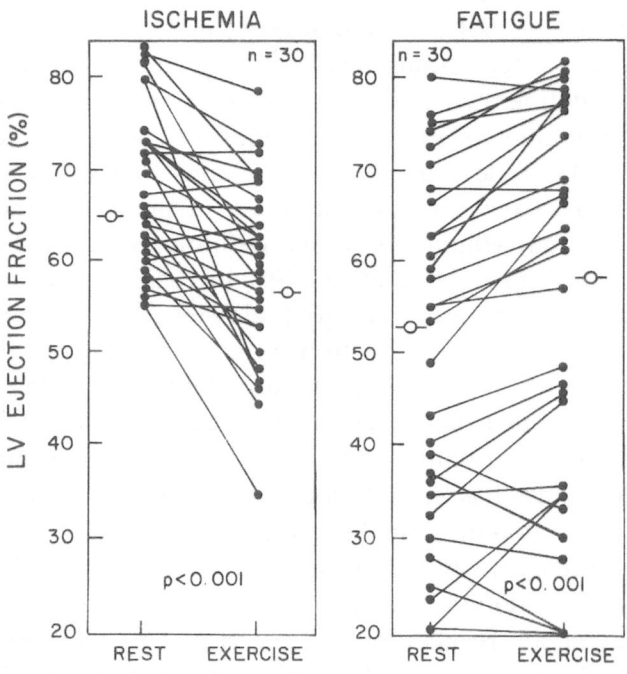

Figure 5. Rest and exercise left ventricular ejection fraction in 60 patients with coronary artery disease. Patients are subdivided into those with electrocardiographic evidence of myocardial ischemia and those who exercized only to an end-point of fatigue. Note that all 30 patients with ischemia had a normal resting ejection fraction but an abnormal ejection fraction response. In contrast, there was a wider range of resting left ventricular ejection fractions in those exercizing to fatigue. In addition, the exercise response was variable. Overall, the sensitivity of exercise radionuclide angiocardiography for detection of coronary artery disease in this patient population was approximately 85%. LV = left ventricle. Reproduced with permission from Berger HJ, Reduto LA, Johnstone DE, et al.: Global and regional left ventricular response to bicycle exercise in coronary artery disease: assessment by quantitative radionuclide angiocardiography. Am J Med 66: 13–21, 1979.

diagnostic value of a negative result has less impact and should be interpreted accordingly.

Exercise-induced regional wall motion abnormalities occur frequently in association with abnormal global responses and left ventricular dilatation. While regional wall motion abnormalities, except of the apex, are relatively specific for coronary artery disease, they occur less frequently than exercise-induced abnormalities in global ventricular performance [71, 72, 73, 74]. In addition, because of the lower technical quality of two-minute gated equilibrium studies, they may be very difficult to appreciate.

Based upon pooled results in the literature since 1978, the sensitivity of exercise radionuclide angiocardiography for detection of coronary artery disease is approximately 85 to 90% [75]. From a pooled analysis of 427 patients initially reported between 1978 and 1980, a specificity of 92% was noted. However, using a multivariate analysis, a subsequent study noted a significantly lower specificity [73]. The precise values obtained for specificity depend upon the criteria used for defining a normal response, as well as the criteria for patient entry. Clearly, stress-induced left ventricular dysfunction is a finding common to many if not most forms of heart disease. In a direct diagnostic comparison of upright exercise radionuclide angiocardiography and treadmill exercise testing, the radionuclide study had a significantly higher diagnostic accuracy for detecting coronary artery disease. The sensitivity of exercise radionuclide ventricular performance studies is highest in patients who exercise maximally to an appropriate endpoint, in those with left main coronary artery stenosis and/or triple vessel disease, and when there is electrocardiographic evidence of myocardial ischemia [71, 73, 76]. The frequency of abnormal ejection fraction responses and the magnitude of fall in left ventricular ejection fraction with exercise increase as the severity of coronary artery disease increases. However, in an individual patient, the extent of exercise-induced left ventricular dysfunction appears to be more a marker of the severity of transient myocardial ischemia rather than the number of coronary arteries involved. By virtue of the amount of myocardium involved, there are many instances in which a single critical left anterior descending coronary stenosis may result in the same ejection fraction response as three angiographically significant coronary lesions.

References

1. Strauss HW, Zaret BL, Hurley PJ, Natarajan TK, Pitt B: A scintiphotographic method for measuring left ventricular ejection fraction in man without cardiac catheterization. Am J Cardiol 28: 575–580, 1971.
2. Zaret BL, Strauss HW, Hurley PJ, Natarajan TK, Pitt B: A noninvasive scintiphotographic method for detecting regional ventricular dysfunction in man. N Engl J Med 284: 1165–1170, 1971.
3. Dyke D van, Anger HO, Sullivan RW, Vetter WR, Yano Y, Parker HG: Cardiac evaluation from radioisotope dynamics. J Nucl Med 13: 585–592, 1972.
4. Zaret B, Berger H: Techniques of nuclear cardiology, In: Hurst JW (ed), The heart. New York, McGraw-Hill, pp 1803–1843, 1981.
5. Berger HJ, Matthay RA, Pytlik LM, Gottschalk A, Zaret BL: First-pass radionuclide assessment of right and left ventricular performance in patients with cardiac and pulmonary disease. Semin Nucl Med 9: 275–295, 1979.
6. Wackers FJ, Giles RW, Hoffer PB, Lange RC, Berger HJ, Zaret BL: Gold-195m, a new generator-produced short-lived radionuclide for sequential assessment of ventricular performance by first-pass radionuclide angiocardiography. Am J Cardiol 50: 89–94, 1982.
7. Holman BL, Neirinckx RD, Treves S, Tow DE: Cardiac imaging with tantalum-178. Radiology 131: 525–526, 1979.
8. Treves S, Cheng C, Samuel A, et al.: Iridium-191 angiocardiography for the detection and quantitation of left-to-right shunting. J Nucl Med 21: 1151–1157, 1980.
9. Wackers FJTh, Stein R, Lange R, et al.: Sequential first-pass assessment of left ventricular performance during upright exercise in man with short half-life gold-195m: combined studies with Tl-201 perfusion imaging. J Am College Cardiol 1: 578, 1983 (abstract).
10. Berger HJ, Matthay RA, Loke J, Marshall RC, Gottschalk A, Zaret BL: Assessment of cardiac performance with quantitative radionuclide angiocardiography: right ventricular ejection fraction with reference to findings in chronic obstructive pulmonary disease. Am J Cardiol 41: 897–905, 1978.
11. Berger HJ, Gottschalk A, Zaret BL: Radionuclide assessment of left and right ventricular performance. Radiol Clin North Am 18: 441–466, 1980.
12. Marshall RC, Berger HJ, Costin JC, et al.: Assessment of cardiac performance with quantitative radionuclide angiocardiography: sequential left ventricular ejection fraction, normalized left ventricular ejection rate, and regional wall motion. Circulation 56: 820–829, 1977.
13. Rerych SK, Scholz PM, Newman GE, Sabiston DC Jr, Jones RH: Cardiac function at rest and during exercise in normals and in patients with coronary heart disease: evaluation by radionuclide angiocardiography. Ann Surg 187: 449–464, 1978.
14. Schelbert HR, Verba JW, Johnson AD, et al.: Nontraumatic determination of left ventricular ejection fraction by radionuclide angiocardiography. Circulation 51: 902–909, 1975.
15. Jengo JA, Oren V, Conant R, et al.: Effects of maximal exercise stress on left ventricular function in patients with coronary artery disease using first-pass radionuclide angiocardiography: a rapid, noninvasive technique for determining ejection fraction and segmental wall motion. Circulation 59: 60–65, 1979.
16. Marshall RC, Berger HJ, Reduto LA, Cohen LS, Gottschalk A, Zaret BL: Assessment of cardiac performance with quantitative radionuclide angiocardiography: effects of oral propranolol on global and regional left ventricular function in coronary artery disease. Circulation 58: 808–814, 1978.
17. Bodenheimer MM, Banka VS, Fooshee CM, Gillespie JA, Helfant RH: Detection of coronary heart disease using radionuclide determined regional ejection fraction at rest and during handgrip exercise: correlation with coronary arteriography. Circulation 58: 640–648, 1978.
18. Scholz PM, Rerych SK, Moran JF, et al.: Quantitative radionuclide angiocardiography. Cathet Cardiovasc Diagn 6: 265–283, 1980.

19. Burow RD, Strauss HW, Singleton R, et al.: Analysis of left ventricular function from mulitple gated acquisition cardiac blood pool imaging: comparison to contrast angiography. Circulation 56: 1024–1028, 1977.

20. Green MV, Ostrow HG, Douglas MA, et al.: High temporal resolution ECG-gated scintigraphic angiocardiography. J Nucl Med 16: 95–98, 1975.

21. Pavel DG, Zimmer AM, Patterson VN: In vivo labeling of red blood cells with ^{99m}Tc: a new approach to blood pool visualization. J Nucl Med 18: 305–308, 1977.

22. Callahan RJ, Froelich JW, McKusick KA, Leppo J, Strauss HW: A modified method for the in vivo labeling of red blood cells with Tc-99m: concise communication. J Nucl Med 23: 315–318, 1982.

23. Bacharach SL, Green MV, Borer JS, Douglas MA, Ostrow HG, Johnston GS: A real-time system for multi-image gated cardiac studies. J Nucl Med 18: 79–84, 1977.

24. Bacharach SL, Green MV, Borer JS: Instrumentation and data processing in cardiovascular nuclear medicine: evaluation of ventricular function. Semin Nucl Med 9: 257–274, 1979.

25. Van Aswegen A, Alderson PO, Nickoloff EL, Householder DF, Wagner HJ Jr: Temporal resolution requirements for left ventricular time-activity curves. Radiology 135: 165–170, 1980.

26. Kelly MJ, Giles RW, Simon TS, et al.: Multigated equilibrium radionuclide angiocardiography: improved detection of left ventricular wall motion abnormalities and aneurysms by the addition of the left lateral view. Radiology 139: 167–173, 1981.

27. Holman BL, Wynne J, Zielonka JS, Iodine JD: A simplified technique for measuring right ventricular ejection fraction using the equilibrium radionuclide angiocardiogram and the slant-hole collimator. Radiology 138: 429–435, 1981.

28. Parker JA, Uren RF, Jones AG, et al.: Radionuclide left ventriculography with the slant hole collimator. J Nucl Med 18: 848–851, 1977.

29. Bourguignon MH, Douglass KH, Links JM, Wagner HN Jr: Fully automated data acquisition, processing, and display in equilibrium radioventriculography. Eur J Nucl Med 6: 343–347, 1981.

30. Chang W, Henkin RE, Hale DJ, Hall D: Methods for detection of left ventricular edges. Semin Nucl Med 10: 39–53, 1980.

31. Goris ML, Briandet PA, Thomas AJ, McKillop JH, Sneed P, Wiklander DP: A thresholding for radionuclide angiocardiography. Invest Radiol 16: 115–119, 1981.

32. Sorensen SG, Ritchie JL, Caldwell JH, Hamilton GW, Kennedy JW: Serial exercise radionuclide angiography. Validation of count-derived changes in cardiac output and quantitation of maximal exercise ventricular volume change after nitroglycerin and propranolol in normal men. Circulation 61: 600–609.

33. Wackers FJ, Berger HJ, Johnstone DE, et al.: Multiple gated cardiac blood pool imaging for left ventricular ejection fraction: validation of the technique and assessment of variability. Am J Cardiol 43: 1159–1166, 1979.

34. Adam WE, Tarkowska A, Bitter F, Stauch M, Geffers H: Equilibrium (gated) radionuclide ventriculography. Cardiovasc Radiol 2: 161–173, 1979.

35. Goris ML, McKillop JH, Briandet PA: A fully automated determination of the left ventricular region of interest in nuclear angiocardiography. Cardiovasc Intervent Radiol 4: 117–123, 1981.

36. Alpert NM, Strauss HW, Tarolli EJ, Chesler DA: Determination of ventricular borders by adaptive filtering. J Nucl Med 21 (6): P47, 1980 (abstract).

37. Maddox DE, Wynne J, Uren R, et al.: Regional ejection fraction: a quantitative radionuclide index of regional left ventricular performance. Circulation 59: 1001–1009, 1979.

38. Papapietro SE, Yester MV, Logic JR, et al.: Method for quantitative analysis of regional left ventricular function with first-pass and gated blood pool scintigraphy. Am J Cardiol 47: 618–625, 1981.

39. Maddoc DE, Holman BL, Wynne J, et al.: Ejection fraction image: a noninvasive index of regional left ventricular wall motion. Am J Cardiol 41: 1230–1238, 1978.

40. Ratib O, Henze E, Schön H, Schelbert HR: Phase analysis of radionuclide ventriculograms for

150

the detection of coronary artery disease. Am Heart J 104: 1–12, 1982.

41. Botvinick E, Dunn R, Frais M, et al.: The phase image: its relationship to patterns of contraction and conduction. Circulation 65: 551–560, 1982.

42. Frais MA, Botvinick EH, Shosa DW, et al.: Phase image characterization of ventricular contraction in left and right bundle branch block. Am J Cardiol 50: 95–105, 1982.

43. Links JM, Douglas KH, Wagner HN Jr: Patterns of ventricular emptying by Fourier analysis of gated blood pool studies. J Nucl Med 21: 978–982, 1980.

44. Turner DA, Von Behren PL, Ruggie NT, et al.: Noninvasive identification of initial site of abnormal ventricular activation by least-square phase analysis of radionuclide cineangiograms. Circularion 65: 1511–1518, 1982.

45. Verba J, Bornstein I, Almasi J, Goliash T, Eisner R, Howak D: The application of three-dimensional Fourier filtering techniques to nuclear cardia studies. J Nucl Med 20 (6): P658, 1979 (abstract).

46. Okada RD, Pohost GM, Kirshenbaum HD, et al.: Radionuclide determined changes in pulmonary blood volume with exercise: improved sensitivity of multigated blood pool scanning in detecting corronary artery disease. N Engl J Med 301: 569–576, 1979.

47. Rutlen D, Wackers F, Zaret B: Radionuclide assessment of peripheral intravascular capacity: a new technique to measure intravascular volume changes in the capacitance circulation in man. Circulation 64: 146–152, 1981.

48. Dehmer GJ, Lewis SE, Hillis LD, et al.: Nongeometric determination of left ventricular volumes from equilibrium blood pool scans. Am J Cardiol 45: 293–300, 1980.

49. Links JM, Becker LC, Shindledecker JG, et al.: Measurement of absolute left ventricular volume from gated blood pool studies. Circulation 65: 82–91, 1982.

50. Slutsky R, Karliner J, Ricci D, et al.: Ventricular volumes by gated equilibrium radionuclide angiography: a new method. Circulation 60: 556–564, 1979.

51. Bough EW, Gandsman EJ, North DL, Shulman RS: Gated radionuclide angiographic evaluation of valve regurgitation. Am J Cardiol 46: 423–428, 1980.

52. Rigo P, Alderson PO, Robertson RM, Becker LC, Wagner HN Jr: Measurement of aortic and mitral regurgitation by gated cardiac blood pool scans. Circulation 60: 306–312, 1979.

53. Sorenson SG, O'Rourke RA, Chaudhuri TK: Noninvasive quantitation of valvular regurgitation by gated equilibrium radionuclide angiography. Circulation 62: 1089–1098, 1980.

54. Lam W, Pavel D, Byrom E, Sheikh A, Best D, Rosen K: Radionuclide regurgitant index: value and limitations. Am J Cardiol 47: 292–298, 1981.

55. Bacharach SL, Green MV, Borer JS, Ostrow HG, Redwood DR, Johnston GS: ECG-gated scintillation probe measurement of left ventricular function. J Nucl Med 18: 1176–1183, 1977.

56. Berger HJ, Davies RA, Batsford WP, Hoffer PB, Gottschalk A, Zaret BL: Beat-to beat left ventricular performance assessed from the equilibrium cardiac blood pool using a computerized nuclear probe. Circulation 63: 133–142, 1981.

57. Wagner HN Jr, Wake R, Nickoloff E, Natarajan TK: The nuclear stethoscope: a simple device for generation of left ventricular volume curves. Am J Cardiol 38: 747–750, 1976.

58. Schneider J, Berger HJ, Sands M, Lachman A, Zaret B: Beat to beat left ventricular performance in artrial fibrillation: radionuclide assessment with the computerized nuclear probe. Am J Cardiol 51: 1189–1195, 1983.

59. Giles RW, Berger HJ, Barash PG, et al.: Continuous monitoring of left ventricular performance with the computerized nuclear probe during laryngoscopy and intubation prior to coronary artery bypass surgery. Am J Cardiol 50: 735–741, 1982.

60. Berger HJ, Byrd W, Giles R, Orphanoudakis S, Zaret BL: Beat-to-beat left ventricular pressure-volume relationships assessed from the equilibrium cardiac blood pool using a computerized nonimaging nuclear probe, In: Computers in Cardiology. New York, IEEE computer Society, pp 55–60, 1982.

61. Marx P, Borkowski H, Sands MJ, Wolfson S, Berger HJ, Zaret BL: Exercise left ventricular

performance in aortic regurgitation: dissimilar responses in supine and upright positions. Circulation 66: II-354, 1982 (abstract).

62. Berger HJ, Reduto LA, Johnstone DE, et al.: Global and regional left ventricular response to bicycle exercise in coronary artery disease: assessment by quantitative radionuclide angiocardiography. Am J Med 66: 13–21, 1979.

63. Borer JS, Bacharach SL, Green MV, Kent KM, Epstein SE, Johnston GS: Real-time radionuclide cineangiography in the noninvasive evaluation of global and regional left ventricular function at rest and during exercise in patients with coronary artery disease. N Engl J Med 296: 839–844, 1977.

64. Caldwell JH, Hamilton GW, Sorensen SG, Ritchie JL, Williams DL, Kennedy JW: The detection of coronary artery disease with radionuclide techniques: a comparison of rest-exercise thallium imaging and ejection fraction response. Circulation 61: 610–619, 1980.

65. Rozanski A, Berman D, Gray R, et al.: Preoperative prediction of reversible myocardial asynergy by postexercise radionuclide ventriculography. N Engl J Med 307: 212–216, 1982.

66. Poliner LR, Dehmer GJ, Lewis SE, Parkey RW, Blomqvist CG, Willerson JT: Left ventricular performance in normal subjects: a comparison of the responses to exercise in the upright and supine positions. Circulation 62: 528–534, 1980.

67. Berger HJ, Sands MJ, Davies RA, et al.: Exercise left ventricular performance in patients with chest pain, ischemic-appearing exercise electrocardiograms, and angiographically normal coronary arteries. Ann Intern Med 94: 186–191, 1981.

68. Brady TJ, Lo K, Thrall JH, Walton JA, Brymer JF, Pitt B: Exercise radionuclide ejection fraction: correlation with exercise contrast ventriculography. Radiology 132: 703–705, 1979.

69. Marshall RC, Wisenberg G, Schelbert HR, Henze E: Effect of oral propranolol on rest, exercise and postexercise left ventricular performance in normal subjects and patients with coronary artery disease. Circulation 63: 572–583, 1981.

70. Borer JS, Bacharach SL, Green MV, Kent KM, Johnston GS, Epstein SE: Effect of nitroglycerin on exercise-induced abnormalities of left ventricular regional function and ejection fraction in coronary artery disease: assessment by radionuclide cineangiography in symptomatic and asymptomatic patients. Circulation 57: 314–320, 1978.

71. Borer JS, Kent KM, Bacharach SL, et al.: Sensitivity, specificity and predictive accuracy of radionuclide cineangiography during exercise in patients with coronary artery disease: comparison with exercise electrocardiography. Circulation 60: 572–580, 1979.

72. Hecht HS, Hopkins JM: Exercise-induced regional wall motion abnormalities on radionuclide angiography. Lack of reliability for detection of coronary artery disease in the presence of valvular heart disease. Am J Cardiol 47: 861–865, 1981.

73. Jones RH, McEwan P, Newman G, et al.: The accuracy of diagnosis of coronary artery disease by radionuclide measurements of left ventricular function during rest and exercise. Circulation 64: 586–601, 1981.

74. Kent KM, Bonow RO, Rosing DR, et al.: Improved myocardial function during exercise after successful percutaneous transluminal coronary angioplasty. N Eng J Med 306: 441–445, 1982.

75. Okada RD, Boucher CA, Strauss HW, Pohost GM: Exercise radionuclide imaging approaches to coronary artery disease. Am J Cardiol 46: 1188–1204, 1980.

76. Newman GF, Rerych SK, Upton MT, Sabiston DC Jr, Jones RH: Comparison of electrocardiographic and left ventricular functional changes during exercise. Circulation 62: 1204–1211, 1980.

8. The detection of intracardiac shunts and valvular regurgitation by radionuclide angiography

Pierre Rigo

Introduction

The value of radionuclide angiography for evaluation of patients with intracardiac shunts or valvular regurgitation has long been recognized [1]. Since both these abnormalities primarily impose a volume overload on the left or the right ventricle, recent advances in the radionuclide angiographic determination of ventricular volumes have enhanced the capabilities of this technique to assess the functional importance of shunts or regurgitation. In addition, radionuclide angiography can be used to measure flow through the heart. Thus theoretically it should be an ideal technique to detect, quantify and assess the functional repercussion of shunts and aortic- or mitral regurgitation [2].

In this review, we will describe the basic techniques of radionuclide angiography as well as the proposed methods for quantitation of left to right and right to left shunts, and for detection and quantitation of valvular regurgitation, together with their clinical indications.

Methodology

Isotopes to be used for radionuclide angiography

Radionuclide techniques for detection of intracardiac shunts and mitral- or aortic regurgitation mainly employ non diffusible tracers that remain in the intravascular space. Technetium labeled serum albumin or preferably labeled red blood cells are mostly used and are mandatory for equilibrium studies. For first pass studies, however, a tracer that diffuses from the intravascular space can be used, provided that diffusion is fast enough to allow separation of the initial and recirculation curves. Technetium pertechnetate and ^{15}O labeled water satisfy these latter requirements [3]. Other new short-lived isotopes such as Iridium-191m, Tantalum-178, or

Gold-195m can also be used for first pass radionuclide angiography. These generator-produced tracers allow significant reduction of the radiation dose to the patient. Furthermore, studies with these tracers can be repeated within a few minutes in order to assess the effect of an intervention, and in case of an inadequate bolus injection [4, 5, 6]. Krypton-81m (13 sec T 1/2), a generator produced diffusible gas (Rb-81 Kr-81m) can be administered intravenously, dissolved in a glucose solution. It is exchanged at the alveolar capillary level and is mostly exhaled. Insignificant amounts remain in the systematic circulation. Therefore, it is an ideal tracer to study the function of the right ventricle and to document right to left shunts [7]. Similarly, technetium labeled macroaggregates or microspheres are useful tracers for quantification of right to left shunting. These particles are normally trapped in the pulmonary capillaries but shunted particles will reach the systemic circulation. Although available data suggest a wide margin of safety, the use of this technique has been limited due to theoretical concern over microembolisation of systemic end-arteries [8].

First pass radionuclide angiography [9]

In this technique, a single small bolus of the tracer is administered intravenously. In order to achieve a discrete bolus in the right atrium, a central venous catheter or jugular vein injection is frequently used. Moreover, in our experience, the use of an antecubital vein is adequate for most purposes. The volume of the tracer should remain as small as possible (less than 1 ml for 20 mCi). Whenever possible, we use a small intravenous catheter and flush the isotope from a prefilled extension tube with 5–20 ml saline, depending on the age of the patient. With this system we can wait until the patient is relaxed before the injection is given in order to avoid Valsalva manoeuvers which can influence the size and direction of the shunt as well as pulmonary blood flow and the shape of the pulmonary curves. The transit of the indicator through the heart and lungs is usually examined by the camera in the anterior projection. That projection is closest to the chest for best resolution and positioning is easy. It provides the best separation between the lungs and the right and left heart cavities. Other projections such as the left anterior oblique projection which provides a better separation of the left and the right ventricles and the RAO projection which better separates the atria and ventricles can also be used. The data are recorded in list or frame mode. Two to four frames per second depending on the heart rate are adequate for left to right shunt evaluation while 20 frames/second or more are required for evaluation of ventricular function. After completion of the study, the quality of the bolus should be checked in a region of interest over the superior vena cava. For left to right shunt studies, a bolus of 2 seconds or less duration is required (FWHM).

Concomitant recording of the electrocardiogram allows for direct (gated first pass) or retrospective synchronisation of the data to produce an average cardiac cycle suitable for evaluation of global and regional systolic left ventricular function. Evaluation of diastolic filling with first pass is difficult since the concentration of the tracer in the heart diastole changes continuously [10]. For assessment of valvular regurgitation during first pass left and right ventricular- as well as atrial time-activity curves can be constructed with appropriate regions of interest. In patients with left to right shunts, evaluation of left ventricular function is frequently inadequate from first pass data, since the temporal separation of the left and right ventricles is blurred as a result of recirculation. The technique for the first pass studies is similar if short-lived isotopes are used. One tracer, $C^{15}O_2$, can be administered by inhalation and results in the labeling of water directly into the pulmonary capillaries thus bypassing the venous circuit and right heart transit. This results in a compact bolus in the left atrium with better separation of the first transit and recirculation peaks for evaluation of left to right shunts. Furthermore, labeled water distributes in the whole body water content, thus systemic recirculation is delayed and diminished and has less influence on the shunt curves [11].

Equilibrium radionuclide angiography [12]

The equilibrium study is performed after equilibration of a vascular tracer, preferably labeled red cells, into the blood pool. The data are acquired as 16–64 frames spanning the entire cardiac cycle. Acquisition is performed for 200 to 600 cardiac cycles (2 to 8 minutes, usually 4 minutes) yielding more than 250 K counts per frame (25 mCi in adults with a LEAP or high sensitivity collimator). Details are discussed in chapters 7 and 9.

The left anterior oblique projection used for evaluation of shunts and regurgitation must provide adequate separation of both ventricles from adjacent structures. We start with 35° LAO with 5–10° of cranio-caudal obliquity, but modify the angulation as needed using the persistence scope. The use of a slanthole collimator can also help to achieve adequate positioning. After acquisition, phase and amplitude images of the first Fourier coefficient of the regional time-activity curves are generated.

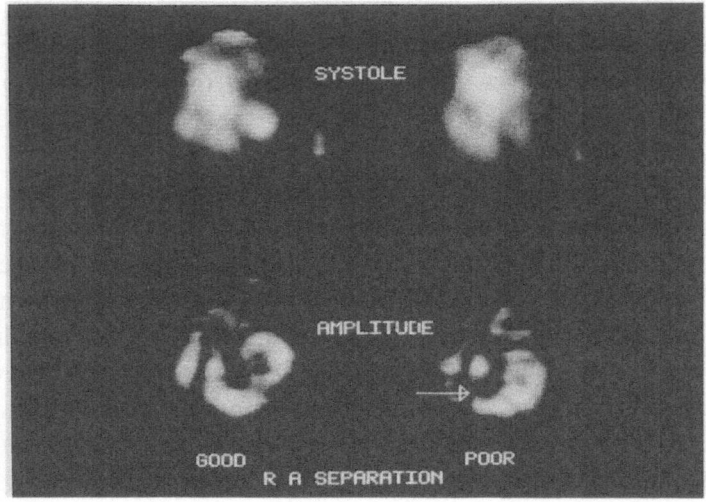

Figure 1. Examples of good and poor positioning with adequate and inadequate right atrial separation. In case of right atrial overlap, a discontinuity in the right ventricular amplitude image is observed (arrow). This overlap causes underestimation of the right ventricular stroke counts and the acquisition should be repeated.

Identification of all 4 cardiac chambers is required for adequate positioning. In cases of significant overlap, for instance if one of the atria is not individualized, or if the right ventricular amplitude image is distorted by the atrial overlap which causes a discontinuity of the external border of the image, acquisition is repeated after repositioning (Figure 1).

Adquate positioning can be obtained in more than 90% of the cases. It is most difficult in patients with marked right ventricular dilatation, in patients with isolated left atrial enlargement, as in mitral stenosis, and in patients with left ventricular septal aneurysm [13].

Measurement of ventricular volumes rely on the count-volume proportionality principle. To estimate ventricular counts, definition of areas of interest over the left and right ventricles and a background region is required. Since the background remains essentially stable during the cardiac cycle, background correction is not necessary for the calculation of stroke counts.

Automatic programs for the definition of areas of interest have been proposed for the left ventricle as described in chapter 9, but none are currently satisfactory for the right ventricle. We therefore prefer to trace the region of interest manually with the help of functional images. Con-

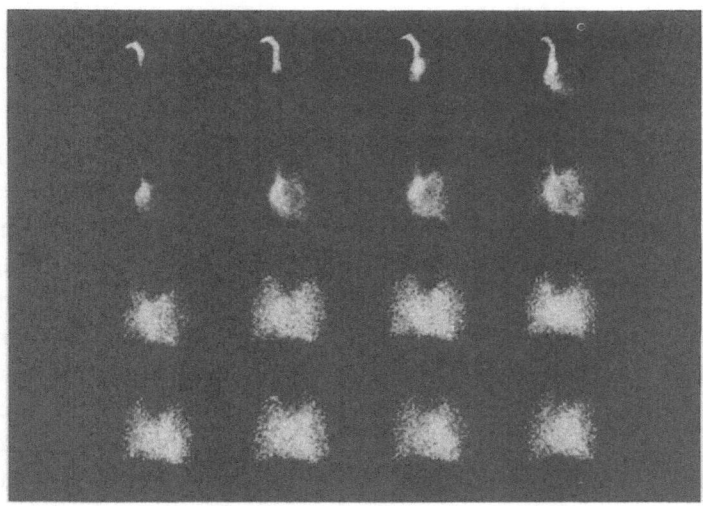

Figure 2. First transit study (one image every 0.5 second) in a patient with atrial septal defect. Persistance of activity in the lungs and poor visualisation of the left ventricle and aorta are suggestive of a left to right shunt.

comitant examination of end-diastolic and end-systolic frames, Fourier amplitude and phase images can help to define the functional limits for an "average" chamber where calculated stroke counts are maximal.

Transformations of the arbitrary units of counts into volume requires normalization for the time of acquisition, radioactive decay, tracer concentration and attenuation. Collection of a blood sample at the time of acquisition gives adequate measurement of tracer concentration, but attenuation correction is more difficult. One proposed method involves calculation of the mean depth of the left ventricle through geometric measurement and of attenuation using a theoretical value for tissue density. Other techniques measure the attenuation factor with the aid of a known source of activity in the right ventricle or oesophagus [14–18]. While these techniques can provide a reasonable estimate of left and probably right ventricular volumes, absolute measurements are not necessary in case of normalized parameters such as ejection fraction, ejection rate, filling rate or left to right stroke volume ratio. However, absolute measurements are necessary to calculate the derived parameters of stroke volume or cardiac output at equilibrium.

Detection of left to right shunts

First pass technique

The technique of choice to assess patients with left to right shunts is first pass radionuclide angiography performed as indicated earlier. Inspection of serial 0.5–1 second images obtained during the initial cardio-pulmonary transit may be diagnostic for left to right shunts by demonstrating persistance of the activity in the lungs and poor visualisation of the left ventricle and aorta. This reflects recirculation of the tracer in the pulmonary circuit (Figure 2). Careful inspection of the images may help to differentiate a patent ductus arteriosus from an atrial septal defect or a ventricular septal defect. Indeed, with patent ductus arteriosus activity returns directly to the pulmonary artery and the right heart is void of activity during shunt recirculation. More precise localization of the shunt requires careful analysis of the time-activity curves at several regions of interest over the superior vena cava, right atrium, right ventricle and lungs [8]. Quantitative analysis has usually been performed on time-activity curves calculated over the lungs, for both practical and theoretical reasons. Regions of interest over the lungs are easy to trace either manually or with the help of a semi-automatic program based on time to peak functional images [19]. The indicator is usually uniformly mixed by passage through mixing chambers and valves, and the counting geometry and efficacy are unchanged during first and recirculating transit. Sampling closer to the level of the shunt would be subject to errors due to poor mixing, especially because a right atrial or right ventricular region of interest can only sample part of these chambers. A more distal sample would further spread the curves and obliterate separation between its components.

Analysis of the pulmonary time-activity curve is performed by calculation of an activity ratio. The C2/C1 ratio first proposed by Folse and Braunwald is the simple ratio between the peak count rate of the first transit curve C1 at a time T1 after the first appearance of the activity (or more reliably when activity reaches some percentage, i.e., 10% of the peak activity) and the count rate C2 on the descending limb of the time-activity curve at a time $T2 = 2 \times T1$ (Figure 3). This method is reliable to discriminate normal patients from those with a shunt. It is not as reliable whenever cardiac abnormalities other than shunts produce a widening of the first transit curve, such as valvular heart disease or cardiomyopathies [20].

CTS/0.5 SEC

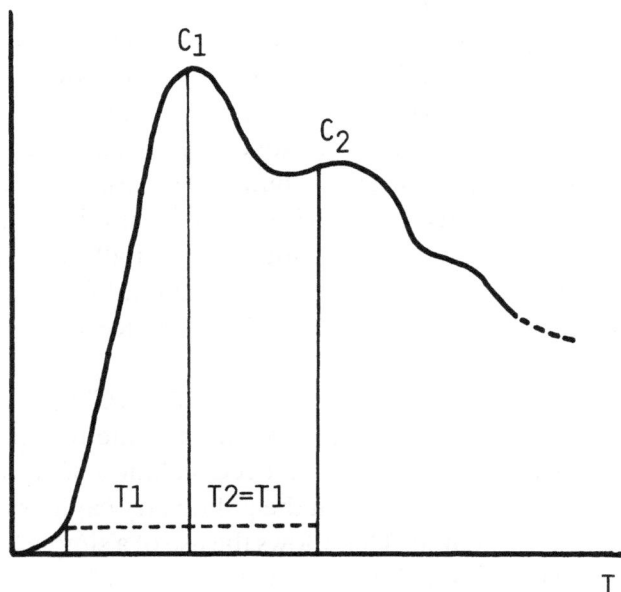

Figure 3. Calculation of the C2/C1 ratio. This is done on the pulmonary time-activity curve (usually of the right lung). The time to peak (T1) and activity at peak (C1) are first determined. The activity C2 at a time occurring after peak at a time T2 (peak to T2 = T1) is then measured and the ratio calculated. See text for further details.

Mathematical curve fitting to the data of the pulmonary time-activity curve reduces the dependence on statistically less reliable values Anderson *et al.* suggested dividing the descending portion of the pulmonary time-activity curve into two sections by extending and exponential function from its peak [21]. The area under the time-activity curve is divided into 2 regions, one above the extrapolated curve (area x) and one below (area y). The ratio of these areas is used to determine the presence and size of a shunt. This technique is a slight modification of a method discussed by Flaherty, which used the overall time-activity curve rather than its descending portion [22]. Maltz and Treves used a computer to fit a gamma variate function to the initial pulmonary transit and then again to the shunt curve calculated as the difference between the areas on the first gamma variate function (A1) and the real data curve [23]. As the geometry and counting efficiency do not change, indicator dilution principles indicate that the area under this second gamma variate function (A2) is proportional to shunt flow while A1 is proportional to the total pulmonary

160

flow. The gamma variate technique thus allow immediate calculation of QP/QS as illustrated in Figure 4.

More recently, a method has been described that utilizes multiple deconvolutions as input function. First, the superior vena cava time-activity curve is deconvolved to correct for the spread of the bolus, and secondly the right ventricular time-activity curve to predict the pulmonary transfer function without shunt. Comparison of the deconvolved pulmonary time-activity curve with the measured pulmonary transfer function allows determination of shunt flow in all patients except those with patent ductus arteriosus in whom the shunt flow does not affect the right ventricle. Unfortunately, clinical experience with this technique is limited as yet [24].

Calculation of the shunt can be simplified when $C^{15}O_2$ is inhaled in order to produce a bolus of $H_2^{15}O$. The separation of the first transit and shunt component is now improved, systemic recirculation of $H_2^{15}O$ is diminished and the disappearance curve from the pulmonary capillary volume is very close to a true exponential. This allows the use of a simple height ratio with a constant factor ($e = 2.72$) representing the influence of the spread produced by the first recirculation, to calculate the shunt fraction and QP/QS [25].

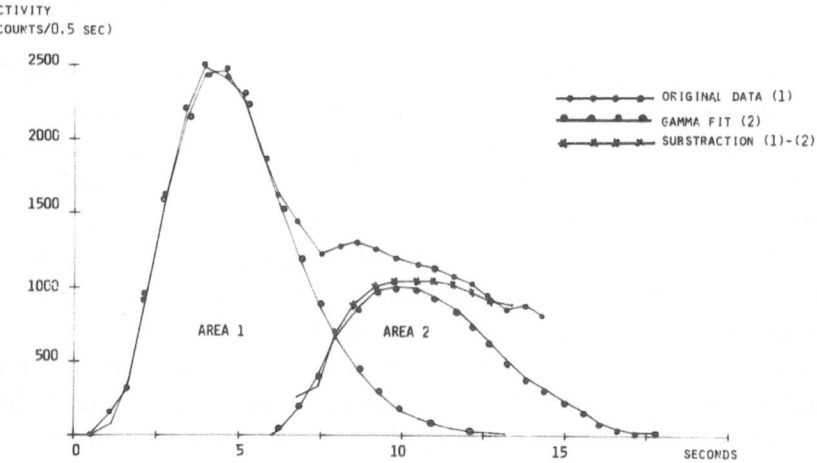

Figure 4. Calculation of the QP/QS using the gamma variate technique of Maltz and Treves (see text). The raw data, the gamma fit to the initial part of the curve, the substracted shunt curve, and the gammafit to the shunt curve are displayed. The area under the first gammafit A1 is proportional to the total pulmonary blood flow, while the area under the second gammafit A2 is proportional to the shunt flow.

Equilibrium technique

Evaluation of shunts at equilibrium relies on the comparison of the left- and right ventricular stroke counts. The results depend on the location of the shunt and on the flow dynamics through the shunt. Partial anomalous pulmonary venous return and an atrial septal defect result in right ventricular overload, patent ductus arteriosus overloads the left ventricle. The situation is more complex in a ventricular septal defect. Shunt flow occurring during systole in a VSD does not produce diastolic volume overload of the right ventricle while left to right shunt flow that occurs during diastole is counted as right ventricular diastolic volume overload only. As both ventricles are overloaded, the equilibrium results reflect the difference between systolic and diastolic shunt flow. Most frequently however, diastolic shunting remains minimal and the left ventricular volume overload appears to reflect the size of the shunt. To facilitate data analysis, the stroke ratio is expressed as right ventricular over left ventricular stroke ratio in patients with left to right shunts and right ventricular volume overload and as left ventricular over right ventricular stroke ratio in patients with left ventricular volume overload [26].

Measurement of shunt size in clinical practice

Satisfactory results of all methods to detect and quantify left to right shunts in children and adults have been reported. The useful range for shunt evaluation is a QP/QS ratio between 1.2 and 3.0. Shunts with a QP/QS ratio over 3.0 are recognized as large [3] but cannot be adequately quantified [23]. The discriminant value published for the C2/C1 ratio varies slightly (from 0.3 to 0.6) depending on the criteria used for initial appearance and on the type of injection. Although more recent reports with a more standardized technique seem to concur for a separation value of around 0.35, it is advised that each laboratory defines its own normal range. The separating value for the area ratio technique of Anderson *et al.* is 0.80. Finally, the other techniques described use an upper normal value of QP/QS = 1.2. Therefore, minimal shunts cannot be reliably detected. False positive results may be encountered in cases of a widened or fragmented bolus; thus, quality control of the bolus is mandatory. While these inadequate studies should be repeated, if possible with a short-lived isotope, it seems possible to recover some of these through deconvolution of the pulmonary curve using the superior vena cava as input function for a widened bolus, or by substraction of a minified and displaced bolus and pulmonary curve from the original data to determine the delay and minification factor on the bolus curve [27–29].

Comparative analysis of area ratio techniques and C2/C1 ratio has been reported by Alderson in a study of 50 children with suspected left to right shunts. All techniques detected all shunts with an oximetry ratio greater than 1.2:1. However, half the patients with heart disease but no shunt were either falsely classified or borderline [30]. In addition, one normal child had a C2/C1 ratio that was borderline abnormal. While both area techniques showed greater specificity, the gamma function technique provided the best discrimination and had the best correlation and lowest standard error as compared with the results of shunt size determination by oximetry.

The reliability of deconvolution analysis was documented by Alderson in dogs and by Ham in patients. Both groups reported improved correlation with the reference method when a deconvolution technique was used in cases of a prolonged bolus. Furthermore, the number of studies that could be processed by the gamma variate technique has increased significantly [28, 29].

Results reported with $C^{15}O_2$ are also excellent with high sensitivity and specificity even in the presence of concommitant cardiac pathology. The ability of this technique to localize shunts is limited since a special camera or collimator are required which limit the sensitivity of the detector [11, 25].

Comparison of QP/QS measurements obtained by oximetry and equilibrium radionuclide angiography reveals a reasonable correlation ($r = .75$) in patients with single lesions. Because of the relatively large range of values obtained in normals however, the equilibrium technique cannot be used to detect or exclude small shunts and should only be used in conjunction with first pass studies. It then provides an independent confirmation of the results and an alternative to reinjection in case of first pass technical problems (fragmented bolus, valsalva, etc.). However, the potential usefulness of the method in patients with complex lesions and biventricular volume overload remains to be evaluated.

The equilibrium technique furthermore provides information on the location of the shunt as it separates shunts with right and left ventricular volume overload. In our study, these results were obtained in all patients (10 with atrial septal defects or anomalous pulmonary venous return, 4 with ventricular septal defects and 2 with ductus arteriosus [26]. Combined first pass and equilibrium studies are mandatory when analysis of left ventricular function needs to be performed simultaneously.

Patients with congenital.abnormalities usually require cardiac catheterization for physiologic and anatomic evaluation prior to surgery. Nevertheless, noninvasive diagnostic techniques are useful in a number of specific clinical situations. In patients and particularly in children with a heart murmur of uncertain etiology, radionuclide techniques can rule out the presence of a shunt. This may help to differentiate atrial septal defects from pulmonary stenosis which may be clinically difficult. Also, these methods can discriminate between the murmur of papillary muscle rupture and ventricular septal rupture in the setting of acute myocardial infarction [31] although echocardiography as right heart catherization is often to be preferred (chapter 1).

Localization of the shunt (e.g., partial anomalous pulmonary venous return, atrial septal defect, ventricular septal defect or patent ductus arteriosus) and accurate quantifaction of shunt flow may be useful to indicate the need for surgery. For instance, small left to right shunts (QP/QS ratio less than 1.5 to 1) with an atrial or ventricular septal defect often do not require surgery. Serial measurements of small ventricular septal defects can aid to document the spontaneous closure of the defect which may occur [8].

In newborn children, radionuclide angiography can aid to separate cardiac- from pulmonary diseases. Indeed in premature infants, patent ductus arteriosus may coexist with a respiratory distress syndrome and represent a complex diagnostic problem. When a patent ductus is present, repeated studies can follow its evolution and the results of therapeutic manipulations with drugs such as Indomethacin to obtain ductus closure.

Noninvasive studies are also useful to follow the results of surgical repair and to assess the need for reoperation if complications occur. Careful use of these studies in selected indications can thus help to avoid cardiac catheterization and angiography in a number of patients [32]. In patients with atrial septal defect, right ventricular hypokinesis and decreased ejection fraction are related to pulmonary hypertension and symptoms. After surgery right ventricular function improves in most patients [33]. Preoperative left ventricular dysfunction at rest in a patient with atrial septal defect is rare but a diminished functional reserve is more frequent. Since it markedly improves after surgery [34] it is partly related to right ventricular volume overload and abnormal septal motion rather than to intrinsic irreversible myocardial dysfunction. Similar studies have not yet been conducted in patients with ventricular septal defects or patent ductus but should be useful to increase our knowledge about the role of surgery and to assist in determining more precisely the indications and timing of the intervention.

Detection of right to left shunts

Right to left shunts will not be covered in detail in this review. Indeed, cardiopathies with right to left shunts are usually more complex and require cardiac catheterization and angiography.

Radionuclide techniques involve injection of labeled particles (microspheres). These are normally trapped by the pulmonary capillaries. In patients with right to left shunts, they will reach the systemic capillary bed in proportion to the flow partition at the level of the shunt. Percent right to left shunts can be calculated by dividing the systemic activity (total body minus lung activity by the total activity). The technique is also useful to measure residual perfusion in the lung after palliative surgical procedures [8].

Right to left shunts can also be measured by first pass radionuclide angiography and analysis of left ventricular or arterial (aorta or carotid artery) curves according to indicator dilution principles [35, 36].

Finally, by the use of intravenous Krypton right to left shunt can be documented as the tracer does not normally reach the systemic circulation. However, experience with this tracer is limited.

Measurement of valvular regurgitation

The most widely used technique for evaluating valvular incompetence with radionuclides involves equilibrium calculation of left and right ventricular stroke counts [37]. A recent paper has shown that a similar principle can be applied to first pass radionuclide angiography performed in the anterior projection [38]. Other semi-quantitative or qualitative techniques have also been proposed based on first pass studies.

First pass techniques

Early studies addressed the detection of aortic regurgitation by radionuclide radiocardiography. De Vernefoul *et al.* observed that analysis of the time-activity curve over the descending aorta could allow detection of severe aortic insufficiency [39]. Kriss *et al.* later described the qualitative distortion in the transit of an indicator through the heart of patients with valvular lesions as observed with their variable time-lapse video-scintiscope [1]. Kirsch *et al.* proposed a computerized first pass technique that required selective injection into the left atrium and data sampling from both left ventricular and left atrial regions of interest [40]. Later, Rösler proposed the use of functional images (trend scintigraphy) obtained during the downslope of the left ventricular time-activity curve to detect mitral regurgitation. This technique however, cannot be used for aortic regurgitation [41]. More recently, Janowitz and Fester adapted the stroke volume ratio method to first pass radionuclide angiography acquired in the anteroposterior projection [38]. They measured the total stroke counts ejected from both ventricules during the transit of the indicator by summation of the individual beat by beat stroke counts. They proposed to use either all identifiable beats or to extrapolate exponentially the stroke counts per heart beat curve (plotted on semi-log paper) to account for loss of data in late cycles due to overlap of both ventricles. The latter method can be used to separate normal subjects with similar left and right stroke counts from patients with left-sided regurgitation in whom the overload ventricle has excessive stroke counts. An excellent correlation has been observed with angiography. The authors claimed that the anterior projection did not result in a difference in attenuation between both ventricles. The same group also proposed a method to estimate mitral- and aortic regurgitation from $C^{15}O_2$ time-activity curves [42].

Equilibrium techniques

As the basic methodology has been described previously, we will only discuss here the details of the stroke counts calculation and further manipulation of the data. We prefer the use of single regions of interest over both ventricles rather than end-systolic and end-diastolic regions of interest. Indeed, we found that the improved accuracy of the latter technique in normal subjects is associated with an increased complexity and a higher measurement variability. This has recently been confirmed by Nicod *et al.* [43]. The use of amplitude and phase images enables us to define the smallest regions of interest that include all stroke counts [44]. However, the calculation should not be done on stroke volume images, as left and right ventricular systoles are frequently not synchroneous. For similar reasons, the amplitude image provides a better reference than the stroke volume image to draw the region of interest (Figure 5).

Attention to positioning is critical. While functional images can help trace the regions of interest and provide guidelines to reject inadequate studies, they will not permit to recover studies in patients with improper positioning. Even adequate positioning cannot prevent some degree of overlap and the stroke counts ratio in normals is not unity (1.2 ± 1.5 in our

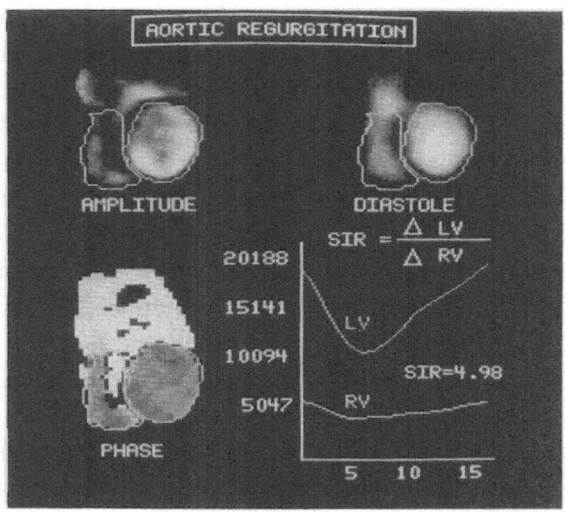

Figure 5. Patient with aortic regurgitation. The diastolic image shows LV dilatation. The Fourier images (amplitude and phase) shows an increase in amplitude over the left ventricle. This is confirmed by the left and right ventricular time-activity curves. The stroke index ratio in this patient was calculated to be 4.98.

laboratory). To account for this systematic error, we calculate the regurgitation fraction as follows:

$$\text{Regurgitant fraction} = \frac{\text{SIR} - 1.2}{\text{SIR}} \tag{1}$$

instead of the original equation:

$$\frac{\text{SIR} - 1}{\text{SIR}} \tag{2}$$

[45]; in which SIR is the stroke index ratio.

It may be expected that in the future rotating tomographic acquisition of the gated blood pool will provide better separation of both ventricles and thus allows more accurate calculation of stroke counts.

It should be pointed out that the relationship between the stroke count ratio and the regurgitation fraction is nonlinear. However, the absolute volumes can be measured and the absolute forward and regurgitation flows can be calculated with the methods described by Slutsky [14] and Dehmer [15] which relate the activity measured in the left ventricle to the activity measured in a blood sample after correction for attenuation [16]. Konstam *et al.* [46] have proposed to obtain the regurgitant fraction by comparison of the total stroke volume with the forward stroke volume as measured by the Fick method or by the standard thermodilution technique. This approach should be particularly useful in cases where the right ventricular stroke volume differs from the systemic stroke volume, such as in the rare patients with both a left to right shunt and regurgitation.

Clinical studies in selected normal subjects

The equilibrium technique for analysis of regurgitant volumes was evaluated in a series of 24 subjects without any sign of valvular heart disease, and in whom an adequate study could be obtained. A mean left ventricular/right ventricular stroke index ratio of 1.20 ± .15 (1 SD) was observed in this group defining our range of normal. Reproducibility of 2 different acquisitions (repeated after 15 minutes with complete repositioning) was excellent. The mean variation in stroke count ratio in 11 patients was only 4%. Nicod *et al.* using the stroke volume image and similar techniques reported normal values of 1.22 ± 0.25 [43]. Janowitz *et al.* using first pass claim a narrower range between 1.00 and 1.13 [38].

Sensitivity and specificity of the routine measurement of the stroke index ratio

To evaluate the cause and incidence of discordant studies in routine radionuclide angiography, we have analyzed the results of 130 consecutive patients studied during a three months period [13].

The stroke index ratio was normal (LV/RV 1.5 and RV/LV 1.2) in 92 of 112 patients without other evidence of ventricular volume overload. A false positive result was thus observed in 20 patients. All were only mildly abnormal (LV/RV 2). The misinterpretations were caused by inadequate positioning (7 patients), an aneurysm involving the septum (8 patients) and right ventricular myocardial infarction with right ventricular and right atrial dilatation (3 patients). In only 2 patients no obvious error or other disease was found. A poor ejection fraction as such was not the cause of discordant results, although this has been reported by Lam [47].

Among 18 patients with independent evidence of ventricular volume overload, 14 had an abnormal index, while 4 remained within the normal range. One of these had biventricular overload, a known pitfall of the technique, while the other had only mild regurgitation.

Results in patients with valvular regurgitation

In our initial study [37] we compared the stroke volume ratio with qualitative angiographic estimates of valvular regurgitation in 20 patients. Patients with moderate regurgitation (mean ratio 2.15) and severe regurgitation (mean ratio 4.02) could be separated from normals and from each other on the basis of the stroke index ratio with little overlap. These observations were confirmed in the experimental animal [48]. Several authors reported a good correlation between the scintigraphic and angiographic regurgitant fractions [49–50]. Urquhart *et al.* [49] also documented the expected decline in the regurgitant fraction one to four months after successful valve replacement. We have studied several patients with persisting or recurrent failure after valve replacement and found the technique useful to differentiate between ventricular dysfunction and correctable residual regurgitation due to valvular leakage or prothesis dysfunction. The technique has also been used to evaluate the effect on regurgitant lesions of interventions such as exercise and vasodilator drugs which decrease the regurgitant fraction of both aortic and mitral regurgitation [51–53]. Application of the stroke index ratio to the study of isolated tricuspid regurgitation has also been described, but these patients are rare as tricuspid regurgitation frequently complicates concomitant left-sided valvular lesions [54]. Phasic count variation of the liver blood pool can also be used to recognize tricuspid regurgitation [55].

Clinical utility of radionuclide angiography in patients with valvular regurgitant lesions

Although the diagnosis is usually evident, clinical evaluation of patients with aortic incompetence and the timing of surgery remains difficult. Indeed, compensatory changes can mask the development of left ventricular dysfunction and delay the apparition of symptoms. Evaluation of left ventricular ejection fraction, regurgitant fraction and especially of left ventricular volume may help to precise the stage of the disease and document its evolution. Such precise determination appears more useful in patients with volume overload and severe left ventricular dysfunction. Concomitant measurement of right ventricular ejection fraction and the regurgitant fraction may indicate the patients most likely to benefit from valve replacement [56] (see also Chapter 1).

At an earlier stage, detection of a diminished left ventricular reserve and of exercise-induced left ventricular dysfunction is important if one wishes to avoid the development of irreversible left ventricular damage before surgery. Borer and several other authors have proposed to study the changes in ejection fraction induced by exercise [57–59]. Indeed, the ejection fraction frequently diminishes even in asymptomatic patients with aortic regurgitation and migh reflect early left ventricular dysfunction. However, the decreased ejection fraction might also result from a decreased end-diastolic volume consecutive to the reduced regurgitant fraction frequently observed with exercise. Comprehensive analysis of left ventricular response to exercise therefore requires analysis of all volumes: end-diastolic volume, end-systolic volume, regurgitant volume and forward stroke volume. It is likely that either the end-systolic volume alone or an end-systolic volume and end-systolic pressure index will prove most useful.

Concomitant analysis of pulmonary blood volume [60] and of right ventricular function during exercise also appears important especially in patients with mitral valve disease. Ventricular volume changes resulting from pacing induced tachycardia should also provide important data on the ventricular response to a diminished regurgitant fraction and preload in aortic regurgitation [61].

After valve replacement, radionuclide angiography is useful to document the extent of postoperative improvement or to assess the cause of failure such as persisting left ventricular dysfunction or recurrent valvular or paravalvular insufficiency [49].

Conclusion

Radionuclide angiography appears to play an increasing role in the clinical evaluation of patients with left to right shunts and valvular regurgitation. Besides its noninvasive character, the increasing ability of this technique to provide precise functional data including ventricular volumes makes it an ideal technique for the serial evaluation of patients before or after surgery.

References

1. Kriss JP, Matin P: Diagnosis of congenital and acquired cardiovascular diseases by radioisotope angiography. Trans Ass Amer Physicians 82: 109–120, 1969.
2. Strauss HW, Pitt B: Evaluation of cardiac function and structure with radioactive tracer tech-

niques. Circulation 57: 645–654, 1978.

3. Adelstein SJ, Maseri A: Radio-indicators for the study of the heart: Principles and applications. Prog Cardiovasc Disease 20: 3–17, 1977.

4. Treves S, Kulprethipanju S, Hnatowick DJ: Angiography with Iridium-191m: an ultrashort-lived radionuclide (T 1/2:4.9 sec). Circulation 54: 275–279, 1976.

5. Neirinckx RD, Jones AG, Davis MA, Harris GI, Holman BL: Tantalum-178, a short-lived nuclide for nuclear medicine: development of a potential generator system. J Nucl Med 19: 514–519, 1978.

6. Wackers FJ, Giles RW, Hoffer PB, Lange RC, Berger HJ, Zaret BL: Gold-195m, a new generator produced short-lived radionuclide for sequential assessment of ventricular performance by first pass radionuclide angiography. Am J Cardiol 50: 89–94, 1982.

7. Knapp WH, Helus F, Lambrecht RM, Elfner R: Kr-81m for determination of right ventricular ejection fraction. Eur J Nucl Med 5: 487–492, 1980.

8. Parker JA, Treves S: Radionuclide detection, localization and quantitation of intracardiac shunts and shunts between the great arteries. Prog Cardiovasc Disease 20: 121–150, 1977.

9. Berger H, Matthay R, Pytlik LO, Gottschalk A, Zaret BL: First pass radionuclide assessment of right and left ventricular performance in patients with cardiac and pulmonary disease. Semin Nucl Med 9: 275–295, 1979.

10. Bonow RO, Bacharach SC, Green MV: First pass technique and diastolic phenomenon. Circulation 65: 640–641, 1982.

11. Chevigné M, Quaglia L, Delfiore G, Peters JM, Rigo P: Evaluation de la fonction ventriculaire gauche et détection des shunts G-D par $C^{15}O_2$: In: Radioaktive Isotope in Klinik und Forschung, Band 15, Höfer R, Bergmann H (ed), H Egermann, Vienna, Austria, pp 31–38, 1982.

12. Strauss HW, McKusick KA, Boucher CA, Bingham JB, Pohost GM: Of linen and laces. The Eight Anniversary of the gated blood pool scan. Sem In Nucl Med 9: 296–309, 1979.

13. Chevigné M, Rigo P: Value of stroke index ratio in routine equilibrium gated scintigraphy. In: Nuclear medicine and biology, Raynaud C (ed), Pergamon Press, Paris, pp 80–82, 1982.

14. Slutsky R, Karliner J, Ricci D, et al.: Left ventricular volumes by gated equilibrium radionuclide angiography: a new method. Circulation 60: 556–564, 1979.

15. Dehmer GJ, Lewis SE, Hillis LD, et al.: Nongeometric determination of left ventricular volumes from equilibrium blood pool scans. Am J Cardiol 45: 293–300, 1980.

16. Links J, Becker LL, Shindledecker JL et al.: Measurement of absolute left ventricular volume from gated blood pool studies. Circulation 65: 82–90, 1982.

17. Schwaiger M, Henze E, Ratib O, Grossman R, Schelbert HR: Accurate determination of left ventricular volumes with gated blood pool studies using a direct measurement of photon attenuation. In: Nuclear medicine and biology, Raynaud C (ed), Pergamon Press, Paris, pp 1297–1300, 1982.

18. Maurer AH, Siegel JH, Deneberg B, Malmud LS, Spann JF: Absolute left ventricular volume by a non-invasive esophageal transmission measurement. In: Nuclear medicine and biology, Raynaud C (ed), Pergamon Press, Paris, pp 1301–1303, 1982.

19. Goris ML, Wallington J, Baum D, Kriss JP: Nuclear angiography: automated selection of regions of interest for the generation of time activity curves and parametric image display and interpretation. Clin Nucl Med 1: 99, 1976.

20. Folse R, Braunwald E: Pulmonary vascular dilution curves recorded by external detection in the diagnosis of left to right shunts. Brit Heart J 24: 166–172, 1962.

21. Anderson PA, Jones RH, Sabiston DC: Quantitation of left-to-right cardiac shunts with radionuclide angiography. Circulation 49: 512–516, 1974.

22. Flaherty JT, Canent RV, Boineau JP et al.: Use of externally recorded radioisotope dilution curves for quantification of left to right shunts. Am J Cardiol 20: 341, 1967.

23. Maltz DL, Treves S: Quantitative radionuclide angiocardiography. Determination of Qp:QS in children. Circulation 47: 1049–1056, 1973.

24. Bourguignon MH, Links J, Douglass K, Alderson PO, Roland J, Wagner HN: Quantification of left to right cardiac shunts by multiple deconvolution analysis. Am J Cardiol 48: 1086–1090, 1981.
25. Watson DD: Shunt detection with the short-lived radioactive gases. Sem Nucl Med 10: 27–38, 1980.
26. Rigo P, Chevigné M: Measurement of left to right shunts by gated radionuclide angiography: Concise communication. J Nucl Med 23: 1070–1075, 1982.
27. Ham HR, Dobbeleir A, Viart P, Piepsz A, Lenaers A: Radionuclide quantitation of left to right cardiac shunts using deconvolution analysis. J Nucl Med 22: 688–692, 1981.
28. Alderson PO, Douglas KH, Mendenhull KG: Deconvolution analysis in radionuclide quantitation of left to right cardiac shunts. J Nucl Med 20: 502–506, 1979.
29. Lis GA, Zubi SM: Removal of bolus fragmentation artefacts from pulmonary curves as applied to QP:QS shunt determination. J Nucl Med 23: 930–933, 1982.
30. Alderson PO, Jost RG, Strauss HW: Radionuclide angiocardiography: improved diagnosis and quantification of left to right shunts using area ration techniques in children. Circulation 51: 1136, 1975.
31. Chevigné M, Rigo P: Evaluation des ruptures septales et des insuffisances mitrales dans l'infarctus aigu du myocarde. In: Non invasive methods in ischemic heart disease, G. Faivre, A. Bertrand, F. Cherrier, M. Amor, J.L, Neimann, (eds), Specia, Nancy, 1982, pp. 327–331.
32. Treves S, Fogle R, Lang P: Radionuclide angiography in congenital heart disease. Am J Cardiol 46: 1247–1255, 1980.
33. Liberthson RR, Boucher CA, Strauss HW, Dinsmore RE, McKusick KA, Pohost GM: Right ventricular function in adult atrial septal defect. Pre- and post-operative assessment and clinical applications. Am J Cardiol 47: 56–60, 1981.
34. Bonow RO, Borer JS, Rosing DR, Bacharach SL, Green MV, Kent KM: Left ventricular function reserve in adult patient with atrial septal defect: Pre- and post-operative studies. Circulation 63: 1315–1322, 1981.
35. Riihimaki E, Heiskanen A, Tahti E: Theory of quantitative determination of infracardiac shunts by external detection. Ann Clin Res 6: 45, 1974.
36. Peter CA, Armstrong BE, Jones RH: Radionuclide quantitation of right to left intracardiac shunts in children. Circulation 64: 572–577, 1981.
37. Rigo P, Alderson PO, Robertson RM, Becker LC, Wagner HNJr: Measurement of aortic and mitral regurgitation by gated cardiac blood pool scans. Circulation 60: 306–312, 1979.
38. Janowitz WE, Fester A: Quantitation of left ventricular regurgitant fraction by first pass radionuclide angiography. Am J Cardiol 49: 85–92, 1982.
39. De Vernejoul P, Fauchet M, Barritault L: Coeur. In: Traité de Médecine Nucléaire, Tome II, Meyniel G (ed), Flammarion, Paris, pp 134–156, 1975.
40. Kirch DL, Metz CE, Steele PP: Quantitation of valvular insufficiency by computerized radionuclide angiocardiography. Am J Cardiol 34: 711–722, 1974.
41. Rösler H, Ramos M, Noelpp U, Salzmann C, Fritschy P: Trend scintigrams in studies of ventricular function. In: Frontiers in nuclear medicine, Horst W, Wagner HNJr and Buchanan JW (eds, Springer Verlag, Berlin-Heidelberg-New York, pp 235–241, 1980.
42. Watson DD, Kenny PJ, Gelband H et al.: A non-invasive technique for the study of cardiac hemodynamics utilizing $C^{15}O_2$ inhalation. Radiology 119: 615, 1976.
43. Nicod P, Corbett JR, Firth BG et al.: Radionuclide techniques for valvular regurgitant index: comparison in patients with normal and depressed ventricular function. J Nucl Med 23: 763–769, 1982.
44. Rigo P, Chevigné M: Measurement of left to right shunts by gated cardiac blood pool scans: a new technique. In: Radioaktive Isotopes in Klinik und Forschung, Band 14, Gasteiner Internationales Symposium. Höfer R, Bergmann H (eds), H Egermann, Vienna, pp 333–343, 1980.
45. Rigo P, Chevigné M: The role of gated cardiac blood pool scans to assess valvular regurgitation and left to right shunts. First international symposium on nuclear cardiology, Tel Aviv, p 163, 1981.

46. Konstam MA, Wynne J, Holman BL, Brown EJ, Weill JM, Kozlowski: Use of equilibrium (gated) radionuclide ventriculography to quantitate left ventricular output in patients with and without left sided valvular regurgitation. Circulation 64: 578–585, 1981.

47. Lam W, Pavel D, Byrom E, Sheikh A, Best D, Rosen K: Radionuclide regurgitant index: Value and limitations. Am J Cardiol 47: 292–298, 1981.

48. Baxter RH, Becker LC, Alderson PO, Rigo P, Wagner HNJr, Weisfeldt ML: Quantification of aortic valvular regurgitation in dogs by nuclear imaging. Circulation 61: 404, 1980.

49. Urquhart J, Patterson RE, Packer M, Goldsmith SJ, Horowitz SF, Litwak R, Gorlin R: Quantification of valve regurgitation by radionuclide angiography before and after valve replacement surgery. Am J Cardiol 47: 287–291, 1981.

50. Sorensen SG, O'Rourke RA, Chaudhuri TK: Non-invasive quantitation of valvular regurgitation by gated equilibrium radionuclide angiography. Circulation 62: 1089–1098, 1980.

51. Besozzi M, Clare J, Santinga A, Thrall J, Pitt B: Exercise LV/RV stroke index ratios measured by gated blood pool scans in aortic regurgitation, pre- and post-valve replacement. J Nucl Med 21: 49, 1980 (abstract).

52. Henze E, Wisenberg C, Schelbert HR: Effects of exercise on regurgitant fraction and right and left ventricular function in aortic and mitral insufficiency. J Nucl Med 21: 47, 1980 (abstract).

53. Horowitz S, Goldman M, Kukin M, Patterson R, Urquhart J, Teicholz L, Armas R, Goldsmith S, Gorlin R: Scintigraphic evaluation of regurgitant index during multi-intervention studies in aortic regurgitation. Circulation 64, IV: 247, 1981 (abstract).

54. Chevigné M, Rigo P: Quantification of isolated tricuspid regurgitation by gated cardiac blood pool scans. Eur J Nucl Med 7: 39–40, 1982.

55. Pavel D, Hawdler B, Lam W, Meyer-Pavel C, Byrom E, Pietras R: A new method for the detection of tricuspid insufficiency. J Nucl Med 22: 4, 1981 (abstract).

56. Boucher CA, Okada RD, Pohost GM: Current status of radionuclide imaging in valvular heart disease. Am J Cardiol 46: 1153–1163, 1980.

57. Borer JS, Bacharach SL, Green MV et al.: Exercise-induced left ventricular dysfunction in symptomatic and asymptomatic patients with aortic regurgitation: assessment with radionuclide cineangiography. Am J Cardiol 42: 351–357, 1978.

58. Dehmer GJ, Firth BG, Hillis LD, Corbett JR, Lewis SE, Parkey RW, Willerson JT: Alterations in left ventricular volumes and ejection fraction at rest and during exercise in patients with aortic regurgitation. Am J Cardiol 48: 18–27, 1981.

59. Iskandrian AS, Hakki A, Kane SA, Segal BL: Quantitative radionuclide angiography in assessment of hemodynamic changes during upright exercise: observations in normal subjects, patients with coronary artery disease and patients with aortic regurgitation. Am J Cardiol 48: 239–246, 1981.

60. Nichols AB, Strauss HW, Moore RH et al.: Acute changes in pulmonary blood volume during upright exercise stress testing in patients with coronary artery disease. Circulation 60: 520–530, 1979.

61. Firth BG, Dehmer GJ, Nicod P, Willerson JT, Hillis DL: Effect of increasing heart rate in patients with aortic regurgitation. Am J Cardiol 49: 1860–1867, 1982.

9. Review of methods for computer analysis of global and regional left ventricular function from equilibrium gated blood pool scintigrams

Johan H.C. Reiber

Introduction

Assuming a homogeneous distribution of the radioactive tracer (tech-netium-99m) in the blood pool, the changes in precordial count rates reflect the cyclic volume changes of the heart cavities. In the mid sixties Hoffmann and Kleine introduced heart studies with a single probe detec-tor system and an ECG gating procedure to measure activity changes during the heart cycle [1]. However, this technique did not allow to differentiate between the left and right ventricles. To solve this problem, Adam *et al.* applied a few years later the gating procedure to a gamma camera and a computer system [2, 3]. To measure and visualize the cyclic changes in geometry and volume of the heart chambers, the data need to be collected over several hundreds of heart cycles. This results in a representative cardiac cycle divided into a number of time segments; the scintigraphic data are stored in computer memory in a corresponding number of frames. Modern computer systems allow the frames to be displayed on a video monitor screen in a closed loop movie format, thus allowing the detection of wall motion abnormalities. Gated equilibrium radionuclide ventriculography with technetium-99m as the radioactive tracer is nowadays a routinely applied noninvasive procedure for the assessment of left ventricular function at rest, stress and different stages of interventions [4].

The generalized use of minicomputers in nuclear medicine applications has resulted in advances towards quantitation of left ventricular function. Absolute values of global and regional ejection fraction (EF) and the changes in these parameters as a function of the intervention, have been used for these purposes most frequently [5, 6]. Initially, regions of interest (ROI's) around the left ventricular (LV) structure and in a background area were drawn manually by the user, but over the years various semi- and fully-automated procedures for the boundary detection of the left ventricular activity structure in one or more frames and the subsequent computation of the ejection fraction have been published. Nearly every manufacturer of nuclear medicine computer systems nowadays offers such a computer program. For such an analysis procedure to be acceptable in clinical practice, several conditions should be fulfilled: (1) the scintigraphic ejection fraction values should be similar to the contrast ejection fraction values obtained from left ventriculograms under similar physiologic conditions, (2) the procedure should be characterized by low inter- and intra-observer variations to appreciate small changes in the results from intervention studies with statistical significance, (3) the analysis procedure should be computationally fast and (4) it should be characterized by a high rate of success under different image qualities.

Besides the computation of global and regional ejection fraction from the gated blood pool scintigrams, Fourier techniques have been introduced as a means to assess wall motion abnormalities from the amplitude and phase images.

It is the purpose of this paper to present an overview on different techniques for data acquisition and analysis of gated blood pool scintigrams. The basic principles for semi- and fully automated boundary detection of the left ventricular activity structure in one or more frames and for the selection of the background ROI are described. Subsequently, methods for the computation of global and regional EF are discussed. An overview from the literature is presented on the comparative data from scintigraphic and contrast left ventricular angiography, as well as on the inter- and intra-observer variations in the analysis of the studies and on the overall reproducibility of the gated blood pool technique. In addition, the value and limitations of exercise gated blood pool scintigraphy are discussed. As a next step, an overview of commercially available state of the art computer programs for the computation of global and regional EF is presented. Finally, the principles and potential clinical values of the Fourier technique will be discussed.

Data acquistition

For gated blood pool scintigraphy 15–25 mCi (555–925 MBq) of technetium-99m labeled human serum albumin or red blood cells labeled, either *in vivo, in vitro* or *semi in vitro* is used [7, 8]. For reasons of convenience, the *in vivo* method is used most frequently. For rest studies, data are usually collected in the LAO45° view modified with a 10° caudal tilt and in the LAO65° and RAO25° views. The modified LAO45° view provides the best separation between the left and right ventricles and least overlap with other cardiac structures. Both low-energy-all-purpose (LEAP) and high sensitivity (HS) parallel hole collimators have been used for these purposes. Several investigators have also applied the 30° slant-hole straight-bore collimator in the modified LAO (MLAO) projection [9, 10].

The data collection period per view ranges from 4 to 10 minutes (typically 6 min with LEAP collimator and 4 min with HS collimator). Matrix size is 64×64 pixels in nonzoom mode for small size gamma cameras or in zoom mode for medium and large size cameras. For a medium field camera with a field-of-view (FOV) of 25 cm in diameter and a zoom factor of $\sqrt{2}$, the pixel size equals 2.8×2.8 mm^2. The number of frames ranges from 12 to 64; for purposes of EF and wall motion assessment, approximately 20 frames per cycle are usually obtained. In terms of temporal resolution requirements, a framing time of 50 msec for rest studies and of 40 msec for exercise studies have been shown to be adequate for the measurement of EF [11]. Higher rates of temporal resolution are required for quantification of other LV function indexes, such as systolic and diastolic intervals, and peak rates of LV emptying and filling. At rest framing times between 25 and 40 msec have been suggested for these purposes and at exercise 20 msec per frame [11, 12]. For statistical reasons each frame of size 64×64 and pixel size 2.8×2.8 mm^2 should contain at least 200,000 counts, if regional details are to be quantitated. Synchronization of the data acquisition during the several hundreds of cardiac cycles is by means of a trigger signal derived from the R-wave of the patient's ECG-signal. The data acquisition can be performed in synchronized frame mode or in list mode (also denoted serial mode) [13].

In synchronized frame mode the average R-R interval is divided into a predefined number of time segments, and an equal number of frames is defined in computer memory. Scintillations detected during a specific time bin are stored at the computed x, y-positions in the corresponding frame. This repetitive cycling of data collection proceeds until the preset total number of counts have been collected or until the preset time has elapsed. The average R-R interval is computed immediately prior to the data acquisition and remains fixed or is updated during data collection by the average value measured over the preceding time period with a duration of, e.g., 30 s. or over a certain number of preceding accepted beats, e.g., 30–40. Advantages of this frame mode technique include: 1) only a modest amount of computer data storage is required; and 2) the data are formatted in real time.

Although frame mode acquisition is used most frequently, the handling of arrhythmia is a major limitation of this technique. By setting a tolerance limit in ms. (e.g., 100 ms.) or in percentages of the average R-R interval (e.g., 10%), beats outside of the tolerance limits can be rejected. Since this beat rejection occurs usually on the fly, the cycle(s) following an unacceptable R-R interval are rejected until an acceptable interval is sensed again. Disadvantage of this technique is the fact that the bad or unacceptable R-R interval has been collected already, while the following cycle, which was rejected, could be a perfectly acceptable beat. As a consequence, the last frames of the study usually contain fewer counts than would be the case using an ideal rejection technique. These problems can be circumvented by buffering the data collected during a cardiac cycle and deciding at the end of the cycle whether the data is to be transferred to computer memory or to be rejected (also denoted real-time list mode). However, there are very few computer systems to date that have that capability [13, 14].

In conventional list mode data acquisition, each event (scintillation) is recorded onto the computer disc as a single entity in chronological order and interspersed with typically 10 msec timing marks [15]. The time of occurrence of the R-wave signal is stored as well. At the end of the data acquisition, the data are framed into images. R-R intervals deviating from the average heart cycle duration by more than for example 10% are rejected, as are also each of their two successors. A running average heart cycle duration at a certain time may be obtained from a range of heart beats before and after that time. R-R interval rejection may also be determined on the basis of the histogram of the acquired R-R intervals (R-R interval spectrum). The R-R window selection may be performed automatically, e.g., a width of $\pm10\%$ with respect to the peak value in the histogram, or manually by the user. The framing of the data is performed by one of three methods designated high time (or temporal) resolution (HTR), high phase resolution (HPR) and reverse framing [13]. The HTR method involves organizing the events into successive time intervals of equal length following the R-wave, similar to the synchronized frame mode. This method also requires certain correction techniques to avoid fall-off at the end of the frame series. The other two methods inherently eliminate or reduce this drop off effect. The HPR approach consists of subdividing each cardiac cycle into a fixed number of intervals of variable length. The entire cardiac cycle is thus uniformly stretched or compressed to exactly fit into the same number of images in each cycle. It has been shown that HPR constructed data showed slightly better results in the calculation of ejection fraction, although for the clinical evaluation there was no evidence that the HPR studies were superior to the HTR studies [16]. The reverse gating or framing method (also denoted forward/backward framing) constructs the equivalent of two gated sequences – one produced forward from the R-wave and one produced backwards in time from the R-wave. These two image sequences are then joined at some point in the forward curve (e.g., 2/3 of the mean cycle length), in such a way that the resulting curve has a length equal to the mean beat length.

The greatest disadvantage of list mode acquisition is the large amount of memory that is required on digital disk to store the raw data, while the count rate capability is limited by the disk access times. Also, reformatting of the data after data acquisition may take some time. However, as faster and larger disks now become economically feasible, these disadvantages will become obsolete.

Stress testing is most frequently performed in a supine position on a stress table specially equipped with shoulder restraints, hand grips and attached bicycle ergometer under the gamma camera. Of particular interest hereby is the change of global ejection fraction as a function of the workload. The preferred orientation therefore is the modified LAO45° view. The exercise protocol starts with a rest study, followed by acquisitions at the different levels of the workload. At the end of the stress test a recovery study is obtained. The acquisition time for each of these studies typically is between 2 and 4 minutes. Because of the short acquisition times it is advantageous to use the HS collimator.

Data analysis

The total number of counts within the left ventricular activity structure, after appropriate background subtraction, provides a direct measure for instantaneous left ventricular volume [17, 18]. Computation of the global or regional ejection fraction thus requires the delineation of the left ventricular boundary and the definition of a background region for correction of background activity. This may be achieved by manual tracing of the outlines or by some kind of semi- or fully-automated contour detection algorithm. The manual procedure is characterized by relatively large inter- and intra-observer variations, which hamper the assessment of effects of interventions, such as exercise or pharmacological therapy, on ejection fraction [19, 20]. Therefore, over the last several years various semi- and fully-automated procedures for the boundary definition of the left ventricular activity structure have been developed. In general, the following steps in such an analysis procedure may be distinguished:

(1) localizing left ventricular structure,
(2) preprocessing of the digital data,
(3) edge enhancement of the left ventricular structure,
(4) contour detection of the left ventricular structure (segmentation),
(5) contour detection in ED and ES frames of the study,
(6) contour detection in all frames of the study,
(7) definition of a background region,
(8) computation of global and regional ejection fraction.

Different implementations of these steps will be described in more detail in the following paragraphs.

(1) Localizing left ventricular structure

For purposes of edge detection of the left ventricular activity structure, the global position of the geometric center or of the point of gravity should be known. Various techniques have been described in the literature. The simplest method consists of requesting the user to place a box around the ventricle using a light pen or joystick; this may be done by setting the lower left hand and upper right hand corners [21]. The centroid of the activity distribution within this box is then defined as the approximate center of the left ventricle.

Douglas *et al.* have described a technique for automated definition of a box encompassing the left ventricle based on the characteristics (or signatures) of the row and column sums of the difference image (ED-ES) [22]. A success rate of 80% has been quoted for 20 patient studies.

The signatures of the column and row sums and the count density distribution in the first frame of a study have been used by Reiber *et al.* for the global definition of the LV center [23]. The center position defined by this method does not necessarily coincide with the geometric center of the left ventricle or with its point of gravity. This does not pose a serious problem for the subsequently applied automated contour detection algorithm, since this approximated center position will be updated once again by the contour algorithm itself. The single aim of this LV center routine is to provide an approximate left ventricular center position; this position will be updated in the subsequent contour detection algorithm. The success rate of this method assessed from 100 rest gated blood pool studies has been found to be 98%.

The ED-ES difference image, also denoted stroke count image, has also been used for the definition of the approximate left ventricular center position. Bourguignon defines the pixel with the maximum counts in the ED image to the left of the gravitational center of the stroke count image as the left ventricular centroid [24].

A slightly different approach has been taken by Links *et al.* [25]. After pre-processing of all the frames in the study, which consists of temporal and spatial smoothing, a stroke count image is formed by subtracting the minimum value of each pixel from its value in the first frame of the study (assumed to be close to ED); negative values are zeroed. The count center of gravity of this image is obtained, which typically lies in the region of the interventricular septum. A point within the left ventricle is then found by searching horizontally to the patient's left of this count center for the first local maximum within a 3×3 neighbourhood in the ED-frame. This point is redefined by searching four points above and below for the absolute maximum within the 3×3 box. This final point is taken as the left ventricular marker. This center position is again updated in the edge enhancement step by the geometric center of detected edge positions along eight equal-angle radii.

Almasi *et al.* derive a kind of stroke count image by computing for each pixel in the 64×64 matrices the magnitude and phase of the first harmonic over the cardiac cycle [26]. The ventricular first harmonic (VFH) mask is then obtained by zeroing all pixels whose phase are outside of a window centered on the R-wave. Finally, the centroid of this VFH image locates the center of the léft ventricle.

De Graaf *et al.* have developed a LV localizing algorithm, which can be characterized as a brute force pattern recognition task [27]. The learn set consists of 867 patterns derived from the same number of gated blood pool studies. A success rate of 100% has been reported for 250 patient studies. Average processing time on a HP 1000F computer equals 22 s.

(2) Preprocessing of the digital data

Because of the quantum-limited characteristics of the data acquisition process, the signal-to-noise ratio in the scintigraphic images is rather low. To obtain reliable edge detection results it is therefore imperative that some kind of preprocessing to there images is applied in an attempt to improve the signal-to-noise ratio, while preserving or augmenting the edge information [28–31]. In practice, this preprocessing is often combined with the edge detection algorithm, but we will cover preprocessing very briefly as a separate topic. Such a process requires the use of a linear or non-linear filter, which should preferably preserve the medium spatial frequencies representing the edge information and attenuate the higher frequencies. Example of filters which attenuate not only the higher spatial frequencies, but also slightly the medium frequencies are the weighted and unweighted nine-point smooth filter, applied spatially or both spatially and temporally and the running average filter.

Examples of filters which attenuate the higher frequencies, while preserving the medium frequencies are the median filter, the V-filter [32], the K-nearest neighbor filter [33] and the two-dimensional least squares polynomial bounding technique [31]. Spatial and/or temporal Fourier filtering attenuates both the low and high frequencies; therefore it would be better to include this technique under the edge-enhancement paragraph.

Following the preprocessing step, a linear or nonlinear edge enhancement procedure is applied to the preprocessed image to extract the most prevalent features of edge, i.e., high derivatives [34]. The value of each pixel in the edge-enhanced image is a measure of edge strength, usually based on some kind of first or second difference function or a combination of the two. The detection of the contour of the object is then achieved by means of a postprocessing step.

(3) Edge-enhancement of the left ventricular structure

In this paragraph the basic principles of the generally used edge enhancement algorithms will be described, independent of the fact whether they are used for contour detection in only one, in two or in all frames of the blood pool study. The additional problems encountered in contour detection in more than one frame will be discussed thereafter.

Edge enhancement algorithms are usually based on some kind of first or second difference (derivative) operator or a combination of the two. In this context, the term operator does not refer to a human being, such as the user of the system, but is defined as a mathematical operation on the image data. In terms of spatial frequencies, the edge-enhancement algorithm magnifies the medium and higher frequenties and attenuates the lower frequencies. The earlier use of isocount contours to enhance certain structures can be discarded as the background count density around the left ventricle is inhomogeneous; particularly, the definition of the interventricular septum by this method is extremely unreliable. A good overview of edge enhancement or detection algorithms can be found in Chang [35].

First-difference function

The often used term "derivative" is actually reserved to analog functions. For digital signals $f(i)$ or images $f(i, j)$ the term difference or gradient should be used. The first difference in the positive x- and y-directions for a position (i, j) is defined by

$$\Delta_x f(i, j) = f(i, j) - f(i + 1, j) \tag{1}$$

and

$$\Delta_y f(i, j) = f(i, j) - f(i, j + 1), \tag{2}$$

respectively.

Since edges may occur in any direction, a first-difference operator should be employed that is equally sensitive in all orientations, i.e. the difference operator should be isotropic. An obvious choice would be to compute for each pixel (i, j) the magnitude of the discrete gradient $\Delta f(i, j)$ as:

$$\Delta f(i, j) = ((\Delta_x f(i, j))^2 + (\Delta_y f(i, j))^2)^{1/2}. \tag{3}$$

Since this operator is very sensitive to noise and boundary irregularities, the matrix is usually first smoothed spatially and/or temporally to reduce the noise contributions (preprocessing step).

Computationally, it is advantageous to approximate the expression in (3) by either the sum operator

$$|\Delta_x f(i, j)| + |\Delta_y f(i, j)| \tag{4}$$

or by the maximum operator

$$\max\{|\Delta_x f(i, j)|, |\Delta_y f(i, j)|\}. \tag{5}$$

In an attempt to reduce the appearance of extraneous points in the difference image due to noise contributions in the original image, a smoothed version of the difference operator can be defined which is based on the difference of the average pixel value of two one-dimensional neighborhoods on opposite sides of a pixel. For the smoothed y-difference the following definition can be used:

$$\Delta_y f(i, j) = \frac{1}{\kappa} \left\{ \sum_{n=1}^{\kappa} f(i, j - n) - \sum_{n=1}^{\kappa} f(i, j + n) \right\} \tag{6}$$

A similar definition is then defined for the x-direction. K is usually chosen as 2 or 3 in a 64×64 matrix. It is clear that such a smoothing difference operator combines a certain degree of preprocessing with the edge enhancement procedure. This technique can easily be extended to two-dimensional neighbourhoods.

A useful two-dimensional technique to determine the magnitude and direction of the gradient consists of convolving the image with gradient masks. Operators in this category are the Roberts, Prewitt and Sobel operators [36, 37]. The Roberts-operator is defined by 2×2 masks:

$$H1 = \begin{bmatrix} 0 & -1 \\ 1 & 0 \end{bmatrix} \qquad H2 = \begin{bmatrix} -1 & 0 \\ 0 & 1 \end{bmatrix} \tag{7}$$

while the Prewitt and Sobel-operators use 3×3 masks:

$$H1 = \begin{bmatrix} 1 & 0 & -1 \\ C & 0 & -C \\ 1 & 0 & -1 \end{bmatrix} \qquad H2 = \begin{bmatrix} -1 & -C & -1 \\ 0 & 0 & 0 \\ 1 & C & 1 \end{bmatrix} \tag{8}$$

For the Prewitt-operator C equals 1, for the Sobel-operator C equals 2. The amplitude of the discrete gradient at a matrix position (i, j) can be obtained similarly as described for the one-dimensional case (equations (3)−(6)). Another type of edge-enhancement operator is the template matching operator; it consists of a set of masks (typically 4 or 8, corresponding with the main compass directions), which approximate ideal edges with different orientations. At each position (i, j) the mask with maximum output determines the amplitude and direction of the edge. The use of these compass gradient masks in edge enhancement have been described in detail by Robinson [38]. This technique has been applied in cardiac scintigrams by Douglas and Kan [22, 39].

Since the left ventricular contour to be detected in the LAO45° view may be assumed to a first approximation to be simply connected closed and almost convex, it is also possible to determine the difference values along radial lines from the center position of the left ventricular activity structure. Each radial line is approximately perpendicular to its local LV contour direction. This approach has been implemented in several of the commercially available systems (Table 5) using either first, second or the combination of first and second difference operators.

It has been our experience and that of others that the resulting contour based on the application of first-difference operators does not encompass the entire left ventricular activity structure, since the maxima of the difference function occur at the inflection points of the activity distribution. The outermost pixels of the left ventricular activity structure remain outside of this contour. On the other hand, the maximum response of the second difference operator occurs at the base of the activity distribution. Although the true boundary is likely to be in between the positions defined by the maximum responses of first and second difference operators, the second difference operator is preferred over the first difference operator if the counts within a region of interest are to be determined. These differences have been clearly demonstrated by Hawman [40].

Second difference operator
Many published methods make use of a second difference operator with the maximum response defining the edge position at the base of the activity distribution functions. However, some methods define the edge positions by the zero-crossing of the 2nd difference functions; these positions basically coincide with the positions defined by the maximum first difference.

A well known operator that is orientation insensitive, is the Laplacian, which can be approximated for digital pictures by

$$\nabla^2 f(i,j) = f(i+1,j) + f(i-1,j) + f(i,j+1) + f(i,j-1) - 4f(i,j) \quad (9)$$

Another second difference operator based on the concept of nonoverlapping neighborhoods has been described by Hawman [40]. The computation of the second difference values of a digital image can also be obtained by applying a first difference operator twice, possibly with an intermediate smoothing step. Along this last direction and with particular reference to the problem of edge definition of the left ventricle, the computation of the second difference can be simplified considerably by resampling the image into a polar coordinate system and determining the second difference along the radial lines [23]. Reiber *et al.* sample the original image along 64 radii with respect to an earlier computed center position of the left ventricle. Along each radial line 32 samples are taken with sample distance equal to the pixel distance in the x, y-matrix. The value of the pixel in the polar matrix is defined by the average of the 3×3 neighborhood of the pixel closest to the sample point in the original image. An example of a polar representation is shown in Figure 1 (top center) together with the original sum image. Enhancement of the edges in the polar image is achieved by applying a first difference operator twice along the horizontal lines in the polar image. For the purpose of contour detection, a cost matrix is computed with the cost of a pixel defined by the second-difference value of that pixel, but with inverse sign. The top right image in Figure 1 is the first-difference image and the bottom left image the cost

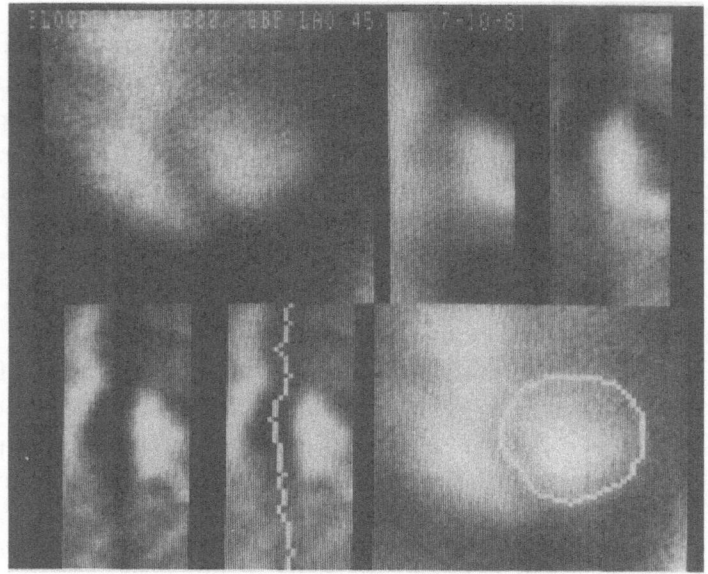

Figure 1. The top images represent from left to right the original sum image, the polar image and the first-difference image, respectively. On the bottom row from left to right the images represent the cost matrix, the detected contour superimposed in the cost matrix and the sum image with the detected contour superimposed, respectively.

matrix. The displayed brightness levels in the cost matrix are proportional to the cost coefficients. The path in which the contour is to be detected is characterized by low costs (low brightness levels) as can be seen in this image.

Combination of first- and second-difference operator
Hawman uses a linear combination of first- and second-difference operators [40]. On the basis of computer simulations of elliptical objects he found that the boundaries defined by the maximum first difference are inside the geometric edge, while those defined by the maximum second-difference are outside of it. If $e_1(i, j)$ and $e_2(i, j)$ denote the first- and second-difference functions, respectively, then

$$e_3(i, j) = a \cdot e_1(i, j) + (1-a) \cdot e_2(i, j) \qquad (10)$$

can be defined as an appropriate combination of the two, with $0 \leq a \leq 1$. An optimal value for a, in the sense of providing contours which closely agree with those drawn by an experienced observer has been found to be $a = 0.4$.

(4) Contour detection on the left ventricular structure (segmentation)

The application of the edge enhancement techniques described above yields a set of pixels with high edge strength. This set may include extraneous elements, but elements truly belonging to the contour may be missing as well. In general, therefore, a postprocessing procedure is required to reject the elements not belonging to the actual contour and to add missing elements. This region identification process is called "segmentation" by the image processing community. Various techniques, either applied alone or in combination, such as thresholding, shrinking and expanding, relaxation, connectivity requirements, ridge tracking, curve matching methods or minimum cost contour detection algorithms have been applied for these purposes. It is beyond the scope of this paper to describe these techniques in detail. A good overview can be found in Pizer [28].

In our institute, we use the minimum cost contour detection algorithm developed by Lie *et al.* [23, 41–43]. Referring to Figure 1, the minimum cost contour is defined as the minimum cost path from the bottom to the top in the cost matrix (lower center). Retransforming to cartesian coordinates and connecting the 64 contour positions results in a connective contour (Figure 1, bottom row right). Since the polar coordinates were computed from the initially defined LV center position, which in general does not coincide with the LV point of gravity, the center position is subsequently updated by the centroid of the bounded left ventricular activity structure and the contour detection process is repeated, resulting in the final LV contour. The use of a two steps iteration in LV contour detection has also been described by Links *et al.* [25].

The approach by Hutton *et al.* is not based on difference operators, but on the definition of a "concavity" value for each pixel in the image computed into two or four directions [44]. The ED and ES LV ROI's are detected on the basis of the binary edge maps in these images derived from the "concavity" data and of user-drawn ROI's. Following the detection of the ED and ES ROI's the computer continues to produce a series of regions for intermediate frames using corresponding edge maps and interpolated regions derived from the ED and ES regions.

(5) Contour detection in ED and ES frames of the study

So far we have discussed different contour detection techniques applied to a single frame, e.g., the end-diastolic frame or the sum-image of a blood pool study. If one is interested in determining the contours in two, non-sequential frames, e.g., the ED and ES frames, the same contour detection algorithm is usually applied to these two frames with minimal or no use of any temporal information present in the series of images.

In the procedure described by Reiber *et al.* the ED and ES frames are selected automatically from the LV time-activity curve computed for the detected contour in the sum image of the study [23]. The LV centroid within this last contour also serves as the initial center point for the ED and ES frames. For each of the frames the earlier described minimum cost contour detection algorithm is applied. To limit the search for the ED contour an expectation window based on the detected contour in the sum image is incorporated in the detection algorithm.

Links *et al.* define the first frame of the gated series as the ED frame. The detected ED contour is used as the seed region for the ES frame, identified as that frame corresponding to the nadir of a time-activity curve from the ED region [25]. Other methods have been described which determine the ED and ES frame numbers by scanning within a manually or automatically set LV box for the images with the maximum and minimum counts, respectively.

(6) Contour detection in all frames of the study

To assess regional wall motion or to compute the actual activity distribution within the separate frames, contour detection in all frames is necessary. To improve the accuracy and reproducibility of the contour detection techniques, information from already detected contours in previous frames may be used to guide the search in the frame under consideration.

The method described by Lie *et al.* starts with a 1-2-1 weighted temporal filtering of the 20 consecutive frames to improve the signal-to-noise ratio in the separate frames [23, 41–43]. For the detection of the left ventricular contour in frame m, the detected contour in frame (m − 1) is used as a model to guide the search, i.e., a narrow expectation window is defined. For each subsequent frame to be analyzed, the centroid of the activity distribution within the region defined by the contour in the previous frame is defined as the new center position. Thus an adaptive process for the definition of the center positions is applied for each of the 20 frames. The minimal cost contour detection procedure, including the expectation window, is then applied to each of the separate frames. In Figure 2 the original first 16 frames of the total of 20 frames of the study are displayed with the detected contours superimposed.

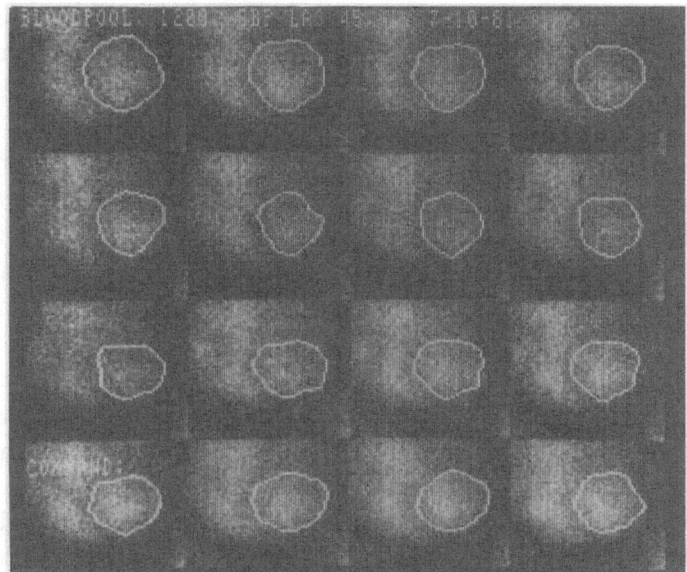

Figure 2. The first 16 frames of the study with the detected contours superimposed.

Hawman *et al.* apply a recursive edge-enhancement scheme for the consecutive frames [40]. A fraction (typically between 10% and 50%) of the edge-enhancement image of the previous frame is added to the current frame's edge enhancement information. Also, the permitted boundary change is restricted through the use of a mask function.

(7) Definition of a background region

Once the boundary of the left ventricle in one or more frames has been determined, the number of counts within the boundary may be computed for each frame. This information comprises the left ventricular time-activity curve. However, the left ventricular counts do not originate exclusively from within the left ventricular cavity, but also from neighboring organs, such as the lungs, liver, from the large vessels and from the vascular activity in the chest wall. To correct for this background activity distribution, a background ROI must be defined.

Numerous approaches have been developed for the definition of a background ROI and for the actual correction of the LV time-activity curves. When selecting a background ROI special attention should be given to the constancy of the background time-activity curve, i.e. no cardiac or vascular structure such as the aortic root should be included. The following techniques for the background ROI have been presented in the literature: 1) defining a small region along the entire or only lower lateral aspect of the left ventricle in the sum- or the ED image [45–47]; 2) defining a small region along the lateral aspect of the left ventricle in the ES image [18, 45, 46] or along the lateral, apical and partly septal aspect in this image [44]; 3) taking the difference in area between the left ventricular contour at end-diastole and the one at end-systole [46]; 4) using for both the ED and ES images a separate small region adjacent to the lateral aspect of the corresponding left ventricular contours [46]; 5) no background correction at all [45]; 6) selecting an "optimal" background region from six automatically generated regions in the directions of 1 through 6 o'clock with respect to the LV center on the basis of minimal variance in the background time-activity curve and lowest mean activity level [23, 43]; 7) using the inclined plane method which corrects for background inhomogeneities [48, 49]; 8) pixel-by-pixel background subtraction using an interpolative technique between inner- and outer-LV perimeters [26], and 9) using computer defined regions centered along the lateral and apical side of a rectangle encompassing the LV and along the lower three-fourths of the septal side [10]. Globally, the implemented techniques for correction of the background contribution range from the computation of average background counts per pixel measured over all frames in the study, through the computation of average background counts per pixel for individual frames to pixel-by-pixel subtraction using interpolative techniques. The various techniques for background correction have been evaluated by several of the authors together with the different LV ROI definition approaches; the ejection fraction computed from contrast left ventriculography has been used as the golden standard. The results will be presented in the section Comparison with X-ray Ventriculography.

No single technique allows the separation of true left ventricular and background counts. All described techniques approximate with more or less success the contribution of background activity. With so many different background ROI methods in use, it is clear that a standardized solution must be found for the computation of LV background contributions.

(8) Global and Regional Ejection Fraction

In the early seventies global EF was assessed using geometric assumptions well known from contrast ventriculography. Strauss *et al.* computed EF on the basis of the area-length method from manually drawn ED and ES contours in the RAO30 projection for equilibrium studies; they found a correlation coefficient of $r = 0.92$ with single plane contrast ventriculography in a group of 20 patients [50]. However, this approach requires accurate boundary definition; because of the underlying geometric assumption and the limited resolution of the scintigraphic images, this method is less likely to be accurate for patients with irregular ventricles and significant wall motion defects. Moreover, a major problem in the RAO30 view is the delineation of the valve planes. An advantage of this geometric approach is that the problem of background correction is avoided. Using the area-length method Folland *et al.*, however, found relatively poor correlations with single plane contrast ventriculography ($r = 0.73$ in the scintigraphic RAO-view, 0.70 in the scintigraphic LAO-view) [51].

With the introduction of the digital computer interfaced to the gamma camera, additional information could be extracted from the acquired scintillations. If an intravenously injected radioactive tracer is uniformly distributed throughout the vascular space, the spatial distribution of absolute tracer is identical to that of the blood. Neglecting scatter contributions, the density (or recorded activity) of each pixel in the resulting image matrix represents the activity of the blood contained within the volume defined by the projection of the pixel area through the patient. The number of detected counts per pixel is then proportional to the total blood volume within the pixel projection. It has been mentioned already in the previous section, that a significant portion of the total activity detected by the left ventricular pixels is contributed by nonventricular, or background, activity. Photons originating from periventricular structure may undergo scattering and be projected into the left ventricular silhouette. Vascular activity in the chest wall interposed between the ventricle and the detector also contributes to apparent left ventricular activity. As a result, total left ventricular activity must be corrected for this nonventricular component. Left ventricular ejection fraction, therefore, can be computed as:

$$EF = \frac{(ED_c - B_d) - (ES_c - B_s)}{ED_c - B_d} \tag{11}$$

where ED_c denotes end-diastolic counts within the left ventricular ROI, ES_c the end-systolic counts within the LV ROI and B_d and B_s the end-diastolic and end-systolic background contributions, respectively. If one further assumes that background activity is constant for end-diastole and end-systole, formula (11) reduces to:

$$EF = \frac{ED_c - ES_c}{ED_c - B_d} \tag{12}$$

Because the ED background contribution is still present in the denominator, accurate determination of background activity is essential to avoid varying degrees of underestimation of EF. Despite the apparent limitations, the use of change in counts appears to be the most widely used method for determining EF. This count-volume method makes no geometric assumptions and is thus unaffected by irregulatories in the shape of the ventricle.

In general, three different methods can be distinguished to compute EF depending on the number of left ventricular regions involved. By the simplest method, denoted fixed ROI, the net ED and ES counts are computed within a single left ventricular ROI determined in the ED or sum image of the study. With the 2 ROI method, the boundaries of the LV in only the ED and ES images are determined and the corresponding counts computed. Following the third method, denoted variable ROI, the left ventricular contours are determined in each of the separate frames of the study and the ED and ES counts computed within the ED and ES ROI's in the corresponding images, respectively.

Although the global EF is the most widely used parameter describing LV function, several approaches have been published on the assessment of regional EF from gated blood pool studies following the count-based technique. However, translation and rotational movement of the heart or overlapping of atria and ventricles may cause changes in regional count density unrelated to regional contraction. For that reason and because of the limited resolution of the regional areas, regional EF has not been applied clinically as widely as global EF.

Silber et al. have divided the end-diastolic LV ROI into twelve radially-ordered sectors of 30° [45]. The radial-segmental EF is then calculated from the respective ED and ES count rates after paracardial background subtraction. The ES segmental count rates are measured within the designated ES LV ROI. The regional values can be displayed in different grey levels as a parametric ("functional") image and plotted as a curve. Normal values have been assessed from a group of 16 healthy control subjects.

Maddox et al. used 3 quadrisecting transverse axes within the manually drawn ED LV contour to obtain eight intraventricular subdivisions; because of overlap with the mitral and aortic valves the upper two regions at the base are excluded for the analysis of regional EF [10]. The 6 remaining intraventricular subdivisions were grouped into 3 anatomic regions. The regional EF is computed from the ED, ES and background counts within the fixed regions; the background counts were estimated using a weighted average of the counts per cell in each of three background regions obtained in the ES frame. Normal values for regional EF in the 3 anatomic regions were determined from the studies of 10 normal subjects. Radionuclide and roentgenographic methods were in agreement as to the presence or absence of abnormal wall motion in 83 of 99 LV regions (84%) in 33 patients evaluated prospectively. The reproducibility determined in 12 patients undergoing repeat radionuclide studies was excellent ($r = 0.98$; $S_{(x, y)} = 5.93$; slope $= 1.0$). Maddox et al. have also proposed the use of the ejection fraction image to assess regional LV wall motion [52]. This EF image represents on a pixel-by-pixel basis the local ejection fraction; it is computed by dividing the difference of the background corrected ED and ES images by the background corrected ED image. Comparison with contrast ventriculography data revealed a 90% agreement regarding presence or absence of wall motion abnormalities.

Reiber et al. compute regional EF for 6 radial segments within the fixed LV ROI automatically detected in the sum image of the study (Figure 3) [23]. The regional EF for segment n is defined by the difference in net ED and ES counts within this region relative to the net ED counts within the entire LV ROI. Background correction is performed by means of the automatically selected background region. As a result, the regional EF values for the 6 regions sum up to the global fixed ROI EF. The local EF for a particular segment is defined by the difference in net ED and ES counts within this region relative to its net ED counts. The range for local EF values is thus from 0 to 100%.

Hutton et al. use 5 radial regions defined with respect to the long axis of the left ventricle in the ED frame [44]. Douglas et al. subdivide the automatically detected ED LV regions into 8 sectors, with equi-angular spacing with respect to the ED geometric center [53]. Regional EF values are computed and compared with normal limits. Finally, for each patient a regional EF deficiency score is computed by summing the deviations from normal of each abnormal sector.

Most of the commercially available software packages provide methods for the computation of regional EF on the basis of a number of pie-shaped regions; the number of regions ranges from 3 to 48 (see Table 5). It appears that in the majority of the cases radial segments are defined with

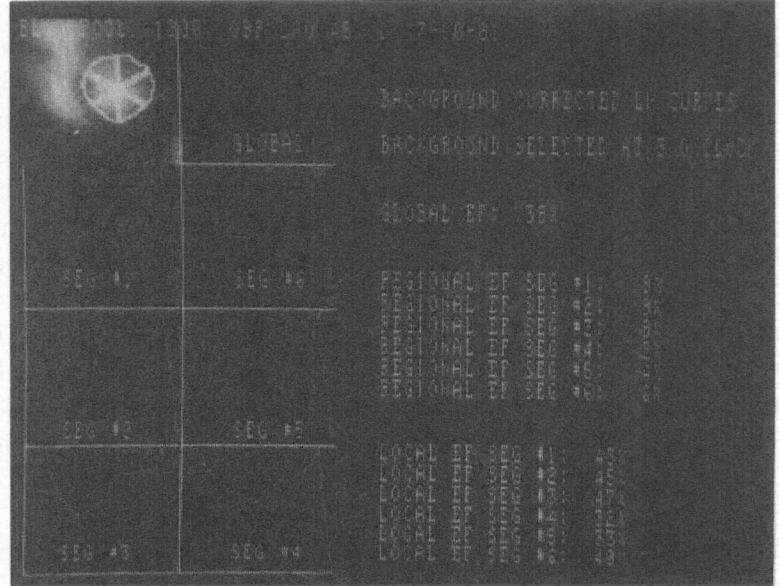

Figure 3. Definition of 6 radial regions for computation of regional and local ejection fractions.

respect to the ED centroid; translation of this point to the ES centroid for the computation of the ES contributions has been implemented in only one program.

The EF and paradox EF functional images are nowadays also supplied by a number of manufacturers. The paradox EF image is usually defined by dividing the difference of the background corrected ES- and ED-images (ES-ED) by the background corrected ES-image.

Besides the global ejection fraction, other parameters may be derived from the LV time activity curve, such as pre-ejection period (PEP), LV-ejection time (LVET), LV- fast filling time (LVFT1), LV- slow filling time (LVFT2), peak ejection rate (PER) and peak filling rate (PFR) [54].

Comparison with contrast ventriculography

Scintigraphic EF values should preferably be similar to the EF values obtained from contrast left ventriculograms under similar physiologic conditions. Several authors have compared the various techniques for the definition of the LV ROI's (fixed, 2 and variable ROI) and of the background region with contrast left ventriculography serving as the standard.

It has been shown that the fixed LV ROI method underestimates the contrast ejection fraction value by at least 10% [18, 19, 46, 47, 55, 56].

On theoretical and practical grounds Bacharach *et al.* have shown that the fixed ROI method is sensitive to background selection, but not to the left ventricular ROI definition. On the other hand, the 2 ROI method is not sensitive to background selection, but it is sensitive to the ES ROI definition [57]. They conclude that for manually drawn ROI's the fixed ROI method is more reproducible, but if the ES ROI can be determined in a highly reliable manner, e.g., by an automated edge detection scheme, the 2 ROI method is to be preferred. This conclusion has been supported by Lie, Gerbrands, Silber and Taylor [23, 43, 45, 46]. It must be clear that with respect to the computation of global EF, the above reasoning applies to the variable ROI method as well.

Evaluation results from the various studies have been tabulated in Table 1. The results are presented by means of the correlation coefficient between the scintigraphic and radiographic techniques and of the stan-dard-error-of-the-estimate (SEE) (if published) given in percent EF units. The number of patients involved in the study is also given, as well as whether the radiographic EF-values were computed from single (S) or biplane (B) cineangiograms. If the left ventricular and background ROI's in the scintigrams were manually defined, this is denoted by M; in one publication the scintigrams were analyzed fully automatically, while in all other instances the images were analyzed with a semi-automated tech-nique, indicated by Semi. It appears that all the fixed and 2 ROI methods, except for the one fully automated procedure, were analyzed manually, while the variable ROI studies were processed semi-automatically. All values of the SEE are below 11%, which seems quite acceptable, if one takes into account that the assessment of the EF by contrast ventriculogra-phy is also hampered by considerable inter- and intraobserver variations [58, 59].

Siber *et al.* compared in a group of 103 patients a total of 12 different scintigraphic methods for the determination of LV EF with the results from biplane contrast ventriculography [45]. Three methods required manual definition of the ED LV boundary only (fixed ROI), while in 3 additional methods the ES boundary was used as well (2 ROI). In three other methods the ED and ES boundaries were defined by means of a computer program on the basis of a first-difference operator and in the final 3 methods on the basis of a second-difference operator. Three different schemes of background definition were used. On the basis of the correlation coefficients Silber found the best correlation with manual

Table 1. Comparison of scintigraphic EF by different LV ROI methods with the data from contrast ventriculography. S: single plane contrast ventriculography; B: biplane contrast ventriculography; M: manual delineation of left ventricular region(s) of interest; Semi: using a semi-automated computer program (name of program)

Reference	No. of patients	Single (S)/ Biplane (B) x-ray	Fixed ROI	2 ROI	Var. ROI	Manual (M)/ (Semi)-automated
Folland [51]	30	S	r = 0.84, SEE = 11			M
Burow [19]	17	S	r = 0.83, SEE = 8			M
* scinti. values mean of 4 obs.					r = 0.92, SEE = 5	Semi
Parker [9] slant-hole coll	22	S	r = 0.94			M
Geffers [48]	30	S		r = 0.91		M
Green [18]	39	S	r = 0.92, SEE = 7			M
Maddahi [60]	35	B			r = 0.93	Semi
Maddox [10] slant-hole coll.	23	S	r = 0.91, SEE = 6			M
Sorensen [55]	20	B	r = 0.95, SEE = 5			M
	51	S	r = 0.72, SEE = 9.3			M
Wackers [61]	26	S			r = 0.83, SEE = 9.1	Semi (MUGE, MDS)
					r = 0.83, SEE = 9.3	Semi (NEW MUGE, MDS)
Pfisterer [62]	24	B			r = 0.84	Semi (MUGE, MDS)
					r = 0.92, SEE = 5.7	
Silber [45]	103	B		r = 0.95		M
Okada [20]	59	S			r = 0.70, sd = 6.2	Semi (MUGE, MDS)
Karsch [56]	37	B	r = 0.90, SEE = 6.7	r = 0.92, SEE = 6.2		M (IMAC, CGR)
						M (IMAC, CGR)
Hutton [44] slant-hole coll.	30	S			r = 0.91	Semi
Reiber [23]	48	S		r = 0.80, SEE = 10		Fully-Automated

designation of the 2 LV ROI's and paracardial background correction using a background ROI selected adjacent to the ED ventricular edge in the apico-lateral region. Only the correlation coefficient for their method of choice has been included in the table.

We have also investigated the effect of 5 different background selection methods on the EF for 3 automatically detected LV ROI methods (fixed, 2 and variable ROI); the results were compared with single plane contrast ventriculography [43]. The 5 background methods were: 1) fixed at 3 o'clock; 2) in a user-defined direction; 3) automatically selected; 4) defined by the difference in area between the ED and ES contours, and 5) no background correction at all. It was concluded from this preliminary evaluation study that the 2 ROI method with automatically selected background was the method of choice. In a final evaluation study only the automated background selection procedure for the 3 different LV ROI methods was considered. The best results were obtained with the 2 ROI method which is characterized by a small average difference of 1.3% EF units with the x-ray EF data and a standard deviation of the differences of 10.4 % EF units; the correlation coefficient equals 0.80 [23].

Based on the presented results and the fact that semi- and fully automated procedures are now widely available (section Overview of commercially available computer programs), it may be concluded that the 2 or variable ROI method should be used for the computation of global EF.

Inter- and intraobserver variations in global EF

When manual or semi-automated computer procedures are used for the computation of left ventricular EF, it is of importance to know the magnitude of the inter- and intraobserver variations. The results on interobserver variations from ten publications are summarized in Table 2. For each reference the number of patient studies involved and the number of observers are given, as well as the kind of LV ROI method used. In addition, the way the patient studies were processed, either entirely manually or with the help of a computer program, is given. Depending on the statistical procedure used, the results in percent EF units are expressed as: (1) the mean value of the standard deviations derived for the individual studies, (2) the mean and standard deviation plus the range of the absolute differences between the observations and (3) the average value of the correlation coefficients and standard-error-of-the-estimate (SEE) values among observers. Table 2 shows that the best results are

Table 2. Interobserver variations in the computation of ejection fraction. M: manual delineation of left ventricular region(s) of interest; Semi: using a semi-automated computer program (name of program). Bkgr: background.

Reference	No. of patients	No. of observers	Fixed ROI	2 ROI	Variable ROI	Manual (M)/ (Semi) automated
Burow [19]	17	4	mean sd = 6.89			M
Green [18]	20	3	r = 0.95, SEE = 6 (mean)		mean sd = 0.78	Semi
Douglas [22]	18	4	mean sd = 3			M
Maddahi [60]	35	2			r = 0.99 (2 min acq.)	Comput. edge detection
Slutsky [63]	18	2			3 ± 2 (range 0-6)	Semi (MUGE, MDS)
Wackers [61]	38	2			1.6 ± 1.5 (range 0-6)	Semi (MUGE, MDS)
Pfisterer [62]	24	2			1.0 ± 0.9 (range 0-3)	Semi (MUGE, MDS)
Taylor [46]	11	5	mean sd = 3.4			Isocount ED contour plus ED bkgr ROI
	11	5		mean sd = 8.1		Isocount contours plus ES bkgr ROI (FRAC, MDS)
	11	5		mean sd = 7.7		Isocount contours plus separate ED and ES bkgr ROI's
Okada [20]	11	5			mean sd = 1.2	Semi (MUGE, MDS)
	59	2			sd = 3	Semi (MUGE, MDS)
					sd = 4.4	Semi (NEW MUGE, MDS)
Hutton [44]	30	2			0.2 ± 2.2	Semi

achieved using semi-automated processing of the studies following the variable ROI technique. For this analysis procedure the values of the standard deviations are all below 5 percent EF units.

The intraobserver variations from 5 different publications are summarized in Table 3. In four studies the measurements were repeated twice, in the fifth one five times. The results in percent EF units are presented in terms of (1) correlation coefficient and SEE and (2) the mean and standard deviation plus the range of the absolute differences between the observations. Again the values of the standard deviations are below 5% EF units. The intraobserver variations in the manually processed studies are also very low, which means that the users were consistent in their drawing of the outlines and the selection of the background ROI's.

Reproducibility of GBP

To date only a limited number of studies have been published in the literature concerning the reproducibility and intrinsic variability of gated cardiac blood pool scintigraphy. The results from eight publications are summarized in Table 4. For each reference is given the number of patients involved, the acquisition period of the study, whether it concerns rest or exercise studies and the interval between the repeat studies. It should be clear that the variability data consists of the variability in repeating the GBP study and of the variability in the analysis of the study. The variability is expressed in terms of the mean $\pm$ standard deviation of the relative differences between serial measurements; for most studies the correlation coefficient is given as well. Wackers *et al.* found significant differences in the serial variability between normal (EF $\geqslant 55\%$) patients and abnormal (EF $<55\%$) patients [61]. The mean serial variability of EF in repeated gated studies on the same day for 22 normal patients was significantly larger than for the 19 abnormal patients (0.7 ± 6.7 versus $-0.6 \pm 2.5\%$, respectively, $p <0.05$). Similarly, the mean serial variability for studies on different days in 15 patients with a normal EF was significantly larger than in those 14 patients with an abnormal value (1.1 ± 7.6 versus $-0.2 \pm 3.4\%$, respectively, $p <0.01$).

The results from all these studies indicate that the overall reproducibility of gated blood pool scintigraphy is good with mean values of relative differences in EF between repeat rest and exercise studies less than 2.2 and 1.9% EF units, respectively and standard deviations of the differences less than 6.1 and 7.3% EF units, respectively.

Table 3. Intraobserver variations in the computation of ejection fraction. M: manual delineation of left ventricular region(s) of interest; Semi: using a semi-automated computer program (name of program)

Reference	No. of patients	No. of repeated meas.	Fixed ROI	2 ROI	Var. ROI	Manual (M)/ (Semi)automated
Sorensen [55]	51	2	$r = 0.98$, SEE = 2.8			M
					$r = 0.94$, SEE = 5.6	Semi (MUGE, MDS)
					$r = 0.97$, SEE = 3.9	Semi (NEW MUGE, MDS)
Slutsky [63]	18	2			2 ± 2 (range 0-5)	Semi (MUGE, MDS)
Wackers [61]	156	2			1.4 ± 1.2 (range 0-5)	Semi (MUGE, MDS)
Okada [20]	59	2			sd = 2.9	Semi (MUGE, MDS)
					sd = 4.4	Semi (NEW MUGE, MDS)
Karsch [56]	3	5	sd = 2.7	sd = 3.2		M (IMAC, CGR)
						M (IMAC, CGR)

Exercise gated blood pool studies

Exercise gated blood pool studies have been used as a noninvasive procedure for the detection of patients with coronary artery disease [5, 67–69]. Slutsky *et al.* have shown that in normal subjects, the end-diastolic volume (EDV) does not change significantly with exercise, while the end-systolic volume (ESV) declines by an average of 56%, thereby accounting for the rise in EF [6]. In patients who develop angina, the EF decreases because of an increase in the ESV, while the EDV remains unchanged. In patients with coronary disease who do not develop angina, the changes in volume tend to vary considerably, but the mean values for this group show little change in EDV, ESV or EF.

Caldwell *et al.* found a specificity of only 54% by using a fixed ROI method for the computation of rest and exercise EF [70]. The sensitivity based on abnormal exercise EF response was 93%. If an abnormal rest study was considered a positive test, even though EF increased with exercise, then a sensitivity of 95% was found. Sorensen *et al.* have shown that falsely abnormal EF responses to exercise radionuclide angiography may occur due to the method of ROI-selection in normal subjects with normal or high ejection fractions [71]. In their study abnormal values were found using the fixed ROI method; these deviations were resolved by using a 2 ROI method. Essentially, the same findings have been reported by Karimeddini *et al.* [72]. Sorensen *et al.* conclude that in patients showing normal exercise duration, normal blood pressure and pulse-rate response, but with an abnormal EF response by the fixed ROI method, repeated analyis with a 2 or varying region method should be carried out.

Data acquisition at exercise is usually performed in the modified LAO45 orientation with the subject in the supine position. Berman *et al.* employ upright bicycle exercise since it represents a more physiologic form of stress. However, they have shown that upright and supine exercise scintigraphic techniques are equally effective in the assessment of stress ventricular function [69, 73]. Studies have been performed with imaging only taking place during maximal exercise for a period of at least two minutes [68], as well as during each step of the workload, with acquisition periods ranging from 2–4 minutes. Matrix sizes of both 64×64 and 32×32 are in use. Green *et al.* proposed a matrix size of 32×32 with 12 images spanning the average cardiac cycle and the use of a high sensitivity collimator [67]. Both low-energy-all-purpose (LEAP) collimators and high-sensitivity (HS) collimators have been used during exercise studies. The great advantage of the HS-collimator, of course, is the fact that

Table 4. Reproducibility of gated blood pool scintigraphy. M: manual delineation of left ventricular region(s) of interest; Semi: using a semi-automated computer program (name of program)

Reference	No. of patients	Acquisition periods	Interval	Fixed ROI	2 ROI	Variable ROI	Manual (M)/ (Semi)-automated
Maddahi [60]	35	2 min; rest	1 hour			5.7 ± 4.8	Computerized edge-detection
		2 min; 6 min rest				$r = 0.99$ (absolute diff.)	
Pfisterer [62]	24	2 min; rest	sequential			$-0.4 \pm 2.1\ r = 0.98$	Semi (MUGE, MDS)
	24	2 min; 5 min rest					
Pfisterer [64]	16	5 min; rest	average 15 days (range 1-66)			-0.2 ± 1.3	Semi (MUGE, MDS)
						$0.3 \pm 3.6\ r = 0.95$	Semi (MUGE, MDS)
		2 min; exer. 2 + 3'				$0.8 \pm 5.4\ r = 0.91$	
		2 min; exer. 5 + 6'				$0.9 \pm 3.4\ r = 0.97$	
		2 min; max exer.				$1.9 \pm 3.6\ r = 0.97$	
		2 min; recov. 2 + 3'				$0.3 \pm 3.9\ r = 0.95$	

	N					M
		2 min; recov. 4 + 5'			0.3 ± 4.5 r = 0.92	
		2 min; recov. 9 + 10'			2.9 ± 4.4 r = 0.91	
Maddox [10] slant-hole coll.	12	1000 cardiac cycles; rest	40-120 min	SEE = 1.5 r = 0.99		
Wackers [61]	41	6 min; rest	1-2 h		0.1 ± 5.2 r = 0.97	Semi (SUP 8 – MUGE, MDS)
Slutsky [63]	29	6 min; rest	1-5 days		0.5 ± 5.9 r = 0.93	Semi (MUGE, MDS)
	25	10 min; rest	1 h		-0.1 ± 4.2 r = 0.97	
			2 h		-0.4 ± 5.2 r = 0.95	
			3 h		0.2 ± 3.8 r = 0.98	
			4 h		-0.2 ± 4.6 r = 0.94	
Hecht [65]	18	2 min; rest	14 days		2.2 ± 6.1 r = 0.90	Semi (MUGE, MDS)
		2 min; exer.	14 days		1.2 ± 7.3 r = 0.93	
Reiber [23]	12	6 min; rest	aver. 27 min (range 15-50 min)	0.3 ± 3.7 r = 0.98		Fully automated
				0.8 ± 4.3 r = 0.98		Fully automated
Melin [66]	10	5 min; rest	aver. 90 min		1.9 ± 5.6 r = 0.96	Semi (Apex, Elscint)

reasonable statistics may be obtained during the short acquisition periods, however, at the cost of resolution. For purposes of calculating EF, this loss of resolution does not seem to pose a great problem. For that reason, an HS collimator is also used in our institute. Our exercise protocol starts with a 4 min. acquisition at rest, followed by 2.5 min. acquisitions at the different work loads. Exercise starts at 40 W and increases every 3 min. with 20 W. At the end of the exercise study a 4 min. recovery scan is obtained.

Okado *et al.* have studied in a group of 59 patients the observer variance in the quantitation of LV EF using rest and exercise gated blood pool scintigrams [20]. Studies were acquired with a high-resolution (HRES) collimator with 3 min acquisition at each stage of the workload. Data were analyzed with the semi-automated MUGE-program of MDS. EF was determined six times by 2 independent observers. Results were analyzed by a two-way analysis of variance and expressed as ± 2 sd. Intraobserver and interobserver variance for exercise EF determinations were ±9.2% and ±9.6%, respectively. According to Okada, an average of at least 2 determinations for both the rest and exercise scintigrams should be used when calculating an exercise-induced change in ejection fraction. Using this technique, an exercise-induced change in EF must exceed 4.6% to be significant at the 95%-confidence level.

Overview of commercially available computer programs

Nine manufacturers of nuclear medicine computer systems were asked to complete a questionnaire on the different aspects of their state-of-the-art semi- or fully-automated computer program for the computation of global and regional EF. The ADAC and Informatek companies did not respond; however, the CGR data may be used as a guideline for ADAC since the hardware and software of these systems are basically identical. The Philips program has not become commercially available at the time of this publication [74]. The results are summarized in Table 5. The procedure developed in our institute on a Dec Gamma-11 computer system, although not commercially available, has been listed in the last column under Thoraxcenter. For more detailed information the reader is referred to the user-manuals and other publications from the vendors. It should be clear that particularly the data on success rates of the fully automated procedures must be interpreted very carefully. The success rate of a procedure depends to a great extent on the count density in the images, the precise criteria used for acceptance and rejection of the results from an analyzed study, the collimator used, the size of the images, the number of frames, etc. An objective comparison is only possible by creating a large data base of patient studies with rest and exercise, acquired with LEAP and HS collimators, different matrix sizes and frame rates, etc. and analyzing all these studies with the various computer programs. The incompatibility between most of the computer systems makes this an enormous task. It would require acquisition in list mode to obtain the raw data to be transferred to the different computer systems.

Another approach, although not entirely representative for the performance of the programs for routine clinical studies, could consist of setting up a great number of different, reproducible studies with a dynamic heart phantom.[‡*] MacIntyre *et al.* have proposed a computer simulated cardiac model to test edge detection and ejection fraction algorithms [75].

When comparing the details of the listed nine acquisition and analysis procedures, it becomes clear that the methods vary considerably. To the author's knowledge, no large scale evaluation study on the intersystem variability in EF measurements has been performed as yet.

Fourier analysis

So far methods have been described to compute global and regional ejection fraction from rest and exercise gated blood pool studies and the variability in the assessment of these parameters have been discussed. However, the gated studies also allow diagnosis, localization and quantitation of left ventricular regional wall motion abnormalities (RWMA). The simplest technique consists of displaying the images in the different views in closed loop cine format and having the observer visually interpret regional wall motion. This approach is hampered by relatively large inter- and intraobserver variations [20]. Semi- or fully-automated detection of the left ventricular boundaries in the LAO45 view in each of the frames of the gated study and displaying the detected boundaries in a movie format facilitates the interpretation of wall motion abnormalities in this projection. However, the motion of nontangential segments of the ventricle remains impossible to assess from such two-dimensional data.

In recent years, it has been shown that information extraction from the

---

‡ Dynamic cardiac function phantom, Model DCP-101, Veenstra Instrumenten BV.
* Vanderbilt cardiac phantom, Capintec Inc.

Table 5. Overview computer programs for acquisition and analysis of gated blood pool studies

Company/Institute	CGR	Elscint	General Electric	MDS	Philips	Siemens Gammasonics	Technicare	Thoraxcenter
Name program	2 EDGE; EF	Apex	PACE	Auto EF	EF; REGEF	ACAP	MICA/GRADIENT	BP
Acquisition								
1. Frame format	64 × 64; byte 128 × 128; byte	64 × 64; word 128 × 128; word	32 × 32; 12 bits 64 × 64	64 × 64; byte or word	64 × 64; byte	64 × 64; byte	64 × 64; 10 bits 128 × 128; 10 bits	64 × 64; word
2. Zoom/non-zoom in x, y	1, 1.5, 3.0	1, 2.0	1, 1.5, 2.0, 2.5	1, 1.14, 1.30, 1.48, 1.69, 1.93, 2.19, 2.50	1, 1.54	1; √2	1; 2	1; √2
3. Frames/RR interval	16 or 32 (64 × 64); 2, 4, 16 (128 × 128); over typically 90% of R-R interval	max 64 (64 × 64) max 16 (128 × 128)	24	16-32	32	16 frames over 75% of R-R-interval	64 (64 × 64) 16 (128 × 128)	20
4. Acquisition mode(s)	– frame mode – list mode	– frame mode	– frame mode – list mode	– serial mode (recommended) – frame mode	– frame mode – list mode	– frame mode	– frame mode	– frame mode
5. Arrhythmia detection	*frame mode:* gate tolerance of ±10% of average R-R interval, which may be held fixed over study period or allowed to vary (running average over 5 accepted beats) *list mode:* user selects R-R window from histogram; forward/backward framing	double buffering (combined list and frame mode)	*frame mode:* real-time arrhythmia rejection; current cycle buffered; R-R interval outside gate tolerance 5-15% with respect to average R-R interval measured over first 10 beats of acquisition *list mode:* Select acceptance interval with ±4% window; forward/backward framing	*serial mode:* R-R window from histogram; weighted sum of forward and backward framing *frame mode:* no arrhythmia det. (work in progress)	*frame mode:* gate tolerance 15-20% of average R-R interval measured over 50-100 beats previous to study (no running average) *list mode:* R-R window from histogram, either manually selected or automatically (±8%) to peak; forward/backward framing	gate tolerance of ±25% of average of previous 4 accepted R-R intervals	gate tolerance of ±10% with respect to average R-R interval measured over previous 30-40 beats	gate tolerance of 100 ms with respect to running average R-R interval (30 s)

	Method 1	Method 2	Method 3	Method 4	Method 5	Method 6	Method 7	Method 8
6. Semi/Fully automatic	Fully automatic	Semi automatic	Fully automatic	Fully automatic	Fully automatic	Fully automatic	Semi automatic	Semi automatic
7. User interaction possible at crucial steps?	yes; LV center, LV contours, Background selection	yes; background region, LV box	yes; select different edge detection weighting factor	no	no; via Batch processor	yes; LV center, LV parameters, Background region		yes; LV box, LV contours, background region
8. Preprocessing	unweighted spatial (3 × 3) and weighted temporal (1, 2, 1) filtering	spatial (9 pts weighted 1, 6, 1) and temporal (1, 2, 1) filtering	spatial filtering (4 × 4)	spatial and temporal (cosine) filtering	spatial (11 × 11) and temporal, both weighted	Fourier filtering; spatial + temporal	optional; weighted spatial (3 × 3) and temporal (1, 2, 1) filtering	optional; weighted spatial (3 × 3, 5 × 5, or 7 × 7) and temporal (3-5 frames) filtering
9. LV identification	Automatic from signatures of row and column sums	User sets first (diastole) LV box	Automatic; searches for 1/4 moon (RV) and circle (LV) in first frame	Automatic from 1) amplitude and phase data; 2) ED-ES	Automatic from stroke count image	Automatic from 1st harmonic amplitude image and ED image	user sets MASTER ROI around LV	user indicates LV center and adjusts, if necessary, system-generated rectangular box
10. Edge-detection	max. 2nd difference in polar coordinates (64 radii); 2 iterations	Following bkgr. subtr., 4 direction max. gradient search per frame from centroid within adaptive LV box	Combination 1st (40%) and 2nd (60%) difference; region growing; recursive boundary detection	Laplacian in 4 directions	Radial search (8 directions); 1st derivative in ED defines seed region; edge defined by zero-crossing 2nd derivative; 2 iterations	2nd derivative zero crossing plus empirical parameters along 48 radii	2nd derivative zero crossing plus computed threshold values; radial search	Laplacian filter; radial (40 radii) search from centroid; 2 iterations
11. EF by Fixed/2Var(iable) ROI	Fixed/2/Var. ROI	Var. ROI	Var. ROI on first 14 frames	2/Var. ROI	Fixed/2/Var. ROI	Var. ROI	Var. ROI	Fixed/2/Var. ROI
12. Background (bkgr) region	Automatic; 'optimal' region chosen from 6 regions along free wall on basis of minimal values of mean and variance over 14 frames	Manual; user draws region during cine display	Automatic; adjacent to ED contour in lower right quadrant	Automatic; 'optimal' region selected from 5 regions along free wall in ES on basis of minimal variance over 32 frames	Automatic; adjacent to free wall in ES image	Automatic; region between inner and outer perimeter of LV defined by 1st and 2nd zero crossing of 2nd deriv., resp.	Automatic; adjacent to free wall in ES image	Manual; indicate 2 end points of bkgr region in ED or ES image

Table 5. Continued.

Company/Institute	CGR	Elscint	General Electric	MDS	Philips	Siemens Gammasonics	Technicare	Thoraxcenter
13. Background (bkgr) correction	Average bkgr counts in selected frame used for correction in all frames	Average ES bkgr counts used for correction in all frames	Per frame pixel-by-pixel subtraction around LV perimeter; interpolative technique	Average bkgr counts/pixel measured in ES frame applied to each frame	Average bkgr counts/pixel measured in ES applied to each frame	Bkgr contribution measured per frame	Average counts/pixel measured over all frames; subtracted per pixel in each frame	Average counts/pixel within optimal region measured over 14 frames applied to each frame
14. Regional EF	8 radial segments from ED and ES centroids	EF and paradox EF functional images	48 wedges	8 radial segments from centroid ED ROI	8 radial segments from centroid of ED ROI	EF and paradox EF functional images	3 regions with respect to manually defined LV long axis; EF + paradox EF images	6 radial segments from centroid of sum-image
15. Processing time	2–6 min (16 ROI's)	global EF: 1 min; regional EF: add. 1 min	7 min	4 min (32 frames); 2 3/4 min with array processor	1.8 min (2 ROI); 4 min (Var. ROI)	3–4 min (depending on size LV)	4 s per frame; 90 s 16 frames incl. preprocessing	70 s Fixed ROI 120 s 2 ROI 185 s Var. ROI
16. Success rate	90%	–	84% on 69 patient sample	90% of routine patient studies	80% (HS coll) 92% (LEAP coll); stress studies	87% on 120 patient studies	95%	92% on 100 rest patient studies
17. Correlation with contrast LV angio	$r = 0.87$ ($N = 20$ patient studies)	–	–	$r = 0.85$	$r = 0.96$ ($N = 60$ biplane LV angio's)	–	$r = 0.92$ ($N = 17$ patient studies)	$r = 0.80$ (single plane angio's, $N = 48$)
18. Correlation with manual proc.	–	–	$r = 0.99$	$r = 0.95$ with semi-autom. technique (MUGE)	–	$r = 0.94$ ($N = 51$ studies)	–	–
19. Inter-/Intra-observer variations	2%	Interobs. var. = 2% ($N = 20$)	none	none	none	none	Interobs. var. = 2% ($N = 32$)	none

gated blood pool scintigrams with particular reference to the detection of local wall motion abnormalities, can be improved by means of Fourier analysis, first proposed by Geffers *et al.* [48]. This technique also allows the evaluation of hemodynamic changes induced by disturbances of electrical activation (conduction abnormalities) [76, 77].

Methods

Fourier analysis is a mathematical technique by means of which any periodic function can be represented as the sum of sine and cosine waves of different frequencies, each frequency characterized by a specific amplitude and phase. The periodic nature of ventricular contraction seems ideally suitable for this technique. In a gated blood pool study, most of the changes in activity within the heart occur at the fundamental frequency, the heart rate. Therefore, to a first approximation, only the first harmonic of the basic frequency needs to be considered; the amplitude of this frequency component represents stroke volume and the phase the onset of systolic wall motion. The coefficients of the sine and cosine of the base frequency for a particular pixel in the image can be obtained as follows [78, 79]:

$$\text{cosine coefficient } C = \frac{2}{N} \sum_{i=1}^{N} A(i) \cdot \cos\left[(i-1) \cdot \frac{2\pi}{N} \right] \tag{13}$$

$$\text{sine coefficient } S = \frac{2}{N} \sum_{i=1}^{N} A(i) \cdot \sin\left[(i-1) \cdot \frac{2\pi}{N} \right] \tag{14}$$

where N is the number of frames per heart cycle and $A(i)$ the count density at time interval i ($1 \leq i \leq N$). The amplitude (FA) and phase (PH) of the base frequency are then defined by

$$FA = \sqrt{C^2 + S^2} \tag{15}$$

and

$$PH = \arctan(-S/C) \tag{16}$$

As $A(i)$ may be described by a Poisson distribution, the standard deviation (sd) for FA values is given by

$$sd = \sqrt{\frac{1}{N} \sum_{i=1}^{N} A(i)} \tag{17}$$

The amplitude can be visualised using an incremental code (color or monochrome). However, the phase is a cyclic parameter; for an unequivocal visualization a cyclic color code is required [80].

Frame formats that have been used for Fourier analysis range from 16 to 64 frames per R-R interval with matrix sizes of 32×32 and 64×64 pixels. Based on the comparison of the amplitude and phase images by the Fourier and Hadamard transform, Bossuyt et al. conclude that 16 frames are sufficient [81]. To assure reliable results a great number of counts should be collected, which favors the use of a HS collimator. For 16 frames/cycle, matrix size 64×64 and pixel size 4×4 mm a total of 6 Mcounts is typical.

It was described in the early part of this paper that the last frames of a gated blood pool study usually are distorted by the drop in count rate due to irregular cardiac rhythm. Before applying the Fourier analysis, these last frames should be time corrected. Provided the entire heart region is within the image matrix, the total number of counts of each individual frame should approximately remain constant over the representative cardiac cycle. With frame mode acquisition the low data frames at the end of the cardiac cycles may be scaled using the average of the total counts in each frame from the first half of the cycle. In our institute each frame is normalized to the frame with the maximal total number of counts within the matrix. Taylor et al., have proposed to derive the correction factors from the time-activity curve of a non-cardiac region in the images, which should be constant with time [82]. Similarly, Vos places during acquisition a small source of 1.5 MBq (40 μCi) Tc-99m in one of the corners of the field of view of the camera [83]. After data acquisition a curve is generated of the activity within a ROI around the source. The count densities in the frames are then corrected for the effect of variations of cycle lengths on the basis of the measured counts within the ROI with respect to the average number of counts within this ROI assessed over the first frames of the study. In list mode acquisition, time correction is also necessary if a forward synchronizing technique for framing is used; this can be avoided by using an additional set of backward synchronized frames, which replaces about the last third part of the forward synchronized frames.

Vos et al. proposed a variable frequency technique for the calculation of the sinusoid [83]. For each study the most suitable frequency is determined on the basis of the Fourier spectrum of the global LV time-activity curve. This procedure usually excludes the last frames of the study. No relevant information is lost, as nearly all information which is necessary for the assessment of ventricular contractility is contained in the systolic and early diastolic time intervals. This technique allows the use of a simple frame mode acquisition.

Prior to taking the Fourier transform of a study, it is useful to apply spatial and temporal filtering to the images to reduce noise and to preserve the smooth flow of data in a periodic manner. For these purposes a 9 points spatial and 3 points temporal smoothing may be used.

Interpretation

Applying the Fourier analysis to a gated study results in the generation of two parametric images, the amplitude (FA) image and the phase (PH) image. The changes in count density for each pixel in the image over the representative cardiac cycle are characterized by its amplitude and phase, thus allowing the assessment of local wall motion abnormalities. The phase image is a temporal "map" of the sequence of cardiovascular chamber emptying. Moving structures as the ventricles and atria show amplitudes which differ significantly from zero (>2 sd) and nonmoving structures have amplitudes less than 2 sd. The phase-information allows to differentiate between ventricles and atria together with the large vessels due to a phase shift of about 180°. In regions with low count variations, the phase image shows large amounts of noise. Since these phase values have no clinical significance, all pixels with an amplitude below a given threshold (e.g., 2 sd) may be set to the black level in the phase display.

Dyskinetic areas can be recognized by a decrease in amplitude, combined with a phase shift of more than 90° with respect to normal contracting regions. Hypokinetic regions show a decrease of amplitude, with a delay less than 90°. Akinesia can be recognized by the absence of amplitude; recognition of akinetic regions belonging to the left ventricle may be facilitated by superimposing the LV boundary in the parametric images. From the amplitude and phase images, an amplitude weighted or unweighted phase distribution function within a particular ROI may be computed.

In addition to the static amplitude and phase images, a dynamic display may be derived, such as a continuous-loop cinematic display of the wave of emptying as it spreads over the cardiac chambers, as proposed by Links *et al.* [84]. From the phase of each pixel, the frame F in which that pixel's fundamental frequency curve is maximally positive is computed. Subsequently, an N-frame study (with N being the number of frames in study) is created in which each pixel is blacked out in its appropriate frame F. This new study, representing the wave of emptying, can be displayed over either the cinematic display of the original gated study or over a static image formed by adding the ED and ES frames, to serve as an anatomical guide. According to Links *et al.* the cinematic display of the wave of emptying together with a distribution histogram of the pixel phase values is useful in the study of motion abnormalities and asynergies.

The parametric images are usually interpreted subjectively. However, quantification of regional wall motion is necessary to assess the extent, grade and statistical significance of wall motion abnormalities. A number of different approaches towards quantification of the amplitude and phase images have been presented in the literature; these will be described briefly in the following paragraphs.

Adam *et al.* have proposed two different ways [78]:

(a) Histograms of the various parameters within the LV area are calculated and compared with histograms of a group of normal subjects.

(b) The ED LV area is divided into segments. The segment sum of various parameters is calculated and compared with the data from a group of normal subjects.

Phases are normalized to the global phase of the normal LV area, whereas the normalization of the amplitude is based upon the EF of the LV. The sensitivity and specificity for the detection of regional wall motion abnormalities on the basis of the FA and PH images were 86.4% and 100%, respectively in a group of 68 patients with suspected or proven coronary artery disease.

The distribution function of the amplitudes and phases over the left ventricle may be analyzed statistically in order to determine the variance, skew, kurtosis, etc. of the distribution [83, 85]. Bacharach *et al.* have investigated in a simulation study the effects of changes in the details of LV time activity curve shape on the phase and amplitude. They found that diastolic events may influence phase changes as strongly as systolic events. Ratib *et al.* studied the phase distribution (unweighted) within the left ventricular ROI at rest and exercise [86]. The histogram of the ventricular peak is described by a mean phase, as well as the standard deviation. Its upper limits of normal at rest and exercise were established in seven normals as the mean +2 sd and were 12 degrees at rest and 10 degrees at exercise. They concluded, that phase analysis not only permits separation of wall motion abnormalities induced by ischemia from those associated with valvular disease, but that it is also an objective, highly sensitive and specific indicator of regional myocardial ischemia. Vos concluded that the mean amplitude (which is stroke volume) over the LV ROI is the most important parameter for quantification of wall motion abnormalities and that the standard deviation of the phase histogram over the LV ROI is a specific parameter in the detection of regional wall motion abnormalities. In addition, heart rate should be taken into account in phase analysis as phase is sensitive for paradoxically moving wall regions; the phase is of no value for the quantification of hypokinetic wall segments. Skewness and kurtosis of the amplitude and phase histogram were found to be of no additional value for wall motion analysis.

Bossuyt compared in a group of 116 patients regional wall motion abnormalities by the Fourier technique with the subjective interpretation from single and biplane contrast ventriculography [81]. The sensitivity of the radionuclide studies for the diagnosis of normal/abnormal wall motion was found to be 93%, the specificity 95%. Complete agreement on the location of all segmental wall motion disturbances was found in 57% of the patients, partial agreement in 24% and total disagreement in 19%. He concluded that nontangential segments are less well visualized on radionuclide ventriculograms, in particular when they are hypokinetic.

Pavel et al. describe the distribution of unweighted phase in the left and right ventricles by means of: $\triangle$ mean (difference between the mean phase of the left and right ventricles); $\triangle$ mode (difference between the modes of their phase histograms); standard deviation and skewness of each phase distribution histogram [77]. They conclude that the phase image is capable of showing differences between patients with electrical activation and a variety of electrical abnormalities.

Recently, Bacharach et al. have presented a method for characterizing functional maps, such as the phase image, by means of a frequency distribution function (DF) [87, 88]. It has been shown that analysis of the DF permits detection of regional abnormalities of LV wall motion and that a single number may be produced as a descriptor of overall organ function.

Bossuyt et al. have proposed an alternative approach for the quantification of wall motion disturbances by an amplitude/phase dependent factor which takes into account all the Fourier frequencies, except the zero-frequency component. For each pixel a time activity curve is generated and a minimal dc value is subtracted such that the activity in each particular pixel becomes zero in one of the images of the series. Based on the pixel-wise subtracted time activity curve within the LV ROI a contractility index Ci is calculated as

$$Ci = \frac{max - min}{max} \tag{18}$$

Over synchronously moving structure the Ci will reach 100%, while the Ci will decrease if the ROI contains pixels which are out of phase [89]. Displaying the pixel-wise subtracted images also results in contrast enhancement as compared to the original images.

From the above it may be concluded that the Fourier technique is gaining acceptance. However, the true clinical values and limitations have not been fully determined as yet. More work needs to be done to standardize on procedures for the quantitative analysis of these images to allow objective characterization of wall motion abnormalities.

Concluding remarks

It may be concluded from the data presented in this paper that gated blood pool scintigraphy is a clinically accepted noninvasive routine procedure for the assessment of left ventricular function at rest and exercise. When using appropriate semi- or fully-automated computer analysis techniques, the resulting ejection fractions by the 2 or variable ROI methods are similar to those from contrast ventriculography (SEE <11% EF units). Such techniques are characterized by relatively low inter- and intraobserver variations in the computation of global ejection fraction (standard deviations of absolute differences below 5% EF units). The overall reproducibility of gated blood pool scintigraphy is good with mean values of relative differences in EF between rest and exercise repeat studies less than 2.2 and 1.9% EF units, respectively and standard deviations of the differences less than 6.1 and 7.3% EF units, respectively.

Nearly every manufacturer of nuclear medicine computer systems nowadays offers a software package for the semi- or fully-automated analysis of the ejection fraction. Since standardization on the basic principles applied in these programs does not exist at this time, a large scale evaluation study on the intersystem variability in EF measurements should be carried out.

Assessment of left ventricular wall motion abnormalities from Fourier analysis seems very promising, but is not yet in wide use. Criteria need to be developed which allow objective quantitative characterization of wall motion abnormalities.

Acknowledgements

The author greatly appreciates the critical reading of this manuscript by
J.J. Gerbrands, C.J. Kooijman, M.L. Simoons and W. Wijns. He wishes
to acknowledge the secretarial assistance of M.J. Kanters-Stam and A.A.
Wagenaar.

References

1. Hoffmann G, Kleine N: Eine neue Methode zur unblutigen Messung des Schlagvolumens am
   Menschen über viele Tage mit Hilfe von radioaktiven Isotopen. Verh Dtsch Ges Kreislaufforsch
   31: 93–96, 1965.
2. Adam WE, Schenk P, Kampmann H, Lorenz WJ, Schneider WG, Ammann W, Bilaniuk L:
   Investigation of cardiac dynamics using scintillation camera and computer. In: Medical radioisotope scintigraphy II, Vienna, IAEA, 77–89, 1969.
3. Adam WE, Tarkowska A, Bitter F, Stauch M, Geffers H: Equilibrium (gated) radionuclide
   ventriculography. Cardiovasc Radiol 2: 161–173, 1979.
4. Bodenheimer MM, Banka VA, Helfant RH: Nuclear cardiology I Radionuclide angiographic
   assessment of left ventricular contraction: uses, limitations and future directions. Amer J Cardiol
   45: 661–673, 1980.
5. Borer JS, Kent KM, Bacharach SL, Green MV, Rosing DR, Seides SF, Epstein SE, Johnston
   GS: Sensitivity, specificity and predictive accuracy of radionuclide cineangiography during exercise in patients with coronary artery disease. Comparison with exercise Electrocardiography.
   Circulation 60, 3: 572–580, 1979.
6. Slutsky R, Karliner J, Ricci D, Schuler G, Pfisterer M, Peterson K, Ashburn W: Response of left
   ventricular volume to exercise in man assessed by radionuclide equilibrium angiography. Circulation 60: 565–571, 1979.
7. Hegge FN, Hamilton GW, Larson SM, Ritchie JL, Richards P: Cardiac chamber imaging: a
   comparison of red blood cells labelled with Tc-99m in vitro and in vivo. J Nucl Med 19: 129–133,
   1978.
8. Vyth A, Raam CFM, Schoot JB van der: Semi in vitro labelling of red blood cells with ^{99m}Tc: a
   comparison with the in vivo labelling. Pharm Weekblad Sci Ed 3: 198–200, 1981.
9. Parker JA, Uren RF, Jones AG, Maddox DE, Zimmerman RE, Neill JM, Holman BL:
   Radionuclide left ventriculography with the slant hole collimator. J Nucl Med 18: 848–851, 1977.
10. Maddox DE, Wynne J, Uren R, Parker JA, Idoine J, Siegel LC, Neill JM, Cohn PF, Holman BL:
    Regional ejection fraction: a quantitative radionuclide index of regional left ventricular perform-
    ance. Circulation 59: 1001–1009, 1979.
11. Bacharach SL, Green MV, Borer JS, Hyde JE, Farkas SP, Johnston GS: Left-ventricular peak
    ejection rate, filling rate, and ejection fraction – Frame rate requirements at rest and exercise:
    concise communication. J Nucl Med 20: 189–193, 1979.
12. Aswegen A van, Alderson PO, Nickoloff EL, Housholder DF, Wagner HN: Temporal resolution
    requirements for left ventricular time-activity curves. Radiology 135: 165–170, 1980.
13. Bacharach SL, Green MV, Borer JS: Instrumentation and data processing in cardiovascular
    nuclear medicine: evaluation of ventricular function. Sem Nucl Med 9: 257–274, 1979.
14. Apex in Nuclear Cardiology: Brochure, Elscint.
15. Green MV, Ostrow HG, Douglas MA, Myers RW, Scott RN, Bailey JJ, Johnston GS: High
    temporal resolution ECG-gated scintigraphic angiocardiography. J Nucl Med 16: 95–98, 1975.
16. Graaf CN de, Rijk PP van: High temporal and high phase resolution construction techniques for

cardiac motion imaging. In: Medical radionuclide imaging. IAEA Vienna, Vol 1, pp 377–384, 1977.

17. Parker JA, Secker-Walker R, Hill R, Siegel BA, Potchen EJ: A new technique for the calculation of left ventricular ejection fraction. J Nucl Med 13: 649–651, 1972.

18. Green MV, Brody WR, Douglas MA, Borer JS, Ostrow HG, Line BR, Bacharach SL, Johnston GS: Ejection fraction by count rate from gated images. J Nucl Med 19: 880–883, 1978.

19. Burow RD, Strauss HW, Singleton R, Pond M, Rehn T, Bailey IK, Griffith LC, Nickoloff E, Pitt B: Analysis of left ventricular function from multiple gated acquisition cardiac blood pool imaging. Comparison to contrast angiography. Circulation 56: 1024–1028, 1977.

20. Okada RD, Kirschenbaum HD, Kushner FG, Strauss HW, Dinsmore RE, Newell JB, Boucher CA, Block PC, Pohost GM: Observer variance in the qualitative evaluation of left ventricular wall motion and the quantitation of left ventricular ejection fraction using rest and exercise multigated blood pool imaging. Circulation 61: 128–136, 1980.

21. Nuclear Medicine Clinical Programs. User Manual, Technicare.

22. Douglas MA, Green MV, Ostrow HG: Evaluation of automatically generated left ventricular regions of interest in computerized ECG-gated radionuclide angiocardiography. Comp in Card: 201–204, 1978.

23. Reiber JHC, Lie SP, Simoons ML, Hoek C, Gerbrands JJ, Wijns W, Bakker WH, Kooy PPM: Clinical validation of fully automated computation of ejection fraction from gated equilibrium blood-pool scintigrams. J Nucl Med 24, 1983 (in press).

24. Bourguignon MH, Douglass KH, Links JM, Wagner HN: Fully automated data acquisition, processing, and display in equilibrium radioventriculography. Eur J Nucl Med 6: 343–347, 1981.

25. Links J, Brown G, Hall D, Becker L, Wagner H Jr: A new method of fully-automated processing of gated blood pool studies. J Nucl Med 23, 1982: P85 (Abstract).

26. Almasi JJ, Bornstein I, Eisner RL, Goliash TJ, Nowak DJ, Verba JW: Enhanced clinical utility of nuclear cardiology through advanced computer processing methods. Comp in Cardiol: 397–400, 1979.

27. Graaf CN de, Douglas MA, Findley SM, Rijk PP van, Bacharach SL, Green MV, Bonow RO: Een algoritme voor het localiseren van structuren in scintigrafische beelden. NGB 4: 42–46, 1982.

28. Pizer SM, Nackman LR: Methods and limitations of edge detection for noisy images. Technical report, Department of computer science, University of North Carolina, Chapel Hill, 1979.

29. Miller TR, Sampathkumaran KS: Digital filtering in nuclear medicine. J Nucl Med 23, 66–72, 1982.

30. Todd-Pokropek A: Image processing in nuclear medicine. IEEE Trans on Nucl Sci, NS-27: 1080–1094, 1980.

31. Bell PR, Dougherty JM: Nonlinear image processing methods. IEEE Trans on Nucl Sci, NS-25: 928–938, 1978.

32. Kuwahara M, Hachimura K, Kinoshita M: Image enhancement and left ventricular contour extraction techniques applied to radioisotope angiocardiograms. Automedica, 3: 107–119, 1980.

33. Nagao M, Matsuyama T: Edge preserving smoothing. Comp Graphics and Image Processing 9: 394–407, 1979.

34. Davis LS: A survey of edge detection techniques. Comp Graphics and Image Processing 4: 248–270, 1975.

35. Chang W, Henkin RE, Hale DJ, Hall D: Methods for detection of left ventricular edges. Sem in Nucl Med 10: 39–53, 1980.

36. Abdou IE, Pratt WK: Quantitative design and evaluation of enhancement/thresholding edge detectors. Proc IEEE 67: 753–763, 1979.

37. Pratt WK: Digital image processing. John Wiley and Sons, New York, 1978.

38. Robinson GS: Edge detection by compass gradient masks. Comp Graph and Image Proc 6: 492–501, 1977.

39. Kan MK, Hopkins GB: Edge enhancement of ECG-gated cardiac images using directional

masks. Radiology 127: 525–528, 1978.

40. Hawman EG: Digital boundary detection techniques for the analysis of gated cardiac scintigrams. Optical Engineering 20: 719–725, 1981.

41. Lie SP, Reiber JHC, Hoek C, Gerbrands JJ, Simoons ML: Automated boundary extraction from cardiac scintigrams. Proceedings VII Int Conf on Image Processing in Medical Imaging, Stanford, 1981: pp 130–328.

42. Gerbrands JJ, Hoek C, Reiber JHC, Lie SP, Simoons ML: Automated left ventricular boundary extraction from technetium-99m gated blood pool scintigrams with fixed or moving regions of interest. 2nd Int Conf on Visual Psychophysics and Medical Imaging. IEEE 1981: pp 155–159.

43. Gerbrands JJ, Hoek C, Reiber JHC, Lie SP, Simoons ML: Minimum cost contour detection in technetium-99m gated cardiac blood pool scintigrams. Comp in Card: 281–284, 1981.

44. Hutton BF, Cormack J, Fulton RR: A software package for the analysis of gated cardiac blood pool studies. Internal report, Dept. of Nuclear Medicine, Royal Prince Alfred Hospital. Camperdown, NSW, Australia.

45. Silber S, Schwaiger M, Klein U, Rudolph W: Quantitative Beurteilung der Linkensventrikulären Funktion mit der Radionuklid-Ventrikulographie. Herz 5: 146–158, 1980.

46. Taylor DN, Garvie NW, Chir B, Harris D, Sharratt GP, Goddard A, Ackery DM: The effect of various background protocols on the measurement of left ventricular ejection fraction in equilibrium radionuclide angiography. Brit J of Radiol 53: 205–209, 1980.

47. Ashburn WL, Schelbert HR, Verba JW: Left ventricular ejection fraction: A review of several radionuclide angiographic approaches using the scintillation camera. Prog Cardiovasc Dis 20: 267–284, 1978.

48. Geffers H, Adam WE, Bitter F, Sigel H, Kampmann H: Data processing and functional imaging in radionuclide ventriculography. 4 Int Conf on Data Processing and Medical Imaging. Nashville, Tenn., June 1977.

49. Geffers H, Adam WE, Bitter F, Sigel H, Strauch M: Radionuklid-Ventrikulographie I Grundlagen und Methoden. Nuklear Medizin 17: 206–210, 1978.

50. Strauss HW, Zaret BL, Hurley PJ, Nataragan TK, Pitt B: A scintigraphic method for measuring left ventricular ejection fraction in man without cardiac catheterization. Amer J Cardiol 28: 575–580, 1971.

51. Folland ED, Hamilton GW, Larson SM, Kennedy JM, Williams DL, Ritchie JL: The radionuclide ejection fraction: a comparison of three radionuclide techniques with contrast angiography. J Nucl Med 18: 1159–1166, 1977.

52. Maddox DE, Holman BL, Wynne J, Idoine J, Parker JA, Uren R, Neill JM, Cohn PF: Ejection fraction image: a noninvasive index of regional left ventricular wall motion. Amer J Cardiol 41: 1230–1238, 1978.

53. Douglass K, Links J, Wagner HN: Fully automated measurement of regional left ventricular ejection fraction. J Nucl Med 23: P24, 1982 (abstract).

54. Bitter F, Adam WE, Geffers H, Weller R, Ellebruch H: Nuclear medicine: synchronized steady state heart investigations. Proceedings Int. Symp. Fundamentals in Technical Progress. III Nuclear Medicine, Liege 1979: 9.1–9.15.

55. Sorensen SG, Hamilton GW, Williams DL, Ritchie JL: R-wave synchronized blood-pool imaging. A comparison of the accuracy and reproducibility of fixed and computer-automated varying regions-of-interest for determining the left ventricular ejection fraction. Radiology 131: 473–478, 1979.

56. Karsch KR, Schicha H, Rentrop P, Kreuzer H, Emrich D: Validity of different gated equilibrium blood pool methods for determination of left ventricular ejection fraction. Eur J Nucl Med 439–445, 1980.

57. Bacharach SL, Green MV, Schiepers CW, Graaf CN de, Johnston GS: Theoretical behavior of fixed and varying ROI methods for calculating EF. J Nucl Med 22: P60, 1981 (abstract).

58. Chaitman BR, DeMots H, Bristow JD, Rosch J, Rahimtoola SH: Objective and subjective

216

analysis of left ventricular angiograms. Circ 52: 420–425, 1975.

59. Rogers WJ, Smith LR, Hood WP, Mantle JA, Rackley CE, Russell RO: Effect of filming projection and interobserver variability on angiographic biplane left ventricular volume determination. Circ 59: 96–104, 1979.

60. Maddahi J, Berman D, Silverberg R, Charuzi Y, Buchbinder N, Gray R, Waxman A, Vas R, Shah PK, Swan HJC: Validation of a two minute technique for multiple gated scintigraphic assessment of left ventricular ejection fraction and regional wall motion. J Nucl Med 19: 669, 1978.

61. Wackers FJTh, Berger HJ, Johnstone DE, Goldman L, Reduto LA, Langou RA, Gottschalk A, Zaret BL: Multiple gated cardiac blood pool imaging for left ventricular ejection fraction: validation of the technique and assessment of variability. Amer J Cardiol 43: 1159–1166, 1979.

62. Pfisterer ME, Ricci DR, Schuler G, Swanson SS, Gordon DG, Peterson KE, Ashburn WL: Validity of left-ventricular ejection fractions measured at rest and peak exercise by equilibrium radionuclide angiography using short acquisition times. J Nucl Med 20: 484–490, 1979.

63. Slutsky R, Karliner J, Battler A, Pfisterer M, Swanson S, Ashburn W: Reproducibility of ejection fraction and ventricular volume by gated radionuclide angiography after myocardial infarction. Radiology 132: 155–159, 1979.

64. Pfisterer ME, Battler A, Swanson SM, Slutsky R, Froelicher V, Ashburn WL: Reproducibility of Ejection-Fraction determinations by equilibrium radionuclide angiography in response to supine bicycle exercise: concise communication. J Nucl Med 20: 491–495, 1979.

65. Hecht HS, Josephson MA, Hopkins JM, Singh BN, Parzen E, Elashoff J: Reproducibility of equilibrium radionuclide ventriculography in patients with coronary artery disease: Response of left ventricular ejection fraction and regional wall motion to supine bicycle exercise. Amer Heart J 104: 567–574, 1982.

66. De Coster PM, Melin JA, Piret L, Beckers C: Personal communication.

67. Green M, Borer JS, Bacharach SL: Radionuclide cineangiography during stress. Nucl Med 17: 229–231, 1978.

68. Borer JS, Bacharach SL, Green MV, Kent KM, Epstein SE, Johnston GS: Real-time radionuclide cineangiography in the noninvasive evaluation of global and regional left ventricular function at rest and during exercise in patients with coronary-artery disease. N Engl J Med 296: 839–844, 1977.

69. Berman D, Maddahi J, Charuzi Y, Gray R, Waxman A, Vas R, Swan HJC, Forrester J: Evaluation of left ventricular function during sitting bicycle exercise by multiple gated scintigraphy: validation and clinical application in coronary disease. J Nucl Med 19: 771, 1978.

70. Caldwell JH, Hamilton GW, Sorensen SG, Ritchie JL. William DL, Kennedy JW: The detection of coronary artery disease with radionuclide techniques: a comparison of rest-exercise thallium imaging and ejection fraction response. Circulation 61: 610–619, 1980.

71. Sorensen SG, Caldwell J, Ritchie J, Hamilton G: "Abnormal" responses of ejection fraction to exercise, in healthy subjects, caused by Region-of-interest selection. J Nucl Med 22: 1–7, 1981.

72. Karimeddini MK, Smith VE: Abnormal false-positive response of exercise ejection fraction due to the ROI: Fixed compared with variable. J Nucl Med 22: 749–750, 1981 (lett. to ed.).

73. Berman DS, Maddahi J, Garcia EV, Freeman MR, Shah PK: Assessment of left and right ventricular function with multiple gated equilibrium cardiac blood pool scintigraphy. In: Clinical Nuclear Cardiology. Berman DS, Mason DT (eds). Grune and Stratton, New York, 1981, pp 224–284.

74. Feser JA: Automatische Bestimmung der Auswurffraktion des linken Herzventrikels. Röntgenstrahlen 47: 4–7, 1982.

75. MacIntyre WJ, Sufka B, Go RT, Cook SA, Napoli C: A computer simulated cardiac model to test edge detection and ejection fraction algorithms. J Nucl Med 23: P23, 1982.

76. Bossuyt A, Deconinck F: Scintigraphic visualisation of the effect of conduction disturbances on the mechanical events of the cardiac cycle. Annals World Assoc Med Inform 1: 1–5, 1981.

77. Pavel D, Byrom E, Swiryn S, Meyer-Pavel C, Rosen K: Normal and abnormal electrical activation of the heart. Imaging patterns obtained by phase analysis of equilibrium cardiac studies. In: Medical Radionuclide Imaging, IAEA-SM-247/211, 1981, pp 253–261.

78. Adam WE, Bitter F: Advances in heart images. In: Medical Radionuclide Imaging, IAEA-SM-247/211, 1981, pp 195–218.

79. Bossuyt A, Deconinck F, Lepoudre R, Jonckheer M: The temporal Fourier transform applied to functional isotopic imaging. In: Information Processing in Medical Imaging. Di Paola R, Kahn E (eds). INSERM 88, 1979, pp 397–408.

80. Deconinck F, Bossuyt A, Hermanne A: A cyclic color scale as an essential requirement in functional imaging of periodic phenomena. Med Phys 6: 331, 1979.

81. Bossuyt A: Amplitude/phase patterns in dynamic scintigraphic imaging. Thesis, Free University Brussels, 1982.

82. Taylor DN, Hawkes DJ, Goddard BA, Garvie N, Ackery DM, Harris D: A simple method for correcting left ventricular equilibrium radionuclide angiography for the effects of arrhythmias. Phys Med Biol 24: 1162–1167, 1979.

83. Vos PH: Nuclear Cardiology. Fourier functional images in left ventricular wall motion analysis and an investigation into lesion detectability in myocardial perfusion scintigraphy. Thesis, Leiden, University, 1982.

84. Links JM, Douglass KH, Wagner HN: Patterns of ventricular emptying by Fourier analysis of gated blood-pool studies. J Nucl Med 21: 978–982, 1980.

85. Bacharach SL, Green MV, Graaf CN de, Rijk PP van, Bonow RO, Johnston GS: Fourier phase distribution maps in the left ventricle: toward an understanding of what they mean. In: Functional Mapping of Organ Systems. Esser PD (ed). Society of Nuclear Medicine, New York, 1981, pp 139–148.

86. Ratib O, Henze E, Schön H, Schelbert HR: Phase analysis of radionuclide ventriculograms for the detection of coronary artery disease. Amer Heart J 104: 1–12, 1982.

87. Bacharach SL, Graaf CN de, Green MV, Rijk PP van, Bonow RO, Schiepers CW, Ying Lie O, Johnston GS: Phase/amplitude distribution functions for objective assessment of LV wall motion. Proceedings Int Conf Inform Processing in Medical Imaging. Stanford, 1981: 171–191.

88. Bacharach SL, Green MV, Bonow RO, Graaf CN de, Johnston GS: A method for objective evalution of functional images. J Nucl Med 23: 285–290, 1982.

89. Bossuyt A, Deconinck F, Lepoudre R, Dewilde Ph, Block P: Quantification of regional wall motion disturbances by means of radionuclide ventriculography. Comp in Card: 539–542, 1982.

10. Probability analysis for noninvasive evaluation of patients with suspected coronary artery disease

Jacques Melin, William Wijns and Jean-Marie Detry

Introduction

The noninvasive evaluation of patients suspected of ischemic heart disease remains difficult despite the development of many diagnostic procedures such as stress ECG, thallium scintigraphy, radionuclide ventriculography and cardiokymography. This is due to the fact that none of these tests is perfect. Thus there is always some overlap between patients with and without disease, due to the so-called false positive and false negative responders. The analysis of several consecutive diagnostic tests in the same patient increases the overall diagnostic accuracy but sometimes results in further diagnostic uncertainty when the results are discordant. Multiple testing is also limited by the additive cost of each procedure.

In this chapter, the limitations of the current analysis of non-invasive tests are reviewed. The physician should realize that the results of any test are critically affected by the prevalence of disease in the population under study or by the prior probability of disease in a given patient. Furthermore, the accuracy of multiple testing is limited by reporting the results categorically as "normal" or "abnormal". Conditional probability analysis giving a statement of statistical probability may offer a solution to these two problems. Finally, we will show that probability analysis may also aid in developing more cost-effective strategies for diagnosing coronary disease in some subsets of patients.

Diagnostic value of exercise ECG and Thallium-201 scintigraphy: a categorical approach

Before the diagnostic value of exercise electrocardiography and Thallium scintigraphy are discussed, the essential characteristics of a test will be reviewed. The efficacy of a diagnostic test is its ability to indicate the presence or absence of a disease and is usually calculated from a binary table as shown in Figure 1. The value of a diagnostic test is first expressed by two parameters, the sensitivity and the specificity. The sensitivity $(a/(a + c))$ is the likelihood of a positive test when the disease is present. The specificity $(d/(b + d))$ is the likelihood of a negative test when the disease is absent. However, in clinical practice, two other parameters are important: the positive predictive value $(a/(a + b))$ and the negative predictive value $(d/(c + d))$. The two relevant clinical questions are indeed: "if the patient has a positive test, how likely is he to have the disease?" or "if the patient has a negative test, how likely is he not to have the disease?". These two parameters (positive and negative predictive values) are not only dependent on sensitivity and specificity, but also on the prevalence of the disease which is $(a + c)/N$, in the population under study.

Exercise ECG and Thallium (Tl-201) scintigraphy are now commonly used for the noninvasive evaluation of the coronary circulation. In terms of both overall sensitivity and specificity, the great majority of published studies show that exercise Tl-201 scintigraphy is superior to conventional exercise ECG for detection of coronary disease [1, 2, 3, 4]. The sensitivity of exercise planar Tl-201 myocardial imaging is approximately 85% as compared to 75% for exercise ECG. The specificity of Tl-201 imaging is also better than that of exercise ECG (approximately 85 to 90% versus 70 to 80%). Given these two original characteristics (sensitivity and specificity) of the tests, the important clinical questions may be answered: which are the positive and negative predictive values?

		DISEASE		
		PRESENT	ABSENT	TOTAL
TEST	POS	a	b	a + b
	NEG	c	d	c + d
TOTAL		a + c	b + d	N

Figure 1. Contingency table:
a = proportion of patients with disease in whom the test will be positive (true positive).
b = proportion of patients without disease in whom the test will be positive (false positive).
c = proportion of patients with disease in whom the test will be negative (false negative).
d = proportion of patients without disease in whom the test will be negative (true negative).

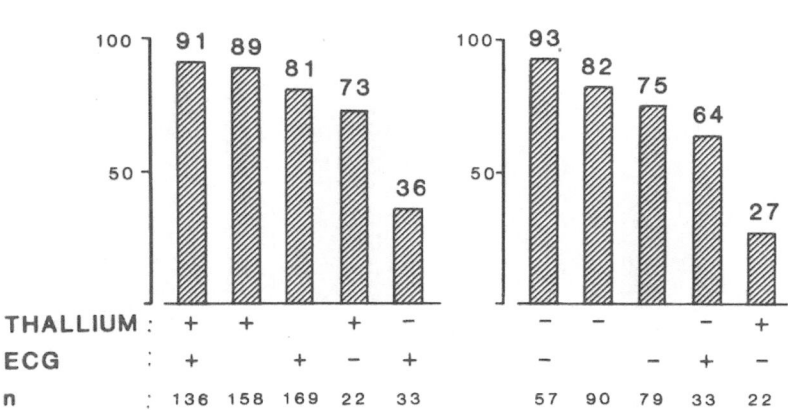

POSITIVE PREDICTIVE VALUE
P(D⁺/T⁺)

NEGATIVE PREDICTIVE VALUE
P(D⁻/T⁻)

Figure 2. Positive and negative predictive values of isolated and combined electrocardiographic and scintigraphic responses to maximal exercise testing in infarct-free patients suspected of coronary disease.

Copyright permission of Clinical Cardiology Publishing Co.

In this respect, the combination of the two tests is particularly important to consider as we have shown in a group of 248 patients suspected of coronary disease without a previous myocardial infarction [5]. In this study, a categorical approach was used; the ECG was reported as abnormal if a $\geqslant 0.1$ mV ST depression was present. The Tl-201 scintigram was abnormal if an area with a relatively reduced $\pm 25\%$ count density in one myocardial segment was observed except the apex. Otherwise the tests were reported as normal. The results are shown in Figure 2. When the results of both tests were in agreement, an abnormal response reliably indicated the presence of coronary disease (positive predictive value: 91%) and a normal scintigram associated with a normal ECG indicated the absence of disease in 93% of the patients (negative predictive value). These predictive values of combined tests were better than those of each test taken individually. When the data provided by the Tl-201 scintigraphy conflicted with the results of the exercise ECG (55 patients; 22% of the group), the interpretation of the tests results had to be very cautious because the predictive values were less satisfactory. In this situation however, Tl-201 scintigram was more reliable than exercise ECG (positive predictive value 73% vs 36% and negative predictive value 64% vs 27%). Very similar results have been shown by Patterson [6]. In this study,

POSITIVE PREDICTIVE VALUE   NEGATIVE PREDICTIVE VALUE

P(D⁺/T⁺)   P(D⁻/T⁻)

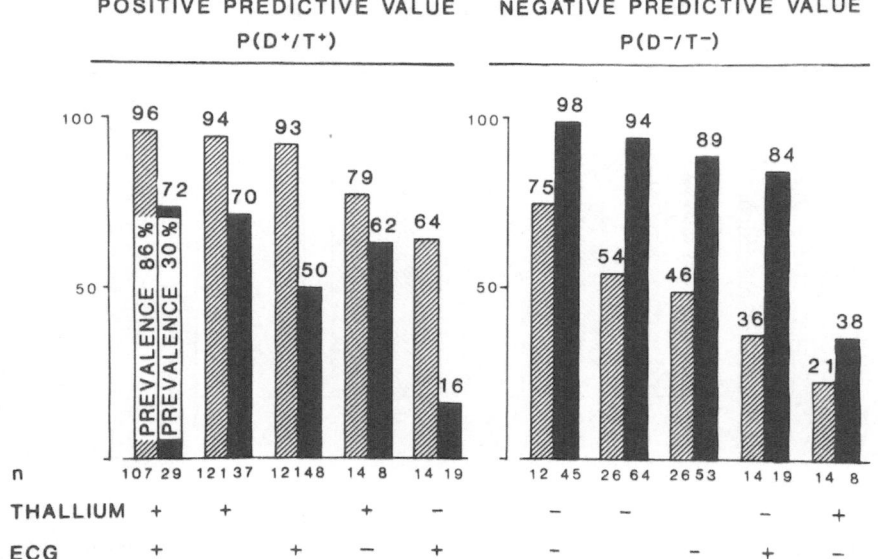

Figure 3. Influence of the prevalence of coronary disease on the predictive values of the responses to maximal exercise testing in patients suspected of coronary disease. The black bars correspond to patients with atypical chest pain, the hatched bars are data for patients with typical angina. See text for further explanation.

negative exercise ECG and Tl-201 scintigram during adequate stress ruled out coronary disease in these patients with considerable reliability (negative predictive value: 94%); the positive predictive value of both positive tests was 90%.

The positive and negative predictive values are influenced by the prevalence of coronary disease. False positive responses to a test are indeed frequent when the prevalence is low and conversely, false negative responses are more frequent when the prevalence is high. The same group of 248 patients [5] was divided according to sex and type of complaints (typical or atypical of angina pectoris). The data collected in 147 men with typical angina pectoris (prevalence of coronary disease: 86%) were compared to those of the 101 other patients (prevalence of disease: 30%). The results are shown in Figure 3. In patients with a high prevalence of coronary disease, an abnormal response to exercise had a high positive predictive value (Tl-201: 94%; ECG: 93%; Tl-201 and ECG: 96%) but in this group, the negative predictive value of a normal response to exercise was low (Tl-201: 54%; ECG: 46%; Tl-201 and ECG: 75%). When the prevalence of coronary disease was low, a normal response to exercise had an excellent predictive negative value (Tl-201: 94%; ECG: 89%; Tl-201 and ECG: 98%); in these patients, an abnormal response to exercise had a low positive predictive value (Tl-201: 70%; ECG: 50%; Tl-201 and ECG: 72%).

When the data of history, ECG and Tl-201 scintigraphy were considered together and gave concordant results ($n = 152$ patients; 62% of the population), the positive (96%) and negative (98%) predictive values were excellent. In 38% of the patients where the information was conflicting, the predictive values were less satisfactory since the overall predictive value was only 70%. This latter observation emphasizes the need of a probabilistic approach for multiple tests in a population with a wide range of disease prevalence.

Use of conditional probability analysis for the evaluation of patients suspected of coronary disease

The predictive value of multiple tests is very high when all results are in agreement but the frequent occurrence of discordant test responses has led to the use of Bayes'theorem of conditional probability [7, 8, 9, 10]. Rather than a categorical and oversimplified statement ("normal" versus "abnormal"), this method of analysis provides an explicit statement of the statistical probability that a given patient has the disease.

What is Bayes'theorem? Essentially, it states (see Bayes' formula in Appendix) that the probability that a patient with a particular set of manifestations of illness (symptoms or test results) has a particular disease ($P(D + /T +)$) depends on the sensitivity and the specificity of this set of findings and on the prevalence of the disease. When multiple tests are analyzed a serial likelihood estimation is done in which the posterior probability after the first test becomes the prior probability for the subsequent test.

In 1959, Hedley and Lusted [11] suggested the use of Bayes'theorem in medicine. In 1977, Rifkin and Hood [7] proposed the use of Bayesian analysis for the interpretation of exercise ECG. In 1979, Diamond and Forrester [8] extended the application of Bayes'theorem in cardiology by combining the prior (pretest) probability of disease based on age, sex and symptoms with the data from four tests for the detection of coronary artery disease: stress ECG, cardiokymography, Tl-201 scintigraphy and cardiac fluoroscopy. The program that they deviced has been expanded to include other data such as gated blood pool imaging and has been incorporated into a commercially available microprocessor computer system (Cadenza [12]). Each of the calculated post-test likelihoods is associated with known confidence limits defined by the statistical variance of the estimate. For practical purposes, a set of tables has been developed [13] and can be easily used by the physician (Tables 1 and 2). The validity of

Table 1. Coronary artery disease post-test likelihood based on age, sex, symptom classification, and exercise induced electro-cardiographic ST segment depression

Age	Typical angina		Atypical angina		Nonanginal chest pain		Asymptomatic	
	Male	Female	Male	Female	Male	Female	Male	Female
≥2.5 mm								
30-39	99	93	92	63	68	24	43	11
40-49	>99	98	97	86	87	53	69	28
50-59	>99	99	98	95	91	78	81	56
60-69	>99	>99	99	98	94	90	85	76
2.0-2.4 mm								
30-39	96	79	76	33	39	8	18	3
40-49	99	93	91	63	65	24	39	10
50-59	99	98	94	84	75	50	54	27
60-69	99	99	96	93	81	72	61	47
1.5-1.9 mm								
30-39	91	59	55	15	19	3	7	1
40-49	97	84	78	39	41	11	20	4
50-59	98	94	86	67	53	28	31	12
60-69	99	98	89	83	62	49	37	25
1.0-1.4 mm								
30-39	83	42	38	9	10	2	4	<1
40-49	94	72	64	25	26	6	11	2
50-59	96	89	75	50	37	16	19	7
60-69	97	95	81	72	45	33	23	15
0.5-0.9 mm								
30-39	68	24	21	4	5	1	2	4
40-49	86	53	44	12	13	3	5	1
50-59	91	78	57	31	20	8	9	3
60-69	94	90	65	52	26	17	11	7
0.0-0.4 mm								
30-39	25	7	6	1	1	<1	<1	<1
40-49	61	22	16	3	4	1	1	<1
50-59	73	47	25	10	6	2	2	1
60-69	79	69	32	21	8	5	3	2

Table 2. Coronary artery disease post-thallium likelihood*

No thallium defect

	0	1	2	3	4	5	6	7	8	9
0		<1	<1	1	1	1	1	1	2	2
10	2	2	2	3	3	3	3	3	4	4
20	4	4	5	5	5	6	6	6	6	7
30	7	7	8	8	8	9	9	9	10	10
40	10	11	11	12	12	13	13	13	14	14
50	15	15	16	17	17	18	18	19	20	20
60	21	22	22	23	24	25	25	26	27	28
70	29	30	31	32	33	35	36	37	38	40
80	41	42	43	46	48	50	52	54	56**	59
90	61	64	67	70	73	77	81	85	90	95

Nonreversible thallium defect

	0	1	2	3	4	5	6	7	8	9
0		1	3	4	6	7	8	10	11	12
10	14	15	16	17	19	20	21	23	24	25
20	26	27	29	30	31	32	33	34	36	37
30	38	39	40	41	42	43	44	45	46	48
40	49	50	51	52	53	54	55	56	57	58
50	59	60	61	62	62	63	64	65	66	67
60	68	69	70	71	72	72	73	74	75	76
70	77	78	78	79	80	81	82	83	83	84
80	85	86	87	87	88	89	90	90	91	92
90	93	93	94	95	96	96	97	98	99	99

Reversible thallium defect

	0	1	2	3	4	5	6	7	8	9
0		10	19	26	33	38	43	47	50	53
10	56	59	61	63	65	67	69	70	72	73
20	74	75	77	78	79	79	80	81	82	83
30	83	84	85	86	86	86	87	87	88	88
40	89	89	89	90	90	90	91	91	91	92
50	92	92	93	93	93	93	94	94	94	94
60	95	95	95	95	95	96	96	96	96	96
70	96	97	97	97	97	97	97	97	98	98
80	98	98	98	98	98	99	99	99	99	99
90	99	99	99	99	99	>99	>99	>99	>99	>99

* The pre-thallium likelihood (or post ECG likelihood) is outside of the table with the 10s on the verticle axis and the 1s on the horizontal axis. Therefore the post-thallium likelihood is determined by reading the column inside the table associated with the pre-thallium likelihood on the margin (example** :pretest likelihood 88%, post-test likelihood 56%).

probability analysis for diagnosing coronary disease has been assessed by comparison of the calculated probability of disease with subsequent coronary angiographic results. Various reports [8, 14, 15, 16] have demonstrated an excellent correlation of posterior probability by Cadenza and angiographic prevalence.

Potential limitations of probability analysis relate to the assessment of likelihood before testing and to the true independence of the individual observations analyzed. The accurate knowledge of the likelihood of disease before testing (based on age, sex and symptoms) is critical for Bayesian analysis. The initial data were obtained by Diamond and Forrester [8] from pooled angiographic and autopsy literature encompassing over 30,000 patients and were thus presumed to contain an element of unknown bias. New information [17] from the CASS study (8157 catheterized patients without previous myocardial infarction) showed a remarkable similarity between these direct observations and the predictions and, therefore, the estimates of the pretest likelihood of disease by Cadenza seem accurate. The fact that the procedures used sequentially are statistically independent has been discussed by Diamond [9, 16]. A limitation of Cadenza is to use a categorical criterion for the interpretation of Thallium scintigraphy. The reason is obviously that no large data base was available at that time. It would be however mandatory that the extent of the Thallium defect would be taken into account.

Posterior probability has been shown not only to serve as an aid for diagnosing coronary disease but also as a predictor of the extent of angiographic disease and of future coronary events [16].

Choice of alternative strategies to diagnose coronary disease

Post-test probabilities given by the Bayesian method might become elements of medical decision making. If one accepts that the diagnostic certainty is sufficient when a post-test probability for coronary disease is greater than 90% or less than 10% (probability threshold) then only the patients with post-test probability between 10 and 90% would need the next diagnostic test in a sequential decision tree. This approach could help to define a diagnostic strategy. It is important to emphasize that there is no agreement among clinicians concerning the appropriate probability threshold for management decisions in coronary disease. With a posterior probability statement, a probability threshold can be defined by each physician according to the clinical situation.

Stason and Fineberg [18] theoretically analyzed different strategies for detection or coronary disease in hypothetical populations in terms of cost-effectiveness. We compared these diagnostic strategies retrospectively in a group of patients with a low disease prevalence: 93 females who all had both exercise Tl-201 scintigraphy and coronary angiogram [19] using conditional probability analysis. The four strategies analyzed were: S_0, no test, the probability of coronary disease is derived from the history and the coronary risk factors; S_1 included stress ECG; S_2 used both stress ECG and Tl-201 in all patients; S_3 when Tl-201 scintigraphy was performed only if the post-ECG probability was between 10 and 90%, in other words, if a sufficient level of certainty was not achieved after the stress ECG. After each of these strategies, a probability estimate was given by Cadenza, the computerized Bayesian algorithm previously described. The four strategies were compared in terms of accuracy and need for diagnostic angiography after the noninvasive tests.

Accuracy was measured by assigning an accuracy score using the coronary angiogram. A general method for measuring the accuracy of probability has been described by Shapiro [20]: the accuracy score is calculated according to the formula described in the Appendix. This accuracy score ranges from 0 to 100 and is highest when the actual outcome is predicted with certainty. The same accuracy score has been used by Hlatky [21] to compare the clinical judgment of 91 cardiologists to the computer of

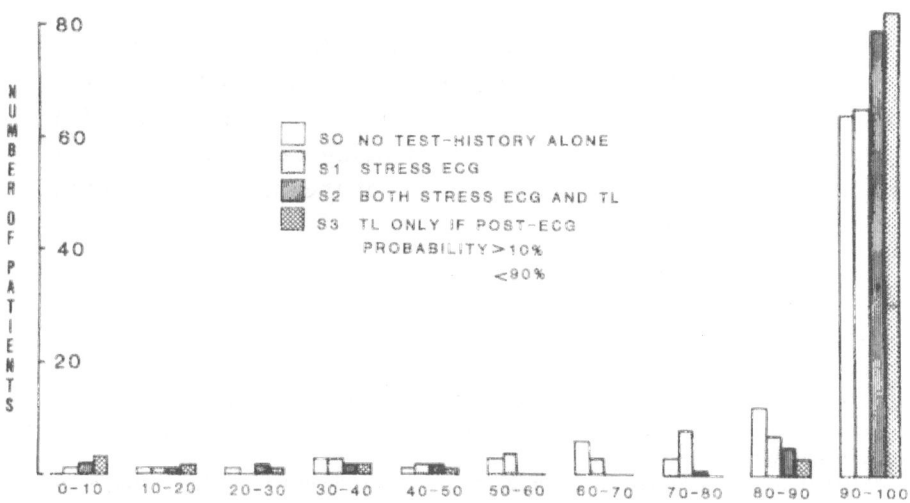

Figure 4. Distribution of accuracy scores of probability estimates after the four diagnostic strategies, as discussed in the text.

Cadenza. The distribution of accuracy scores of probability estimates after the four diagnostic strategies is shown in Figure 4. Seventy-eight of the patients (84%) with S_2 and eighty-one (87%) with S_3 had an accuracy score between 90 and 100. The difference in accuracy scores between the 4 diagnostic strategies were tested statistically by analysis of variance with orthogonal contrast. There was a difference ($p<0.05$) between S_0 and S_1 versus S_2 and S_3. No difference was noticed between S_2 and S_3. However, with S_3, 44% of the Tl-201 scintigrams were avoided.

The need for diagnostic angiography after the 4 strategies was defined by the percentage of patients in whom sufficient diagnostic certainty was not achieved after the 4 strategies, i.e. the probability estimate at the end of the strategy was between 10 and 90%. After S_1, 56% of the patients would have needed a diagnostic catheterization versus 29% after S_2 and 21% after S_3 (S_1 versus S_3: $p<0.001$; S_2 versus S_3: $p<0.05$).

Thus in this group of women, the strategy (S_3) based on ECG and a threshold cutoff probability to guide the use of Tl-201 scintigram was the most cost-effective strategy: without loss of accuracy, Tl-201 scintigram could have been avoided in 44% of the patients and diagnostic catheterization in 79% of the patients.

Conclusion

Bayes'theorem of conditional probability is a useful tool for integrating the results of multiple, even discordant test results relative to the diagnosis of angiographic coronary artery disease. This method may also aid in developing more cost-effective means for the diagnosis of coronary disease. Conditional probability allows choice of the best strategy for a variety of patients' subsets.

References

1. Bailey IK, Griffith LSC, Rouleau J, Strauss HW, Pitt B: Thallium[201] myocardial perfusion imaging at rest and exercise: comparative sensitivity to electrocardiography in coronary artery disease. Circulation 55: 79–87, 1977.
2. Okada RD, Boucher CA, Strauss HW, Pohost GM: Exercise radionuclide imaging approaches to coronary artery disease. Am J Cardiol 46: 1188–1204, 1980.
3. Melin JA, Piret LJ, Vanbutsele RJM, Rousseau MF, Cosyns J, Brasseur LA, Beckers C, Detry JMR: Diagnostic value of exercise electrocardiography and thallium myocardial scintigraphy in patients without previous myocardial infarction: a Bayesian approach. Circulation 63: 1019–1024, 1981.

4. Massie BM, Botvinick EH, Bristow JD: Myocardial perfusion scintigraphy with thallium-201: current status and future prospects. In: Progress in Cardiology, vol. 11. Paul N.Yu (ed), John F Goodwin, Lea Febiger, Philadelphia, 1982, pp. 19–55.

5. Wijns W, Melin J, Piret LJ, Rousseau MF, Vanbutsele RJ, Detry JMR: Diagnostic value of stress myocardial Thallium scintigraphy in patients suspected of coronary artery disease. In: Noninvasive methods in ischemic heart disease. Gabriel Faivre, Alain Bertrand, François Cherrier, Max Amor, Jean-Louis Neimann (eds), Specia, Nancy, 1982, pp. 135–141.

6. Patterson RE, Horowitz SF, Eng C, Rudin A, Meller J, Halgash DA, Pichard AD, Goldsmith SJ, Herman MV, Gorlin R: Can exercise electrocardiography and Thallium-201 myocardial imaging exclude the diagnosis of coronary artery disease? Am J Cardiol 49: 1127–1135, 1982.

7. Rifkin RD, Hood WB: Bayesian analysis of electrocardiographic exercise testing. N Engl J Med 297: 681–686, 1977.

8. Diamond GA, Forrester JS: Analysis of probability as an aid in the clinical diagnosis of coronary artery disease. N Engl J Med 300: 1350–1358, 1979.

9. Diamond GA, Forrester JS, Hirsch M, Staniloff HM, Vas R, Berman DS, Swan HJC: Application of conditional probability analysis to the clinical diagnosis of coronary artery disease. J Clin Invest 65A: 1210–1221, 1980.

10. Epstein SE: Implications of probability analysis on the strategy used for non invasive detection of coronary artery disease. Amer J Cardiol 46: 491–499, 1980.

11. Ledley RS, Lusted LB: Reasoning foundations of medical diagnosis. Science 130: 9–21, 1959.

12. Diamond GA (in collaboration with Forrester JS): CADENZA: Computer-assisted diagnosis and evaluation of coronary artery disease. 1979. Cardiokinetics, Seattle, Washington (software and documentation magnetic tape).

13. Staniloff HM, Diamond GA, Freeman MR, Berman DS, Forrester JS: Simplified application of Bayesian analysis to multiple cardiologic tests. Clin Cardiol 5: 630–636, 1982.

14. Wong DF, Tibits P, O'Donnell J, Collison H, LaFrance H, Han S, Otto A, Karam M, Camargo EE, Wagner HN: Computer-assisted Bayesian analysis of the diagnosis of coronary artery disease (abstr). J Nucl Med 23: P83, 1982.

15. Dans PE, Weiner JP, Melin JA, Becker LC: The use of conditional probability in the diagnosis of coronary artery disease (abstr.). Clinical Research 30: 297A, 1982.

16. Diamond GA, Saniloff HM, Forrester JS, Pollock BH, Swan HJC: Computer-assisted diagnosis in the noninvasive evaluation of patients with suspected coronary artery disease. J Am Coll Cardiol 1(2): 444–455, 1983.

17. Chaitman BR, Bourassa MG, Davis K, Rogers WJ, Tyras DH, Berger R, Kennedy JW, Fisher L, Judkins MP, Mock MB, Killip T: Angiographic prevalence of high-risk coronary artery disease in patient subsets (CASS). Circulation 64: 360–367, 1981.

18. Stason WB, Fineberg HV: Implications of alternative strategies to diagnose coronary artery disease. Circulation 66 (Suppl III): 80–86, 1982.

19. Melin JA, Wijns W, Vanbutsele R, Decoster PM, Beckers C, Detry JM: Choice of optimal strategies to diagnose coronary artery disease in women. In: Abstractbook, European Society of Cardiology, Working group on use of isotopes in Cardiology, Rotterdam, 1983, p 15.

20. Shapiro AR: The evaluation of clinical predictions. A method and initial application. N Engl J Med 226: 1509–1514, 1977.

21. Hlatky M, Botvinick E, Brundage B: Diagnostic accuracy of cardiologists compared with probability calculations using Bayes'rule. Am J Cardiol 49: 1927–1931, 1982.

Appendix

Symbols used in Bayes' formula

Probability notation	*Common name*	*Meaning*
P(D+/T+)	Positive predictive value	Frequency of disease when test is positive
P(D+)	Prevalence or prior probability of disease	Frequency of disease in the population
P(T+/D+)	Sensitivity; true positive	Probability that test is positive when disease is present
P(T+/D−)	False positive	Probability that test is positive when disease is absent
P(T−/D−)	Specificity; true negative	Probability that test is negative when disease is absent
P(D−)	Prevalence or prior probability of no disease	Frequency of no disease in the population
P(T−/D+)	False negative	Probability that test is negative when disease is present

Derivation of Bayes' theorem from horizontal assessment of data from the binary table

Binary table displaying test data

	DISEASE	
	PRESENT P(D+)	ABSENT P(D−)
POS **TEST**	a True positive TP P(T+/D+)	b False positive FP P(T+/D−)
NEG	c False negative FN P(T−/D+)	d True negative TN P(T−/D−)

Bayes' formula

Positive predictive value P(D+/T+) =

$$= \frac{a}{a+b} = \frac{TP}{TP+FP}$$

$$= \frac{P(D+) \cdot P(T+/D+)}{P(D+) \cdot P(T+/D+) + P(D-) \cdot P(T+/D-)}$$

$$= \frac{(\text{prevalence}) \cdot (\text{sensitivity})}{(\text{prevalence}) \cdot (\text{sensitivity}) + (1 - \text{prevalence}) \cdot (1 - \text{specificity})}$$

Negative predictive value $P(D-/T-) =$

$$= \frac{d}{d+c} = \frac{TN}{TN + FN}$$

$$= \frac{P(D-) \cdot P(T-/D-)}{P(D-) \cdot P(T-/D-) + P(D+) \cdot P(T-/D+)}$$

$$= \frac{(1 - \text{prevalence}) \cdot (\text{specificity})}{(1 - \text{prevalence}) \cdot (\text{specificity}) + (1 - \text{prevalence}) \cdot (1 - \text{specificity})}$$

The accuracy score:

$$s_i: ([(1 + x_i) \log (1 + p_i) + (2 - x_i) \log (2 - p_i) - \log (2)]/ \log (2)) \times 100$$

Where:
p_i = the estimated probability of coronary disease in patient "i";
s_i = the accuracy of this estimate;
x_i = 1 if patient "i" has coronary disease and,
x_i = 0 if patient "i" does not have disease.

11. Standards for acquisition, data analysis and interpretation of myocardial scintigraphy and blood pool scintigraphy

Duncan S. Dymond

Introduction

The perfect image is one that is indistinguishable from the original object under the same viewing conditions. Unfortunately, there is no nuclear medicine image that meets this criterion, and interpretation of cardiac scintigrams is hampered by the limited resolution of our imaging systems, compounded by the fact that unlike other organs the heart moves while being imaged. Nevertheless, with careful attention to technical detail and by employing rigorous standards for the three major facets of nuclear cardiology, namely, acquisition, analysis and interpretation of data, the very imperfect nuclear cardiology images can be of major clinical value. The requirements for these facets vary greatly, from the simple gamma camera equipped with a persistence oscilloscope and a polaroid camera for qualitative interpretation of analogue thallium scans, to highly sophisticated camera-computer systems for quantitative analysis of static or dynamic data.

Thallium scintigraphy

Thallium-201 is a potassium analogue which after intravenous injection is distributed throughout the body in proportion to regional cardiac output, according to the Sapirstein principle [1]. Areas of reduced perfusion appear on the images as areas of decreased thallium uptake when compared to areas of normal perfusion. Although most defects on thallium scans are due to paucity of flow, the uptake by the myocardium is related also to the efficiency of extraction by the organ, a process dependent on the Na-K-ATPase system. If 2 mCi of thallium are administered, then assuming the heart receives approximately 3% of cardiac output, and an extraction efficiency by the myocardium of 85% (2), there will be only 50–60 microcuries in the heart, providing a low target to background ratio.

The low 69–83 keV photon energy of thallium-201 leads to a great deal of attenuation and patient scatter, particularly from the back of the heart. These two factors, combined with the motion of the heart, point to thallium scintigrams being low resolution images. Although there has been no universal agreement among thallium users as to the best standards for minimising artefacts and inter-laboratory discrepancies in image interpretation [3], there are certain basic requirements needed to overcome the problems. Since the major use of thallium scintigraphy is to demonstrate stress-induced differences in regional myocardial perfusion in patients with known or suspected coronary artery disease, this review will concentrate on aspects of exercise or pharmacological stress as well as on the technical and physical sides of imaging.

Production of thallium-201

The production process yields small quantities of thallium-200 (half-life 26 hours) and thallium-202 (half-life 288 hours) in addition to thallium-201. It is therefore prudent to allow a short delay in use to permit decay of thallium-202 relative to thallium-201. A delay of more than 2 to 3 days allows the percentage of thallium-202 to increase to an unacceptable level. The optimum time for use will depend on the exact levels of the impurities from each production site.

Exercise protocols

Either treadmill or bicycle exercise may be used [3] but many patients will not be able to achieve the same levels of exercise on a bicycle as on a treadmill, due either to unfamiliarity between man and machine, or leg muscle weakness. Evaluation of patients' functional capacity is more easily achieved with treadmill exercise because of the relationship of exercise performance during a Bruce or Naughton protocol to maximum oxygen consumption. Algorithms have recently been described for converting bicycle performance into multiples of resting oxygen uptake or METS [4]. Exercise must be graded and consist of gradual increments in stages, ideally preceded by a warm-up stage without load. Each stage should be of at least 2 minutes [3]. There is no doubt that symptom-limited exercise provides a greater yield of detected perfusion defects than does less severe exercise [5].

The tracer is injected at maximum exercise, and the patients should be exhorted to continue their exercise for at least 30, preferably 60 seconds after injection. This maintains the perfusion gradient while the tracer is being extracted by the myocardium and helps to increase the sensitivity of the technique. In addition, if the patients are fasting at the time of the exercise study then the hepatic and splanchnic uptake of tracer are reduced and subsequent interpretation of the images is facilitated. Unlike exercise electrocardiography and radionuclide angiography (see below), where it is advisable to withold beta-blocking drugs to reduce the incidence of false negative tests, thallium scintigraphy does not seem to be affected by beta-blockade [3]. Propranolol does not affect the extraction fraction by the myocardium although hypoxia does [6].

Dipyridamole imaging

Vasodilator stress with dipyridamole is becoming more widely used as an alternative to dynamic exercise. The drug is a powerful vasodilator, and the principle behind its use with thallium is that dipyridamole will induce differential increases in coronary blood flow in regions supplied by normal and stenotic coronary arteries to a degree that will be appreciated as differences in regional perfusion on a thallium scan. Regions subtended by critically stenosed coronary arteries will receive an increase in flow, but substantially less than that enjoyed by normally perfused regions [7]. The protocol employs infusion of the drug at a dose of 0.15 mg/Kg/min for 4 minutes, with heart rate and blood pressure being carefully monitored. Aminophylline, a dipyridamole antagonist, must be readily available during the infusion to counteract any serious side effects, particularly angina. Following infusion, the patients walk in place for 60 seconds, thallium is administered, walking is continued for a further 4 to 5 minutes and imaging is then performed.

The advantages of this technique over exercise are:

1. A greater increase in coronary flow is achieved.
2. Higher myocardial to background ratios are obtained, and the increase is due to a rise in myocardial counts rather than to the fall in background counts which occurs with exercise.
3. Less time and equipment are required.
4. There is a less rapid decrease in coronary flow after cessation.
5. It is suitable for patients who cannot exercise due to other disabilities.

The disadvantages of vasodilator stress are:

1. Lack of functional assessment of exercise tolerance or of diagnostic ECG changes.
2. Occasional severe side effects such as hypotension or angina.

Oral dipyridamole has not been tested adequately, but preliminary reports suggest it does not provide the image quality produced by intravenous administration. The sensitivity of dipyridamole imaging appears to be equal to that of exercise studies [7] and similarity is not altered by beta-blockade.

Imaging technique

Imaging should be performed with a modern generation camera with at least 37 photomultiplier tubes [3]. A 20% window is usually used, centred over the 75 keV X-ray peak. If multiple energy analysers are available the use of the 135 keV and 167 keV photons reduces imaging time. At least 300,000 counts per image should be obtained, which provides more than 50,000 counts in the heart. For computer acquisition, a 64 × 64 (word mode) or 128 × 128 (byte mode) matrix is used. With a large field of view camera, 128 × 128 may be preferable to increase the number of pixels in the cardiac image, but with a standard field, or in "zoom" mode 64 × 64 should be adequate. The theoretical benefits of increased spatial resolution with 128 × 128 may not be apparent with thallium scintigraphy due to the resolution-limiting factors discussed previously.

Three main types of collimator have been used [3]. The medium resolution, low energy, all purpose (LEAP) collimator has gained wide popularity because of its increased sensitivity compared to high resolution, low energy collimators. Once again, the physical limitations imposed by a moving heart restrict the advantages of high resolution collimators. One way of overcoming the problem of cardiac motion is the use of gated scintigrams whereby imaging is carried out for only the 50 msec associated with each end diastole. Statistically reliable images take approximately 30 minutes to acquire, even with a high sensitivity collimator [8]. The resolution of these images is greater than that of unsynchronised images and it is worth collecting these in 128 × 128 for this reason. With 30 minutes per view, multiple projections of exercise scans are not practicable, but adequate "stop action" diastolic images can be obtained with a larger window than 50 msec, with consequent shortening of acquisition time [3]. Gated images may enhance perception of perfusion defects in difficult cases.

Multiple views are mandatory to extract the maximum information from the scans. This is because small lesions are best seen in tangent or face on, and may be missed if below a certain size. Mueller *et al.* [9] found that in the dog the smallest defect that could be consistently detected was equivalent to an area of muscle with a mass of 6 grams and a perfusion decrease of 40% compared to normal myocardium. Most people recommend the use of anterior (ANT), a shallow and steep left anterior oblique (LAO), and a left lateral view. The exact angulation of the LAO views is not critical, with most workers choosing two projections between 30 and 70 degrees. Usually the images are obtained with the patient supine and the camera rotated. The left lateral view may be better performed with the patient on his side instead. This allows the heart to take up a more vertical position and the apex and posterior wall of the left ventricle to be a similar distance from the collimator. This may produce a more uniform appearance on the image, which otherwise often shows considerable attenuation posteriorly [3].

The timing of imaging after injection is important. Imaging should be delayed for about 5 to 10 minutes after injection to allow myocardial to background levels to rise. Because the distribution of thallium in the potassium pool is not static, but changes rapidly as ischaemia resolves, imaging must be completed within 40 minutes if the images are to represent the status of regional perfusion during ischaemia. Redistribution, which involves the loss of thallium from normal myocardium and increased extraction from the blood pool by areas that were transiently ischaemic, begins immediately [10], but does not interfere clinically with image interpretation until 40 minutes or so. Comparison of stress images with images taken under basal conditions is obligatory in order to characterise the nature of abnormalities on the stress images. Redistribution images are therefore obtained 3 to 4 hours after stress, and the patient serves as his own control for image interpretation. The use of redistribution images seems to be an acceptable substitute for true rest images [11] which would involve a separate injection of tracer on another occasion and increase the radiation burden to the patient. A defect present on the redistribution scans does not always indicate a scar, however, and it is probably true to say that redistribution images overestimate the "fixed" component compared to rest scans [12]. It follows that redistribution scans should not be used to assess the presence of viable myocardium.

Image interpretation

Although the human eye is very skilled at detecting different intensities on an image, most workers agree that some form of objective evaluation of the images is preferable to a global qualitative inspection of analogue images on polaroid or X-ray film. A form of segmental analysis, whereby each image is divided into 5 to 7 segments, is a simple method for comparing regional tracer uptake at rest and under stress, as well as allowing comparison with coronary anatomy. Defects in the anterior wall and septum correspond well with disease in the left anterior descending artery, and inferior wall defects with disease in the right coronary, but defects in the apex correlate less well with specific coronary anatomy [13]. In addition, because the scans reflect relative differences in regional perfusion, rather than absolute coronary flow, the images will identify only the most severely ischaemic regions as abnormal: hence the reduced sensitivity for detecting individual lesions in multi-vessel disease [13]. As a corollary to this, conventional thallium scans are not reliable in detecting multi-vessel disease [14] and are therefore of limited value in patients with typical angina pectoris. A promising indirect method of quantification involves comparison of lung thallium activity with that in the mediastinum [15]. Increased lung uptake correlates well with exercise induced left ventricular dysfunction, which in turn relates to the amount of ischaemic myocardium.

Computer processing of data may quantify changes in tracer distribution, but as yet no ideal method for quantification has been agreed. The first stage in quantification is background subtraction. The simplest approach is a fixed percentage subtraction, but this has varied between 10% and 50% [3]. An interpolative correction using a matrix from pixels surrounding the cardiac region makes allowances for non-uniform background levels [16], and this may be weighted to cause a more rapid fall-off of the background reference plane as it moves beneath the heart away from a region of intense extracardiac activity, such as liver or spleen [17]. Various methods for quantification include:

1. The use of isocount levels to define areas of normality and abnormality [18].
2. The use of average counts per segment compared to previously defined normal ranges [19].
3. Counts per unit area of the image compared to maximum counts per unit area in the same image [20].
4. Space-time quantification using the maximum myocardial counts along 60 six degree radials at exercise and redistribution [17].
5. Statistical image analysis [21].

None of these methods overcome the problem of photon attenuation which is the major obstacle to true quantification. The use of the seven-pinhole collimator attachment to carry out longitudinal tomography does not appear to provide any major advantages over a quantitative approach to planar images [22].

There are important pitfalls in qualitative or quantitative interpretation of the images, which are set out in Table 1, and some of which are illustrated in Figure 1. It is important to be aware of these if the cardinal error of over-reporting of abnormalities is to be avoided. Although most of these are due to physical and anatomical constraints, Okada *et al.* [23] have suggested that the inter-observer variance may be reduced by multiple observers reporting the studies, or by the use of inter-observer variance analysis. Finally, the interpretation of thallium scintigrams *must* take into account the prevalence of the disease in the population under study (pre-test probability of disease). A negative test in a middle-aged man with typical angina pectoris is of little diagnostic value, as is a positive scan in a teenage girl with no symptoms [24].

First pass radionuclide angiography

By definition, such studies involve the acquisition of dynamic data for the short time needed for an intravenously injected tracer to pass through the central circulation for the first time. This usually takes 30 to 50 seconds at rest. Current first pass studies differ from the original Prinzmetal radio-cardiograms [25] in that they are shown as images, not just curves. In addition to the detailed examination of left and right ventricular function

Table 1. Pitfalls in interpretation of thallium scans

1. Breast attenuation. This may cause apparent defects especially in the lateral projection.

2. Apical thinning. This is a normal variant, and apparent apical defects on the ANT view may be due to reduced muscle density, not reduced counts/unit area.

3. Tapering of activity in the upper septum in the LAO view, due to the aortic valve plane.

4. Tapering of activity in the upper posterolateral segment in the LAO view, due to mitral valve plane and left atrium.

5. Overestimation of 'fixed defects' by redistribution scans.

6. Lack of quantitative assessment of coronary disease.

7. Reduced sensitivity for detecting remote coronary disease in patients with prior anterior myocardial infarction.

8. Considerable inter-observer variance in qualitative interpretation.

240

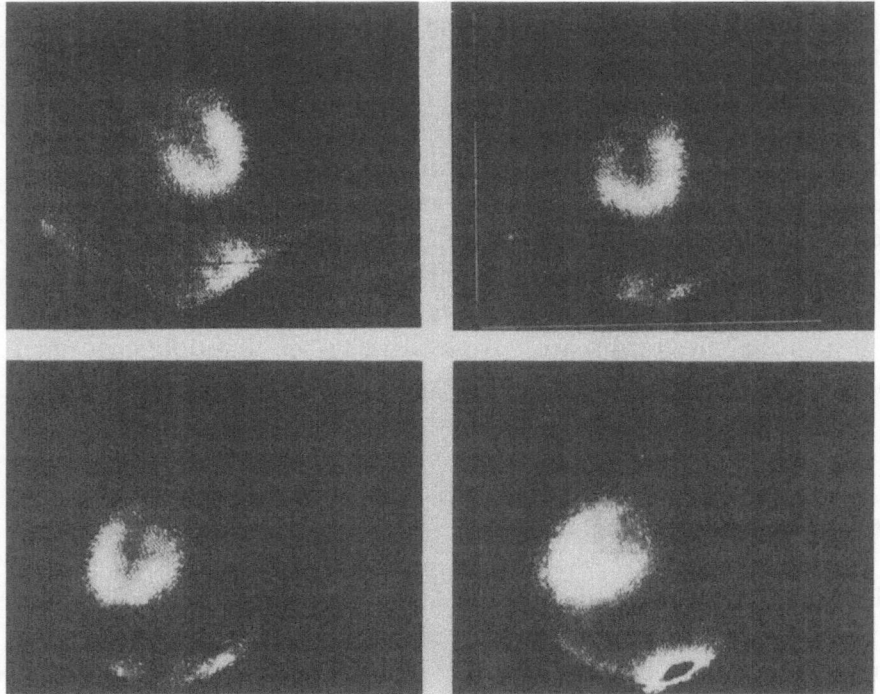

Figure 1. Normal thallium scintigram in (from top left clockwise) ANT, 30 degree LAO, 70 degree LAO, and left lateral projections. The images have been smoothed and background subtracted. Note the apparent defects in the upper septum on the shallow LAO and in the postero-lateral wall on the steep LAO views. These are due to aortic and mitral valve planes and left atrium.

that is possible with correctly performed studies, the first pass technique permits evaluation of intracardiac shunts and chamber to chamber transit times on the basis of well-established indicator dilution principles [26]. The success of first pass studies depends upon achieving good spatial and temporal separation of the chambers and upon obtaining enough counts to make the studies statistically reliable.

Technical requirements

1. The studies are usually performed with 15 to 20 mCi of technetium-99m as free pertechnetate or as DTPA. It does not need to be bound to an intravascular marker as it has to remain in the vascular space for only a short time. DTPA is preferable where rest and intervention studies are contemplated, as the clearance from the blood pool is quicker, which lessens the residual blood pool activity against which subsequent studies

are performed, as well as reducing radiation to the patient. With the development of new, short half-life agents such as gold-195m, the capacity for multiple examinations has increased [27].

2. The radiopharmaceutical should be injected as a bolus in as small a volume as possible, preferably less than 0.5 ml. The small bolus aids in temporal separation of the cardiac chambers and reproducibility of data is intimately related to bolus integrity [28]. A rapid saline flush usually of 20 ml, at approximately 8 mls/second, is required to inject the bolus. It is not necessary to resort to other injection techniques such as the Oldendorf method. Although the choice of right or left arm is not crucial, it is preferable to choose a medial basilic vein rather than a lateral vein. This is because the former have a more direct path to the right side of the heart whereas the latter often take a prolonged course via collaterals, and the bolus may fragment. It is not necessary in most cases to use a central or jugular injection, both of which detract from the noninvasive nature of the test. As the bolus is injected, the arm should not be hyperextended, and patients should be encouraged not to "hunch" the shoulders. Valsava manoeuvre should be avoided. Neglect of these small but important details may lead to a poor bolus and a sub-standard study.

Paradoxically, a good bolus may not be desirable for studies of right ventricular function. The right atrium is a poor mixing chamber and the bolus may "stream" across the tricuspid valve into the right ventricular outflow tract without filling the right ventricle. This is especially likely with the leading edge of the bolus. Changes in activity may therefore reflect concentration changes rather than volume changes. The use of as many cardiac cycles as possible from the later parts of the right ventricular time-activity curve may lessen this.

3. The first pass technique affords a flexibility of choice of projection not available with other methods. For comparison of radionuclide with contrast angiographic data, the RAO view has been extensively used. When comparison with contrast data and area-length measurements are not required, the anterior view provides information comparable to the RAO, and as the detector may be positioned closer to the patients in the ANT view, technetium dosages can be reduced.

For studies of right ventricular function, the best separation between the right atrium and right ventricle is achieved in the RAO view, and a first pass study in this projection provides probably the best method for quantitative assessment of the right ventricle.

Imaging requirements

Adequate count density is a prerequisite for accurate dynamic studies. As there is only a short time available for first pass data acquisition, and there are only a few [5–10] cardiac cycles involved in the first pass, instruments with high count-rate capabilities are ideally needed. At present, the multicrystal camera (Baird Corporation, Bedford, Mass.) is the best instrument for this [26–28], with count-rates in excess of 350,000 counts per second. The count-rate potential of single crystal instruments is increasing, and modern generation cameras are now more suitable for first pass studies [29] than older systems were.

Assuming adequate count-rates, the temporal resolution must be good enough to resolve the rapidly changing phases of the cardiac cycle. If data are collected in frame mode, there must be enough frames per cardiac cycle to avoid blurring the cycle and assigning early diastolic components to a frame thought to represent end systole. The minimum framing rate required is 20 frames/second for resting studies, probably 30 frames/second for exercise studies. Where rapid framing rates are not readily available, list mode acquisition may be used with flexible frame formatting carried out after acquisition, although this may be time consuming [30]. Framing rate is equally important where ejection phase and filling phase indices are desired. These are usually obtained by a curve or line fitted to the systolic and diastolic portions of the time-volume curve. At faster heart rates there will be fewer data points per cardiac cycle, and errors may therefore occur in the fitting. Table 2 shows the number of frames per cardiac cycle at various heart rates, and it is apparent that low framing rates at fast heart rates are inadequate for curve fitting.

As each chamber contains most of the injected radioactivity during the passage of the bolus through that chamber, the target to background ratio is high. A time-activity curve generated from the left ventricular region of

Table 2. Number of frames per cardiac cycle at various heart rates and framing rates

Heart rate	Frames per second			
	10	20	50	100
60	10	20	50	100
90	6.7	13.3	33.3	66.7
120	5	10	25	50
150	4	8	20	40

interest will display the diastoles and systoles of the individual cardiac cycles as "peaks and troughs" [31]. It is therefore not necessary to record an ECG signal to gate the images as the studies are "intrinsically gated".

Quality control

1. Patient positioning is crucial. If a dose of activity is injected and the heart is incompletely shown in the field of view, then a dose of radioactive material has been administered with no useful gain. This is especially prone to happen with small field of view cameras. It is the author's policy to inject a 1.0 mCi "siting" dose to prevent malpositioning.

2. Quality of injected boluses may be checked by entering a region of interest over the superior vena cava and generating a time-activity curve of the bolus. The full width at half maximum of the bolus, expressed in seconds, provides a quantitative measure of bolus integrity [28]. Reproducibility of ejection fraction measurements is not critically dependent on bolus integrity, but that of shunt or transit time measurements is.

3. Attention to statistics is important. Usually the individual cycles in the first pass are summed by the computer to produce a statistically dense representative cardiac cycle [28, 31]. Statistical fluctuations in first pass studies may also be reduced by temporal smoothing of data [32], or by the application of a root mean square analysis [33]. Large errors may be introduced into ejection fraction calculations due to low counts. Table 3 shows the percentage errors that can occur, related to a series of true ejection fractions at a variety of left ventricular end diastolic counts. For example, if a patient with a true ejection fraction of 60% is imaged and a total of only 500 counts are present in the summed left ventricular end diastolic frame after background correction, the measured ejection frac-

Table 3. Percent error (expressed as percent of true ejection fraction) in ejection fraction calculation at different left ventricular end diastolic count levels, related to true ejection fraction

ED counts	True ejection fraction		
	40%	60%	80%
100	57	39	30
500	25	17	13
1000	18	12	10
2000	13	9	7
5000	8	5	4
10000	6	4	3

tion is subject to a 17% error. This means that the result could vary from 50% to 70%. Similarly, if an intervention study is performed, an observed change in ejection fraction from 70% to 50%, which would be regarded as abnormal, could be entirely due to statistical error at those count levels. With 5000 counts in the end diastolic image the error would only be 5.5%, and the measured ejection fraction would only vary from 57% to 63% due to statistics. A constant check on the observed count rates in the left ventricular end diastolic frame is a simple method for quality control of first pass data.

Analysis

A region of interest may be entered over left or right ventricles and a time-activity curve generated. The curve contains counts not only from the chamber but also from background, extraventricular regions, and the first step in analysis is to correct for this. Background in right heart, lungs and left atrium changes with time as the activity washes out of those structures into the left ventricle, and therefore background corrections should be time-dependent. In addition, the background around the left ventricle is not a uniform ramp, but varies spatially around different left ventricular regions. The background contribution from the basal segments is higher than that from the apex and algorithms which allow background to vary with time and with space are available [31, 32]. Other forms of correction use a circular sampling around the left ventricle [34]. The corrected time-activity curve is then used to calculate ejection fraction in the standard, count-based, geometry independent manner. Although background correction techniques vary from institution to institution, most reports testify to the good agreement between first pass ejection fractions and contrast angiographic values [31–34].

The methods available for regional wall motion analysis will be briefly discussed below.

From the practical standpoint, the major advantages of the first pass technique are the short data acquisition time, particularly valuable for maximal exercise studies, the high target to background ratios in each chamber, and the flexibility of projection. Apart from the need for a separate injection of tracer for each angiogram, the main disadvantages are that the analysis of left ventricular function depends on the function of the right heart being adequate to eject the bolus compactly enough to allow separation of right from left hearts. In the presence of severe right ventricular failure, pulmonary hypertension or tricuspid regurgitation, first pass studies may not be possible from peripheral venous injections. Under these circumstances, the choice rests between a first pass study through a Swan-Ganz catheter, or preferably a gated study in the LAO view. In addition, the limited number of cardiac cycles available makes rejection of ectopic beats difficult, as statistics will be compromised. Similarly, in the presence of atrial fibrillation the representative cycle is an average of beats of different quality. A full discussion of the advantages and disadvantages of the techniques may be found in the report by Knapp *et al.* [35].

Equilibrium gated blood pool imaging

This technique requires that a non-diffusible indicator be injected into the bloodstream and allowed to equilibrate in the entire vascular space before imaging is begun. The method cannot therefore be used for shunt detection or transit time measurements. No specific injection technique is required for these studies.

Technical requirements

The radiopharmaceutical is usually 15 to 25 mCi Tc-99m tagged to the patients' own red blood cells. With *in-vivo* labelling, the use of heparinised catheters is best avoided as the efficiency of labelling is reduced. Red cells are superior to human serum albumin (HSA) which not only leaks from the vascular space with time, but also may denature during labelling and localise in the liver. This increases background counts and reduces the activity available in the heart. With Tc-red cells, the limiting factor in imaging is the half-life of the radiolabel rather than the localisation properties of the tracer. With exercise however, the red cell count may increase and this may cause spurious increases in measured activity [36]. It is therefore important to measure blood activity before and after the intervention before changes in left ventricular activity can be attributed to changes in left ventricular volume.

Because radioactivity is present in all the cardiac chambers at the same time, temporal separation of the chambers is not available. Spatial separation between right and left ventricles is achieved by the use of the left anterior oblique projection, and the exact degree of obliquity varies from institution to institution. Many workers individualise the projection for each patient, using the projection which best separates the right and left ventricles, and in which the interventricular septum is best seen en face. A 10 to 15 degree caudal tilt of the detector aids in separation of left ventricle from left atrium. The use of the RAO view may lead to substantial overlap of the inferior and medial segments of the left ventricle by right ventricle, particularly where the right ventricle is dilated.

Imaging requirements

As radioactivity is at equilibrium in the blood pool and remains so for several hours after injection, there are no time constraints on the collection of data. Therefore high count-rate devices are not necessary and these studies may be performed on any modern single crystal camera interfaced to a computer. As only a fraction of the injected activity is in the left ventricle, "extrinsic gating" is required to resolve the events of the cardiac cycle temporally. Initially, this was achieved using the ECG signal and a gating device to enable and disable the computer so data were only recorded at the ECG-determined end systole and end diastole. Now, multiple gated acquisition allows the cardiac cycle to be divided into multiple slices and the corresponding phases of several hundred cycles are summed to provide a statistically reliable representative image of each respective part of the cycle [35, 37]. The cardiac cycle may be divided into time slices, so that the number of phases in the cycle will vary according to the heart rate, or phase slices, where the time of each slice varies and the number of phases per cycle remains constant. In practice, phase slices are preferable to keep the number of segments per cycle constant [35]. Twenty phases per cardiac cycle are adequate. Data collection should not terminate until each frame contains at least 20,000 counts in the whole image.

Both frame mode and list mode acquisition have been used. Frame mode, where the incoming scintillation data are organised into images in the computer memory immediately, is economical in terms of time and of storage space in the computer, but is less flexible in terms of beat rejection. If flexibility of formatting is required, which is particularly valuable in patients with irregular heart rates, list mode acquisition allows not only beat rejection but also separate formatting of, for example, sinus beats and ectopic beats after acquisition. Unfortunately, list mode requires more time and more storage space [30, 38].

For rest studies, a low energy, parallel hole, all purpose or high resolution collimator is adequate. For exercise studies, or where transient changes need to be detected, a high sensitivity collimator reduces data acquisition time.

Quality control

A "beat length histogram" that displays the frequency distribution of cycle lengths should be obtained to aid in the choice of selection of acceptable cycles. The ability of the camera-computer system to recognise the division of the cardiac cycle into equal slices should be tested by imaging a uniform flood source with a normal or simulated ECG signal as the trigger. The time-activity curve from the resulting gated images should be a straight line. Deviation from this indicates that the process of division of the cardiac cycle into equal segments is faulty.

Analysis

Time-activity curves may be generated from any of the cardiac chambers as with the first pass method. However, background counts are high outside the chamber of interest. Background correction most commonly involves the selection of a horseshoe or crescent-shaped region of interest remote from the end systolic or end diastolic edge of the ventricle. The average counts per channel in the background zone are subtracted from each channel in the left ventricular region of interest [35]. Again, many reports have described the good agreement with ejection fraction from gated studies with those from contrast angiograms [35, 37].

For right ventricular analysis, the problem of overlap of right atrium and right ventricle throughout the cardiac cycle in the LAO view may be partly overcome by the use of variable regions of interest [39].

The major advantages of this technique are the ability to carry out serial imaging over a period of hours after one injection of technetium, the ability to surmount the problem of statistics by increasing the imaging time, and the ability to cope with irregularities of heart rhythm. The disadvantages include the limitations of choice of projection and the long acquisition time, the latter making end-point exercise studies more difficult.

Cardiac measurements

1. *Ejection fraction.* This has been the single most measured index of cardiac function using radionuclide techniques. Although the literature is full of comparisons between contrast and radionuclide angiographic measurements, it must be remembered that the two techniques are never

likely to agree perfectly. Large differences may occur particularly in enlarged, distorted ventricles whose shape deviates from the desired geometric model. Under these circumstances, the geometry-independent radionuclide value may be the more accurate measurement. Each laboratory is obliged to establish its own values for normality and abnormality at the inception of a clinical programme. Reliance on reported values in the literature is not recommended, as small differences in data processing techniques may well alter the values [32]. Both first pass and gated values are highly reproducible, although inter-observer variations of up to 10% may occur [28, 40], and it is recommended that the same observer process the rest and intervention studies in any patient to minimise such errors [32, 41].

2. *Regional wall motion.* Several methods are available for assessment of regional left ventricular function. The contour approach, originally used for contrast angiograms, has been successfully adapted by using computer-generated ventricular outlines of end systolic and end diastolic images and superimposing them [28, 31]. The drawback with this is the difficulty of defining the true edge of the ventricle [35]. Wall motion may be evaluated by the use of the cinematic format, displaying the heart motion on an endless loop.

Neither of these displays make full use of the three-dimensional nature of radionuclide data. The contour images in particular are limited in the detection of akinetic segments in regions that are not tangential to the detector [42]. This has led to the use of functional or parametric cardiac imaging, where "stroke volume images", "regional ejection fraction images", and "phase images" are generated from pixel-by-pixel time activity curves from within the left ventricle [35, 42].

3. *Ventricular volumes.* As with ejection fraction, the earlier attempts to measure volumes used the area-length formulae applied to the contours of the radionuclide images. The problems with edge detection limit this method where small changes in volumes need to be detected. Recently, methods have been described which allow non-geometric calculation of volumes [43, 44] and such measurements provide a lower standard error than geometric values.

4. *Exercise imaging.* The same standards outlined in the section on stress thallium scintigraphy apply to dynamic exercise imaging. There is no doubt that the exercise protocol chosen, especially for first pass studies, has a profound effect on the results of the procedure [45]. Protocols representing less than maximal stress lead to higher exercise ejection fractions, and protocols that provide a supermaximal stress depress ejec-

tion fraction spuriously. An inadequate level of stress reduces the sensitivity of the test for detection of coronary artery disease to only about 60%, compared to 90% in those who achieve adequate exercise [46]. Similarly, a normal exercise response in a patient on a beta-blocking drug does not exclude artery disease, largely due to the blunting of the exercise heart rate response [47]. Naturally, bicycle exercise is the stress of choice, and as mentioned previously, it is possible to assess functional capacity [4]. Although motion artefact is undoubtedly present, it does not seem to invalidate the results of the tests.

The ejection fraction response to exercise is probably not the most specific marker of coronary artery disease [48], and it is important to include an assessment of regional wall motion in the procedure. Another index of left ventricular performance, the peak systolic blood pressure/ end systolic volume ratio appears to be more sensitive than the ejection fraction response [49]. For patients who cannot exercise, other forms of stress such as the cold pressor test or isometric handgrip have been recommended, but the success of such interventions as an alternative to bicycle exercise has been variable [50–52]. Once again, the definition of a normal and abnormal exercise response should be determined in individual laboratories, and attention to the prevalence of the disease in the population under investigation is mandatory [24].

Although there is no doubt that the exercise radionuclide angiogram is a sensitive technique for the detection of coronary artery disease [46, 49, 53, 54], it is not surprising that the results do not always match what might be expected from the coronary arteriogram. The physiological information from the radionuclide studies provides an independent assessment of the impact of anatomically demonstrated coronary stenoses, and should not be judged against the arteriogram. Rather, the information should be complementary to the arteriographic data, and this is especially useful in cases where the severity or clinical importance of a stenosis is in doubt [55]. Finally, the degree of exercise-induced abnormality reflects the amount of myocardium in jeopardy, and although this may roughly correlate with the number of diseased vessels [54], it is also related to the site of stenosis and the dominance of the vessel involved [56]. The potential to relate the extent of jeopardised myocardium to prognosis is an exciting new area in nuclear cardiology.

References

1. Sapirstein LA: Regional blood flow by fractionational distribution of indicators. Am J Physiol 193: 161, 1958.
2. L'Abbate A, Biagini A, Michelassi C, Maseri A: Myocardial kinetics of thallium and potassium in man. Circulation 60: 776, 1979.
3. Rigo P, Reiber HC, Dressler J: Stress thallium-201 myocardial scintigraphy. Review of methodological problems and proposal for standardisation. Eur Heart J 1: 81, 1980.
4. Foster C, Pollock ML, Rod JL, Dymond DS, Wible G, Schmidt DH: Evaluation of functional capacity during exercise radionuclide angiography. Cardiology, in press 1983.
5. McLaughlin PR, Martin RP, Doherty P, Daspit S, Goris M, Haskell W, Lewis S, Kriss JP, Harrison DC: Reproducibility of thallium-201 myocardial imaging. Circulation 55: 497, 1977.
6. Weich HF, Strauss HW, Pitt B: The extraction of thallium-201 by the myocardium. Circulation 56: 188, 1977.
7. Albro PC, Gould KL, Westcott RJ, Hamilton GW, Ritchie JL, Williams DL: Noninvasive assessment of coronary stenoses by myocardial imaging during pharmacologic coronary vasodilatation. III. Clinical trial. Am J Cardiol 42: 751, 1978.
8. Hamilton GW, Narahara KA, Trobaugh GB, Ritchie JL, Williams DL: Thallium-201 myocardial imaging: characterisation of the ECG-synchronised images. J Nucl Med 19: 1103, 1978.
9. Mueller TM, Marcus ML, Ehrhardt JC, Chaudhuri T, Abboud FM: Limitations of thallium-201 myocardial perfusion scintigrams. Circulation 54: 640, 1976.
10. Schwartz JS, Ponto R, Carlyle P, Forstrom L, Cohn JN: Early redistribution of thallium-201 after temporary ischaemia. Circulation 57: 332, 1978.
11. Pohost GM, Zir LM, Moore RH, McKusick KA, Guiney TE, Beller GA: Differentiation of transiently ischaemic from infarcted myocardium by serial imaging after a single dose of thallium-201. Circulation 55: 294, 1977.
12. Blood DK, McCarthy DM, Sciacca RR, Cannon PJ: Comparison of single-dose and double-dose thallium-201 myocardial perfusion scintigraphy for the detection of coronary artery disease and prior myocardial infarction. Circulation 58: 777, 1978.
13. Rigo P, Bailey IK, Griffith LSC, Pitt B, Burow RD, Wagner HJ, Becker LC: Value and limitations of segmental analysis of stress thallium myocardial imaging for localisation of coronary artery disease. Circulation 61: 973, 1980.
14. McKillop JH, Murray RG, Turner JG, Bessent RG, Lorimer AR, Greig WR: Can the extent of coronary artery disease be predicted from thallium-201 myocardial images? J Nucl Med 20: 715, 1979.
15. Kushner FG, Okada RD, Kirshenbaum HD, Boucher CA, Strauss HW, Pohost GM: Lung thallium-201 uptake after stress testing in patients with coronary artery disease. Circulation 63: 341, 1981.
16. Goris ML, Daspit SG, McLaughlin P, Kriss JP: Interpolative background subtraction. J Nucl Med 17: 744, 1976.
17. Watson DD, Campbell NP, Read EK, Gibson RS, Teates CD, Beller GA: Spatial and temporal quantitation of plane thallium myocardial images. J Nucl Med 22: 577, 1981.
18. Lenaers A, Block P, van Thiel E, Lebedelle M, Becquevort P, Erbsmann F, Ermans AM: Segmental analysis of Tl-201 stress myocardial scintigraphy. J Nucl Med 18: 509, 1976.
19. Wainwright RJ, Brennand-Roper DA, Maisey MN, Sowton E: Exercise thallium-201 myocardial scintigraphy in the follow-up of aortocoronary bypass graft surgery. Br Heart J 43: 56, 1980.
20. Murray RG, McKillop JH, Bessent RG, Turner JG, Lorimer AR, Hutton IH, Greig WR, Lawrie TDV: Evaluation of thallium-201 exercise scintigraphy in coronary heart disease. Br Heart J 41: 568, 1979.
21. Faris JV, Burt RW, Graham MC, Knoebel SB: Thallium-201 myocardial scintigraphy: improved sensitivity, specificity and predictive accuracy by application of a statistical image analysis

algorithm. Am J Cardiol 49: 733, 1982.

22. Ritchie JL, Williams DL, Caldwell JH, Stratton JR, Harp GD, Vogel RA, Hamilton GW: Seven-pinhole emission tomography with thallium-201 in patients with prior myocardial infarction. J Nucl Med 22: 107, 1981.

23. Okada RA, Boucher CA, Kirshenbaum HK, Kushner FG, Strauss HW, Block PC, McKusick KA, Pohost GM: Improved diagnostic accuracy of thallium-201 stress test using multiple observers and criteria derived from interobserver analysis of variance. Am J Cardiol 46: 619, 1980.

24. Diamond GA, Forrester JS: Analysis of probability as an aid in the clinical diagnosis of coronary artery disease. N Engl J Med 300: 1350, 1979.

25. Prinzmetal M, Corday E, Bergman HC, Schwartz L, Spritzler RJ: Radiocardiography: a new method for studying the blood flow through the chambers of the heart in human beings. Science 108: 340, 1948.

26. Jones RH, Sabiston DC, Bates BB, Morris JJ, Anderson PAW, Goodrich JK: Quantitative radionuclide angiocardiography for determination of chamber to chamber cardiac transit times. Am J Cardiol 30: 855, 1972.

27. Dymond DS, Elliott AT, Flatman W, Stone D, Bett R, Cuninghame G, Sims H: Clinical validation of gold-195m: a new short half-life radiopharmaceutical for rapid, sequential, first pass angiocardiography in man. J Am Coll Cardiol, in press, 1983.

28. Dymond DS, Elliott AT, Stone D, Hendrix G, Spurrell RAJ: Factors that affect the reproducibility of measurements of left ventricular function from first pass radionuclide angiograms. Circulation 65: 311, 1982.

29. Flatman WD, Dymond DS, Dyke L, O'Keefe J, Short MD: A performance assessment of a mobile digital gamma camera with particular emphasis on its high count-rate performance. Nuc Med Comm, in press, 1983.

30. Lieberman DE: Acquisition of nuclear medicine data. In: Computer methods, the fundamentals of digital nuclear medicine. St. Louis, Mosby CV, 1977, pp 41–57.

31. Marshall RC, Berger HJ, Costin JC, Freedman GS, Wolberg J, Cohen LS, Gottschalk A, Zaret BL: Assessment of cardiac performance with quantitative radionuclide angiography. Circulation 56: 820, 1977.

32. Dymond DS, Halama J, Schmidt DH: Right anterior oblique first-pass radionuclide angiography ejection fractions: effects of temporal smoothing and of various background corrections. J Nucl Med 23: 1, 1982.

33. Schelbert HR, Verba JW, Johnston AD, Brock GW, Alazraki NP, Rose FJ, Ashburn WL: Non-traumatic determination of left ventricular ejection fraction by radionuclide angiocardiography. Circulation 51: 902, 1975.

34. Van Dyke D, Anger HO, Sullivan RW, Vetter WR, Yano Y, Parker HG: Cardiac evaluation from radioisotope dynamics. J Nucl Med 13: 585, 1972.

35. Knapp WH, Dymond DS, Malfanti PL, Ogris E, Pachinger O, Sochor H, Vyska K, Walton S: Radionuclide methods for the evaluation of ventricular function. Eur Heart J 2: 97, 1981.

36. Konstam MA, Tu'meh S, Wynne J, Beck JB, Kozlowski J, Holman BL: Effect of exercise on erythrocyte count and blood activity concentration after technetium-99m *in vivo* red blood cell labelling. Circulation 66: 638, 1982.

37. Burow RD, Strauss HW, Singleton R, Pond M, Rehn T, Bailey IK, Griffith LC, Nickoloff E, Pitt B: Analysis of left ventricular function from multiple gated acquisition cardiac blood pool imaging. Circulation 56: 1024, 1977.

38. Bacharach SL, Green MV, Borer JS, Douglas MA, Ostrow HG, Johnston GS: A real-time system for multi-image gated cardiac studies. J Nucl Med 18: 79, 1977.

39. Maddahi J, Berman DS, Matsuoka DT, Waxman AD, Stankus KE, Forrester JS, Swan HJC: A new technique for assessing right ventricular ejection fraction using rapid multiple-gated equilibrium cardiac blood pool scintigraphy. Circulation 60: 581, 1979.

40. Wackers FJTh, Berger HJ, Johnstone DE, Goldman L, Reduto LA, Langou RA, Gottschalk A,

Zaret BL: Multiple gated cardiac blood pool imaging for left ventricular ejection fraction: validation of the technique and assessment of variability. Am J Cardiol 43: 1159, 1979.

41. Cohn PF, Levine JA, Bergerson GA, Gorlin R: Reproducibility of the angiographic left ventricular ejection fraction in patients with coronary artery disease. Am Heart J 88: 713, 1974.

42. Adam WE, Tarkowska A, Bitter F, Stauch M, Geffers H: Equilibrium (gated) radionuclide ventriculography. In: Cardiac Nuclear Medicine. Holman BL, Abrams HL, Zeitler E. (eds) Berlin, Springer-Verlag, 1979, pp 21–33.

43. Slutsky R, Karliner J, Ricci D, Kaiser R, Pfisterer M, Gordon D, Peterson K, Ashburn W: Left ventricular volumes by gated equilibrium radionuclide angiography: a new method. Circulation 60: 556, 1979.

44. Massie BM, Kramer BL, Gertz EW, Henderson SG: Radionuclide measurement of left ventricular volume: comparison of geometric and count-based methods. Circulation 65: 725, 1982.

45. Foster C, Dymond DS, Anholm JD, Pollock ML, Schmidt DH: Effect of exercise protocol on the left ventricular response to exercise. Am J Cardiol 51: 859, 1983.

46. Brady TJ, Thrall JH, Lo K, Pitt B: The importance of adequate exercise in the detection of coronary heart disease by radionuclide ventriculography. J Nucl Med 21: 1125, 1980.

47. Battler A, Ross J, Slutsky R, Pfisterer M, Ashburn W, Froelicher V: Improvement of exercise-induced left ventricular dysfunction with oral propranolol in patients with coronary heart disease. Am J Cardiol 44: 318, 1979.

48. Gibbons RJ, Lee KL, Cobb F, Jones RH: Ejection fraction response to exercise in patients with chest pain and normal coronary arteriograms. Circulation 64: 952, 1981.

49. Slutsky R, Karliner J, Gerber K, Battler A, Froelicher V, Gregoratos G, Peterson K, Ashburn W: Peak systolic blood pressure/end systolic volume ratio: assessment at rest and during exercise in normal subjects and patients with coronary heart disease. Am J Cardiol 46: 813, 1980.

50. Wynne J, Holman BL, Mudge GH, Borow KM: Clinical utility of cold pressor radionuclide ventriculography in coronary artery disease (abstr). Am J Cardiol 47: 444, 1981.

51. Verani MS, Zacca NM, DeBauche TL, Miller RR, Chahine RA: Comparison of cold pressor and exercise radionuclide angiocardiography in coronary artery disease. J Nucl Med 23: 770, 1982.

52. Bodenheimer MM, Banka VS, Fooshee CM, Gillespie JA, Helfant RH: Detection of coronary heart disease using radionuclide determined regional ejection fraction at rest and during handgrip exercise: correlation with coronary arteriography. Circulation 58: 640, 1978.

53. Berger HJ, Reduto LA, Johnstone DE, Borkowski H, Sands M, Cohen LS, Langou RA, Gottschalk A, Zaret BL: Global and regional left ventricular response to bicycle exercise in coronary artery disease: assessment by quantitative radionuclide angiocardiography. Am J Med 66: 13, 1979.

54. Stone DL, Dymond DS, Elliott AT, Britton KE, Banim SO, Spurrell RAJ: Exercise first pass radionuclide ventriculography detection of patients with coronary artery disease. Br Heart J 44: 208, 1980.

55. Gutman J, Rozanski A, Garcia E, Maddahi J, Miyamoto A, Berman D: Complementary roles of scintigraphic and angiographic techniques in assessment of the extent of coronary artery disease. Am Heart J 104: 653, 1982.

56. Leong K, Jones RH: Influence of the location of left anterior descending coronary artery stenosis on left ventricular function during exercise. Circulation 65: 109, 1982.

Index of subjects